# MORE 4U!

# theclinics.com

## This Clinics series is available online.

Here's what you get:

- Full text of EVERY issue from 2002 to NOW
- Figures, tables, drawings, references and more
- Searchable: find what you need fast

Search | All Clinics ▼ | for | | GO |

- Linked to MEDLINE and Elsevier journals
- E-alerts

## INDIVIDUAL SUBSCRIBERS

## LOG ON TODAY. IT'S FAST AND EASY.

Click **Register** and follow instructions

You'll need your account number

Your subscriber account number is on your mailing label →

This is your copy of:

THE CLINICS OF NORTH AMERICA

CXXX    **2296532-2**    2    Mar 05

J.H. DOE, MD
531 MAIN STREET
CENTER CITY, NY  10001-001

**BOUGHT A SINGLE ISSUE?** Sorry, you won't be able to access full text online. Please subscribe today to get complete content by contacting customer service at 800 645 2452 (US and Canada) or 407 345 4000 (outside US and Canada) or via email at elsols@elsevier.com.

## NEW!

## Now also available for INSTITUTIONS

**ELSEVIER**

Works/Integrates with MD Consult
Available in a variety of packages: Collections containing 14, 31 or 50 Clinics titles
Or Collection upgrade for existing MD Consult customers

Call today! 877-857-1047 or e-mail: mdc.groupinfo@elsevier.com

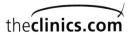

# PSYCHIATRIC CLINICS

# OF NORTH AMERICA

## Neuropsychiatry

GUEST EDITOR
Silvana Riggio, MD

September 2005 • Volume 28 • Number 3

**SAUNDERS**

An Imprint of Elsevier, Inc.
PHILADELPHIA   LONDON   TORONTO   MONTREAL   SYDNEY   TOKYO

**W.B. SAUNDERS COMPANY**
*A Division of Elsevier Inc.*

1600 John F. Kennedy Boulevard • Suite 1800 • Philadelphia, PA 19103-2899

http://www.theclinics.com

| | |
|---|---|
| THE PSYCHIATRIC CLINICS OF NORTH AMERICA | Volume 28, Number 3 |
| September 2005 | ISSN 0193-953X |
| Editor: Sarah E. Barth | ISBN 1-4160-2680-0 |

The ideas and opinions expressed in *The Psychiatric Clinics of North America* do not necessarily reflect those of the Publisher. The Publisher does not assume any responsibility for any injury and/or damage to persons or property arising out of or related to any use of the material contained in this periodical. The reader is advised to check the appropriate medical literature and the product information currently provided by the manufacturer of each drug to be administered, to verify the dosage, the method and duration of administration, or contraindications. It is the responsibility of the treating physician or other health care professional, relying on independent experience and knowledge of the patient, to determine drug dosages and the best treatment for the patient. Mention of any product in this issue should not be construed as endorsement by the contributors, editors, or the Publisher of the product or manufacturers' claims.

*The Psychiatric Clinics of North America* (ISSN 0193-953X) is published quarterly by the W.B. Saunders Company. Corporate and editorial offices: Elsevier, Inc., 1600 John F. Kennedy Boulevard, Suite 1800, Philadelphia, PA 19103-2899. Accounting and circulation offices: 6277 Sea Harbor Drive, Orlando, FL 32887-4800. Periodicals postage paid at Orlando, FL 32862, and additional mailing offices. Subscription prices are $170.00 per year (US individuals), $288.00 per year (US institutions), $85.00 per year (US students/residents), $205.00 per year (Canadian individuals), $349.00 per year (Canadian Institutions), $240.00 per year (foreign individuals), $349.00 per year (foreign institutions), and $120.00 per year (international & Canadian students/residents). Foreign air speed delivery is included in all *Clinics'* subscription prices. All prices are subject to change without notice. POSTMASTER: Send address changes to *The Psychiatric Clinics of North America*, W.B. Saunders Company, Periodicals Fulfillment, Orlando, FL 32887−4800. **Customer Service: 1-800-654-2452 (US). From outside of the US, call 1-407-345-4000.**

*The Psychiatric Clinics of North America* is covered in *Index Medicus, Current Contents/Social and Behavioral Sciences, Social Science Citation Index, Embase/Excerpta Medica,* and PsycINFO.

Printed in the United States of America.

# GUEST EDITOR

**SILVANA RIGGIO, MD,** Associate Professor, Department of Psychiatry, Mount Sinai School of Medicine, and Bronx Veterans Medical Center, New York, New York

# CONTRIBUTORS

**DMITRI BOUGAKOV, PhD,** Department of Neurology, New York University School of Medicine, New York, New York

**MONA BOULES, PhD,** Research Associate, Neuropsychopharmacology Laboratory, Mayo Clinic, Jacksonville, Florida

**CHRISTOPHER R. BOWIE, PhD,** Instructor, Department of Psychiatry, Mount Sinai School of Medicine, New York, New York

**DANIEL F. BRODERICK, MD,** Assistant Professor of Medicine, Mayo Clinic College of Medicine, Mayo Clinic, Jacksonville, Florida

**TODD E. FEINBERG, MD,** Professor of Clinical Psychiatry and Behavioral Sciences and Clinical Neurology, Albert Einstein College of Medicine; and Division Chief, Yarmon Neurobehavior and Alzheimer's Disease Center, Bernstein Pavilion, Beth Israel Medical Center, New York, New York

**CHRISTOPHER M. FILLEY, MD,** Departments of Neurology and Psychiatry, University of Colorado School of Medicine; and Denver Veterans Affairs Medical Center, Denver, Colorado

**PAUL FREDRICKSON, MD,** Associate Professor of Psychiatry, Mayo Clinic College of Medicine, Jacksonville, Florida

**ELKHONON GOLDBERG, PhD,** Clinical Professor of Neurology, Department of Neurology, New York University School of Medicine, New York, New York

**MARTIN ADAM GOLDSTEIN, MD,** Instructor (Neurology), Division of Cognitive and Behavioral Neurology, Department of Neurology, Mount Sinai School of Medicine, Mount Sinai Medical Center, New York, New York

**BRIAN HAINLINE, MD,** Clinical Associate Professor of Neurology, New York University School of Medicine, New York; and Chief, Neurology and Integrative Pain Medicine, ProHEALTH Care Associates, Lake Success, New York

**PHILIP D. HARVEY, PhD,** Professor, Department of Psychiatry, Mount Sinai School of Medicine, New York, New York

**BARBARA C. JOBST, MD,** Assistant Professor of Medicine (Neurology), Dartmouth Medical School; and Section of Neurology, Dartmouth Epilepsy Program, Dartmouth-Hitchcock Medical Center, Lebanon, New Hampshire

**SIONG-CHI LIN, MD,** Assistant Professor of Psychiatry, Mayo Clinic College of Medicine, Jacksonville, Florida

**JOHN A. LUCAS, PhD, ABPP/ABCN,** Associate Professor of Psychology, Department of Psychiatry and Psychology, Mayo Clinic, Jacksonville, Florida

**BRENDA MILNER, ScD,** Professor, Department of Neurology and Neurosurgery, McGill University; and Dorothy J. Killam Professor of Cognitive Neuroscience, Montreal Neurological Institute, Montreal, Quebec, Canada

**JORGE R. PETIT, MD,** Assistant Clinical Professor, Department of Psychiatry, Mount Sinai School of Medicine; and Associate Commissioner, Bureau of Program Services, The New York City Department of Health and Mental Hygiene, New York, New York

**ELLIOTT RICHELSON, MD,** Professor of Psychiatry and Pharmacology, Mayo Clinic College of Medicine, Jacksonville, Florida

**SILVANA RIGGIO, MD,** Associate Professor, Department of Psychiatry, Mount Sinai School of Medicine, and Bronx Veterans Medical Center, New York, New York

**DAVID M. ROANE, MD,** Associate Professor of Clinical Psychiatry, Albert Einstein College of Medicine; and Chief, Division of Geriatric Medicine, Beth Israel Medical Center, New York, New York.

**MICHAEL E. SILVERMAN, PhD,** Assistant Professor (Psychiatry), Division of Cognitive and Behavioral Neurology, Department of Psychiatry, Mount Sinai School of Medicine, Mount Sinai Medical Center, New York, New York

**PETER D. WILLIAMSON, MD,** Professor of Medicine (Neurology), Dartmouth Medical School; and Section of Neurology, Dartmouth Epilepsy Program, Dartmouth-Hitchcock Medical Center, Lebanon, New Hampshire

# CONTENTS

neuropsychologic measures assessing various aspects of the frontal lobe function exist. Because the executive control system is an over-arching construct, a combination of neuropsychologic measures of executive control is appropriate when assessing the frontal lobe function. Some revisions of the concept of executive control are needed. This article discusses several innovative tests capable of tapping such revised aspects of the executive control.

This article provides an overview of the cognitive processes and neural bases of human memory functioning. Common conceptual classifications of memory processes from the cognitive neuro-science literature are presented, and the principal neuronal mechanisms associated with creating, storing, and accessing mem-ories are reviewed. A brief introduction to the brain regions impor-tant to memory functioning is also provided. The article concludes with a review of common clinical syndromes and diseases that typically are characterized by disordered memory.

Memory forms a bridge between past and present and implies the existence of enduring changes in the brain. This historical review reviews memory research in the 1950s and shows how the system-atic study of a few patients with profound anterograde amnesia, resulting from bilateral damage to the medial structures of the tem-poral lobe, provided early evidence for the existence of multiple memory systems in the human brain. Acceptance of these findings hinged on the subsequent discovery of an appropriate animal mod-el, with convergent findings from neurobehavioral studies in hu-man and nonhuman primates. This collaborative work of neuropsychologists, neuroanatomists, and neurosurgeons points to the value of a cross-disciplinary approach.

Impaired cognitive functioning is now recognized as a core feature of schizophrenia and one of the most important predictors of func-tioning across occupational, social, and adaptive domains. The study of cognition in schizophrenia continues to be a major inter-est, with new methods and data illuminating ever-more-precise deficits. This article reviews the literature on cognition in schizo-phrenia, focusing on the most recent data. It provides new insights into the study of the relationship between cognition and functional outcome and suggests future directions.

on the concept of distributed neural networks in which white matter connectivity is crucial.

## Management of the Acutely Violent Patient
Jorge R. Petit

Violence in the work place is a growing problem, and it is likely that a psychiatrist will have an encounter with a violent patient. It is important to be aware of predictors and associated factors in violence and to have a well-defined strategy in approaching the acutely violent patient. Ensuring patient, staff, and personal safety is the most important first intervention in the management of these patients. Restraints, seclusion, and psychopharmacologic interventions are important components of the management. A structured and coordinated team approach is warranted and necessary to care for the acutely violent patient and to ensure safety for all involved.

## Chronic Pain: Physiological, Diagnostic, and Management Considerations
Brian Hainline

Chronic pain is pain that persists more than 1 month longer than might be reasonably expected after tissue insult. Chronic pain, a term interchangeable with neuropathic pain, is sustained by aberrant somatosensory processing within the nervous system. As such, chronic pain is a disorder of physiology, and successful diagnosis and management spring from an appreciation of this point. The complex physiologic processes that drive chronic pain require individualized, multidisciplinary patient care. This article provides an overview of the physiology, diagnosis, and management of chronic pain.

## Neurobiologic Basis of Nicotine Addiction and Psychostimulant Abuse: a Role for Neurotensin?
Paul Fredrickson, Mona Boules, Siong-Chi Lin, and Elliott Richelson

Addiction to psychostimulants such as nicotine, amphetamine, and cocaine represents a serious public health problem for which treatment remains difficult, particularly in patients with comorbid psychiatric illness. This article reviews neurochemical correlates of addiction, including a role for neurotensin, a neuropeptide that colocalizes and interacts with dopaminergic systems implicated in psychosis and addiction. Neurotensin has been termed an endogenous neuroleptic, and neurotensin systems in the brain are promising targets for treatment of psychosis and addiction.

## Index

# FORTHCOMING ISSUES

# RECENT ISSUES

PSYCHIATRIC
CLINICS
OF NORTH AMERICA

Psychiatr Clin N Am 28 (2005) xi–xii

## Preface

# Neuropsychiatry

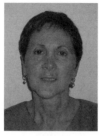

Silvana Riggio, MD
*Guest Editor*

It was with great pleasure that I accepted the role of editor for this issue of the *Psychiatric Clinics of North America* on neuropsychiatry. As a neurologist and a psychiatrist who has collaborated with colleagues in both specialties for many years, I embraced this project as a wonderful opportunity to focus on an area of interest and to work closely with some of the experts in these disciplines. My goal was to present the reader with the spectrum of challenges we confront in our daily practices as they relate to neuropsychiatry and, in doing so, to emphasize the importance of a multidisciplinary approach.

The conviction in the importance of a multidisciplinary approach to health care, not only within the fields of neurology and psychiatry but within all specialties, has led to various projects with my husband, an emergency medicine physician with a strong interest in psychiatry and neurology. Some of these projects, published by the WB Saunders Co. in the *Emergency Medicine Clinics of North America*, include issues on the "Management of Seizures in the Emergency Department" and "Psychiatric Emergencies." This collaboration has allowed us and our patients to benefit from our different perspectives as they relate to neuropsychiatric complaints.

In 1993, I had the opportunity to organize a conference with Drs. Herbert Jasper and Patricia Goldman-Rakic on "Epilepsy and the Functional Anatomy of the Frontal Lobe," which led to a book on this subject. This issue of the *Psychiatric Clinics of North America* is a continuation of the work that started at that conference and, indeed, four of the participants are contributing authors in this issue.

Over the years, my work has given me the firm conviction that neurology and psychiatry cannot exist as two separate disciplines but rather are intertwined. This perspective has been consolidated even further by my recent work in schizophrenia. The goal of this issue was to gather a group of experts in the fields of neurology, psychiatry, neuroradiology, and neuropsychology and provide the framework in which they would focus on the neurobiologic basis of psychiatric disorders and on the clinical and behavioral manifestations of neurologic disorders. My hope is that the reader will become engaged in the relationship between neurology and psychiatry as well as be inspired to pursue future investigation. As we continue searching for an understanding of the many challenges that the field of neuropsychiatry offers, we will also hopefully learn new ways to improve the diagnosis, treatment, and outcome for the many patients who suffer from a neuropsychiatric condition.

Silvana Riggio, MD
*Department of Psychiatry*
*Mount Sinai School of Medicine and Bronx Veterans Medical Center*
*One Gustave L. Levy Place, Box 1230*
*New York, NY 10029, USA*

*E-mail address:* silvana.riggio@mssm.edu

ELSEVIER
SAUNDERS

PSYCHIATRIC
CLINICS
OF NORTH AMERICA

Psychiatr Clin N Am 28 (2005) 507–547

# Neuropsychiatric Assessment

Martin Adam Goldstein, MD[a],*,
Michael E. Silverman, PhD[b]

[a]Division of Cognitive and Behavioral Neurology, Department of Neurology,
Mount Sinai School of Medicine, Mount Sinai Medical Center,
One Gustave L. Levy Place, New York, NY 10029, USA
[b]Division of Cognitive and Behavioral Neurology, Department of Psychiatry,
Mount Sinai School of Medicine, Mount Sinai Medical Center,
One Gustave L. Levy Place, New York, NY 10029, USA

## Historical foundations

Modern neuropsychiatric assessment represents the realization of an integrated approach to mind, brain, and behavior originally advocated by forefathers of modern clinical neuroscience, including Freud, Kraepelin, Charcot, and Alzheimer. Freud, a formally trained neurologist, of course later founded psychoanalysis, among the most complex theories of mind ever developed. Alois Alzheimer, a psychiatrist, described the neurodegenerative disease bearing his name while attempting to correlate changes in brain structure with mental illness. Despite the schism between neurology and psychiatry in the early twentieth century, the original integrated ambitions of early clinical neuro-psychiatrists are being realized by the rapprochement facilitated by neuroscience in the late twentieth century [1,2].

Two fundamental forces are making the comprehensive approach of neuropsychiatry to mental/brain disease compelling. First, there is increasing appreciation of the spectrum complexity of mental/brain disease states (ie, many neurologic states have important psychiatric features, and the reverse) [3]. For example, Parkinson's disease, conventionally conceptualized and managed as a primary neurologic disorder, has cognitive and emotional features that are not merely complicating comorbidities but are intrinsic components of core phenomenology. Second, as psychiatry moves toward etiologically based nosology, there is increasing recognition that the same neural circuitry underlies clinical syndromes with previously distinct neurologic and psychiatric classifications [4]. For example, the abulia of

---

* Corresponding author.
   *E-mail address:* martin.goldstein@mssm.edu (M.A. Goldstein).

0193-953X/05/$ - see front matter © 2005 Elsevier Inc. All rights reserved.
doi:10.1016/j.psc.2005.05.006
*psych.theclinics.com*

fronto-temporal lobar dementia represents dysfunction of the same neural circuitry as that underlying the apathy of psychomotorically retarded depression. Neuropsychiatry therefore stands as an integrative discipline honestly grappling with the complex spectrum of mind/brain phenomenology [5].

## Contemporary approach

### Phenomenological scope

Although the metaphor has well-known limitations, in neuroscience as in computer science, dysfunction can involve "software," "hardware," or some combination thereof. In addition, because of the often intricately interacting processes of neurodevelopment, neurodegeneration, and psychologic function, pathology in different domains can interact complexly, yielding an essentially infinite array of clinical neuropsychiatric permutations. Further, the temporal sequence of clinical manifestations can vary. For example, a neurodevelopmental abnormality such as a nonverbal learning disorder can precipitate psychodynamic maladaptation yielding interpersonal social dysfunction eventually contributing to genesis of depression. Therefore, for many neuropsychiatric states, multiple potential mechanistic admixtures can exist, requiring both broad scope and in-depth analysis to disentangle.

Because of the breadth and complexity of its target substrate, neuropsychiatric examination comprises one of the most challenging assessment procedures in clinical medicine. Proper neuropsychiatric assessment requires drawing on a multidisciplinary knowledge base, strategically employing a wide range of examination skills, integrating complex and layered clinical data into a coherent formulation, and interfacing with clinicians of multiple disciplines. The contemporaneously integrated approach of neuropsychiatry, encompassing the full clinical spectrum of brain/mind illness, facilitates more comprehensive and accurate diagnosis.

### Conceptual foundations

Commensurate with the breadth of its phenomenologic scope, neuropsychiatry relies on a wide range of conceptual foundations, summarized in Box 1. The requirement for broadening the conceptual base in clinical neuroscience is especially evident in the evolution of contemporary behavioral neurology, which, having traversed a path from localizationism and connectionism (eg, Broca and Wernicke) to hierarchical holism (eg, Jackson) to Geschwindian disconnectionism, now draws from the entirety of cognitive and affective neurosciences.

### Clinical components

Because neuropsychiatric pathology can be protean, the range of neuropsychiatric examination comprises not only behavior and mentation

---

**Box 1. Conceptual foundations of neuropsychiatric assessment**

*Neurology*
Neurogenetics
Neurodevelopment
Neuroanatomy
Neurophysiology
Neuropathology

*Neurology and psychiatry*
Neuroimmunology
Neuroendocrinology
Neuropsychology
Neurochemistry
Neurotoxicology
Nutrition

*Psychiatry*
Psychopharmacology
Psychodynamics
Psychodevelopment

---

but also elementary neurologic and medical function. Hence, at least in some ways, neuropsychiatric assessment represents the ultimate integrated implementation of the multiaxial diagnostic approach developed for the *Diagnostic and Statistical Manual of Mental Disorders* (*DSM*) [6]. An inventory of neuropsychiatric assessment is given in Box 2.

*Principles of organization*

Neuropsychiatric assessment is labor-intensive by definition, requiring detailed review of often-extensive medical records, comprehensive physical examination (literally head to toe), and interpretation of multisystem/ multimodal diagnostic test performance and results. Certain overarching principles can help organize the clinical approach.

*Hierarchy*

Brain functions tend to have a hierarchical organization. That is, certain brain functions are basic to others. For example, it is pointless to comment on a patient's anterograde memory function if ancillary processes subservient to memory performance (eg, attention) are so severely impaired that memory formation is disabled. This hierarchy should be reflected in the structure and performance of neuropsychiatric assessment.

---

**Box 2. Neuropsychiatric assessment inventory**

Consciousness
Orientation
Attention
Language
Memory
Executive function
Praxis
Affect
Thought content
Thought processes
Perception
Speech
Comportment
Elementary neurologic function
General medical status

---

*Domain overlap*

Conventional distinctions drawn among cognitive domains are, in fact, somewhat arbitrary, because practically no cognitive function exists in isolation. For example, so-called "pure" measures of verbal memory require patients to sustain attention to and process linguistic stimuli. Consequently, attention or language impairment obfuscates patient performance on measures of memory. Because most assessment instruments de facto test more than one cognitive skill, neuropsychiatric assessment batteries typically rely on a combination of measures within and across cognitive domains to eliminate potential confounds systematically. Quality neuropsychiatric formulation therefore requires supracomponent synthesis, using subtraction and conjunction analyses of individual test results to pinpoint specific cognitive domain deficits precisely.

*Levels of assessment*

Like other medical examinations, neuropsychiatric assessment can be performed with a range of detail and comprehensiveness. The scope and depth of neuropsychiatric phenomenology yields the potential for lengthy and arduous examination. Neuropsychiatric assessment can and should be sculpted to suit clinical context and examination venue to optimize diagnostic efficiency and utility. Accordingly, in reviewing the domains of neuropsychiatric examination, the authors distinguish assessment strategies according to three general levels: (1) emergency room/bedside, (2) clinic/office, and (3) neuropsychologic testing. A variety of standardized assessment inventories exist (summarized in Table 1), and for certain neuropsy-

Table 1
Standardized assessment instruments

| Instrument | Domains assayed |
| --- | --- |
| Mini-Mental Status Examination (MMSE) [9] | Orientation<br>Simple attention<br>Comprehension<br>Simple calculation<br>Visual construction<br>Memory |
| Neuropsychiatric Inventory (NPI) [10] | Thought disturbance<br>Perceptual disturbance (eg, hallucinations)<br>Affect<br>Abulia<br>Agitation/aggression<br>Disinhibition<br>Appetite<br>Sleeping pattern<br>Aberrant motor activity |
| Executive Interview (EXIT) [11] | Executive functions |
| Clinical Dementia Rating Scale (CDRS) [12] | Orientation<br>Memory<br>Problem solving<br>Activities of daily living<br>Social interactions |
| Mattis Dementia Rating Scale (MDRS) [13] | Attention<br>Initiation<br>Perseveration<br>Conceptualization<br>Construction<br>Memory |

chiatric disease states (eg, dementia), there are practice guidelines issued by various professional organizations [7,8]. For most neuropsychiatric syndromes, however, it is the responsibility of individual clinicians to conduct a well-reasoned, methodical diagnostic approach.

Neuropsychology has long cultivated a coalescence of neurologic and psychiatric principles. Neuropsychologic testing represents the reference standard of cognitive assessment (discussed elsewhere in this volume). Here it is important to contextualize the usefulness of neuropsychologic testing within neuropsychiatric assessment, especially regarding indications for its requisition. Purposes of neuropsychologic testing include:

1. More sensitive detection of deficits potentially missed by screening devices (mental status screens frequently have a ceiling effect; results within normal range may still reflect considerable decline compared with premorbid performance).
2. Providing a quantitative account of individual cognitive domain dysfunction by means of standardized and normed assessment.

3. Delineating specific impairment profiles by means of systematic multi-domain assessment.
4. Quantitatively tracking changes over time by means of serial evaluations.

Neuropsychologic testing can substantially inform treatment planning and, by defining areas of relative resilience, facilitate customization of rehabilitation strategies.

## Maintaining diagnostic humility

Because neuropsychiatric pathologies are complex and can be extremely protean, it is important to maintain diagnostic humility when performing assessment. Accordingly, it is crucial to describe clinical phenomenology in as diagnostically conservative terms as possible before attempting formulation of a unifying diagnosis.

## Neuropsychiatric clinical history

### Patient history

Performing a thorough clinical history is an essential component of neuropsychiatric assessment. A detailed history can help narrow the differential diagnosis by facilitating etiologic pattern recognition. Box 3 provides an inventory of key history features.

### Informants

For certain neuropsychiatric states (eg, incipient dementias), family, friends, or colleagues often note clinical manifestations long before the patient would self-present with a complaint. Cognitive, affective, and comportmental function should be reviewed with a reliable informant when clinically indicated.

## Cognitive/affective/behavioral assessment constructs

### Consciousness

Characterization and assessment of consciousness represents one of the most challenging areas of contemporary neuroscience [14]. Accurate evaluation requires conceptual distinction and independent examination of consciousness components.

### Arousal
Conceptual foundations. Arousal represents an essential (but insufficient) component of consciousness. Often defined as equivalent to wakefulness, it

## Box 3. Clinical history survey

*Developmental history*
  Perinatal history
  Developmental milestone history

*Review of systems*
Neurovegetative
  Sleeping pattern
  Appetite
Elementary neurologic
  Visual changes?
  Hearing changes?
  Olfactory changes?
  Taste changes?
  Speech problems?
  Headaches?
  Dizziness/lightheadedness?
  Weakness?
  Numbness?
  Paresthesias?
  Head trauma?
  Seizures?
Neuropsychiatric
  Cognitive changes
  Difficulty concentrating?
  Difficulty finding words?
  Memory problems?
  Difficulty navigating?
  Difficulty completing tasks?
  Mood changes?
  Behavioral changes?
  Stressors?
Cardiovascular
  Hypertension?
  Cardiac disease?
  Peripheral vascular disease?
Respiratory
  Sleep apnea?
Urinary
  Bladder dysfunction?
Gastrointestinal
  Bowel dysfunction?

Endocrine
  Thyroid dysfunction?
  Diabetes?
Dermatologic
  Pigmentation?
  Skin rashes?
Oncologic history
  Cancer history?
Infectious history
  Exposure risk factors?

*Medication*
  Compliance
  Side effects
  Herbal supplements

*Nutrition*

*Sexual history*

*Travel history*

*Toxic exposure*
  Alcohol
  Tobacco
  Illicit drugs
  Industrial toxins, heavy metals

*Personal history*
  Education
  Employment
  Social relationships

*Current adaptation*
  Activities of daily living
    Self-care
    Financial management
  Occupational performance
  Family function
  Social function

*Family medical history*
  Neurologic
  Psychiatric

is colloquially analogized as "power supply," or clinically answering the question, "Are the lights on?" Arousal is subserved by an evolutionarily old set of structures, principally composed of the ascending reticular activating system, thalamus, and thalamo-cortical relays. Arousal does not require coordinated cortical function.

*Assessment.* Clinical definitions of arousal are less than universal. It is therefore best to characterize patient arousal according to observed phenomenology (eg, "opens eyes to tactile stimuli"). Nevertheless, terms with some commonality of acceptance are listed in Table 2.

*Awareness*
*Conceptual foundation.* Awareness has been characterized as the content of consciousness. If arousal can be analogized to, "Are the lights on?", awareness can be analogized to, "Is anyone at home?" Awareness requires coordinated function of distributed polymodal cortical association areas to enable emergence of two key components commonly regarded as essential qualia of consciousness: (1) meaningful processing of exteroceptive and interoceptive stimuli, and (2) capacity for meaningful response to those stimuli.

*Assessment.* Assessment of awareness involves graduated stimulus delivery and observation of patient response. The primary goal is to probe coordinated integration of cortical sensory function. Awareness is modulated fundamentally by arousal level and comprises multimodal sensory and cognitive functions. No specific assessment criteria have been established; awareness assessment is essentially qualitative. Consequently, like arousal, awareness is best characterized phenomenologically (eg, "follows complex commands across midline"). Common assessment techniques are summarized in Box 4.

*Hemispheric dominance*

Because many of the neural substrates of neuropsychiatric functions above consciousness have lateralized characteristics, an essential organizing

Table 2
Arousal clinical terminology

| Level of arousal | Operational definition |
| --- | --- |
| Awake | Full wakefulness |
| Drowsy | Able to be stimulated to full arousal by non-noxious stimuli (eg, auditory/light, tactile) |
| Lethargic | Responds to non-noxious stimuli but unable to be brought to full arousal |
| Stuporous | Requires noxious stimuli to raise level of arousal |
| Coma | No/reflexive response to all stimuli |

---

**Box 4. Awareness assessment: sample criteria**

*Orientation*
  Person
  Place
  Time
  Social context

*Follows complex commands*
  Crosses midline
  Unilateral

*Follows simple commands*

*Visual tracking*
  *Localizes tactile stimuli*
    With limb contralateral to sensory stimulus (demonstrates
      integrated interhemispheric function)
    With limb ipsilateral to sensory stimulus
  *Localizes noxious stimuli*
    With limb contralateral to sensory stimulus (demonstrates
      integrated inter-hemispheric function)
    With limb ipsilateral to sensory stimulus

---

principle for neuropsychiatric examination is hemispheric dominance. Clinically, hemispheric dominance customarily is inferred by handedness, which is used as a peripheral indicator of cerebral hemispheric language lateralization. Handedness exists as a continuum, extending from extreme unilateral hand dominance to ambidexterity. Semiquantitative assessment of handedness can include the Edinburgh Handedness Inventory [15]. Because handedness has been recognized as less of a dichotomous and more of a spectrum entity, the relationship between handedness and language lateralization has been revised. Recent research suggests a linear relationship between handedness and language dominance [16]. For general clinical applications, the following approximations typically suffice. At least 90% of the human population is right-handed [17]. Of right-handers, at least 95% are left-hemisphere dominant for language [18]. Approximately 10% of human population is left-handed. Of left-handers, at least 60% are left-hemisphere dominant for language [18]. Left-handers are more likely to have bilateral language representation.

*Attention*

*Conceptual foundations*

Attention is a complex cognitive construct invoking a layered set of cognitive functions. Consequently, efforts to define and clinically assess attention unidimensionally are inevitably inadequate. Nonetheless, conceptually differentiating attentional components, even though they overlap, facilitates diagnostic assessment. This differentiation is summarized in Box 5.

Simple attention comprises the ability to devote sustained awareness to a specific stimulus or mental set. Select attention is the ability to apply focused awareness to a specific stimulus/mental set while excluding extraneous stimuli/mentation. Complex or divided attention comprises the act of manipulating focused awareness among multiple stimulus/mental sets, permitting simultaneous or proficient alternating processing of these sets. Sustained attention is essentially what is commonly termed concentration.

Neural substrates of attention are the subject of intense investigation by contemporary neuropsychiatric methodologies that are helping determine attention's neuroanatomy and define component operations more empirically. Partly because attentional processes are complex and continue to be defined empirically, a functional neuroanatomic account of attention remains incomplete. Nonetheless, consensus has emerged regarding key neural substrates subserving principal attentional processes. Supramodal (ie, sensory modality–independent) attentional substrates probably include the anterior cingulate and dorsolateral prefrontal cortex; in visual attention, the nondominant parietal cortex, striatal, and select brain stem regions seem to be crucial.

*Assessment*

Attentional assessment tasks are summarized in Table 3.

Attentional dysfunction can be characterized according to features outlined in Box 6.

---

**Box 5. Attentional components**

*Attentional dimensions*
    Attentional demand source
        Externally/stimulus driven
        Internally driven
    Substrate modality
        Bottom-up/modality-dependent
        Top-down/supramodel
    Complexity
        Simple/focused
        Select
        Complex/divided

Table 3
Tests of attention

| Clinical setting | Assessment task |
| --- | --- |
| Emergency room/bedside | Forward/reverse digit span |
| | Spatial span |
| | Backwards spelling |
| | Serial subtraction reverse days / months |
| Office/clinic | Trails A* |
| | Trails B* |
| | Continuous performance tasks |
| | Alternating category lists |
| Neuropsychologic testing | Wechsler Memory Scale III |
| | Letter-number sequencing |
| | Paced serial addition task (PASAT) |
| | Dichotic listening |

* See Mesulam MM. Principles of behavioral and cognitive neurology. New York: Oxford University Press; 2000.

## Language

### Conceptual foundations

Language was the prototype cognitive domain for a modular approach to functional neuroanatomy, demonstrating the explanatory power of the localizationist approach as promulgated by Broca and Wernicke. Contemporary behavioral neurology and neuropsychology have revealed that the distributed network subserving linguistic function is more complicated than the traditional modular model of linguistic function suggested. Nevertheless, because the classic modular model of linguistic neuroanatomy remains clinically powerful, it is summarized in Table 4 and Fig. 1.

### Assessment

An inventory of linguistic assessment procedures is outlined in Table 5. They are applicable in all examination venues; neuropsychologic testing

---

**Box 6. Attentional syndromes**

*Modality-independent*
  Distractibility
  Loss of set

*Modality-dependent*
Visual
  Neglect
Tactile
  Extinction

Table 4
Functional neuroanatomic modules of linguistic function

| Linguistic functional modules | | Neuroanatomy | Dysphasia |
|---|---|---|---|
| Comprehension | Lower-level (eg, phonemic) | Wernicke's area of posterior superior temporal cortex (Brodmann area 22) | Wernicke |
| | Higher-level (eg, semantic) | Temporal–parietal association cortex | Transcortical sensory |
| Expression | Lower-level (eg, motor innervatory patterns) | Broca's area of inferior frontal gyrus (Brodmann area 44) | Broca |
| | Higher-level (eg, syntax) | Frontal association cortex | Transcortical motor |
| Repetition | | Arcuate fasciculus | Conductive |

Table 5
Linguistic assessment tasks

| Linguistic domain | Assessment task | | |
|---|---|---|---|
| Fluency | Rate | | |
| | Phrase length | | |
| | Relational/function word proficiency | | |
| | Generativity | Letter/phonemic fluency | |
| | | Category/semantic fluency | |
| Lexicon | Confrontation naming | Objects | High-frequency items |
| | | | Low-frequency items |
| | | Concepts | High-frequency items |
| | | | Low-frequency items |
| Comprehension | 1,2,3 step commands | | |
| | Relational commands | | |
| Repetition | Simple phrase (eg, "Today is a sunny day.") | | |

should be ordered for patients with subtle language deficits to qualify these deficits precisely and facilitate quantitative tracking.

Individual dysphasias are characterized by a discrete set of clinical features that are outlined in Figs. 2 through 7. In actuality, clinical dysphasias often involve a mixture of phenomenology.

## Paralinguistic communication

Communication involves more than linguistic content. Nonverbal communication, including the emotional valence of spoken language and facial expression, constitutes important expressive and receptive communicative elements. These elements are summarized in Table 6, along with screening assessment guidelines.

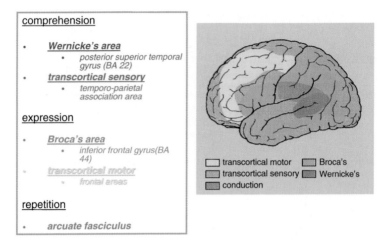

comprehension

- **Wernicke's area**
  - *posterior superior temporal gyrus (BA 22)*
- **transcortical sensory**
  - *temporo-parietal association area*

expression

- **Broca's area**
  - *inferior frontal gyrus(BA 44)*
- *transcortical motor*
  - *frontal areas*

repetition

- **arcuate fasciculus**

transcortical motor □ Broca's
transcortical sensory □ Wernicke's
conduction

Fig. 1. Linguistic neuroanatomic modules. (*Adapted from* Perkin GD. Mosby's color atlas and text of neurology. St. Louis (MO): Mosby; 1998. p. 104; with permission.)

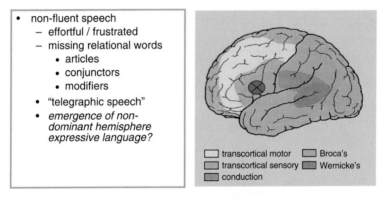

- non-fluent speech
  - effortful / frustrated
  - missing relational words
    - articles
    - conjunctors
    - modifiers
  - "telegraphic speech"
  - *emergence of non-dominant hemisphere expressive language?*

transcortical motor □ Broca's
transcortical sensory □ Wernicke's
conduction

Fig. 2. Broca's aphasia. (*Adapted from* Perkin GD. Mosby's color atlas and text of neurology. St. Louis (MO): Mosby; 1998. p. 104; with permission.)

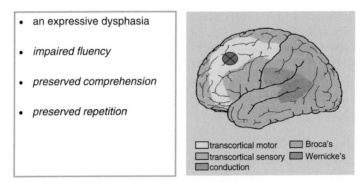

- an expressive dysphasia

- *impaired fluency*

- *preserved comprehension*

- *preserved repetition*

transcortical motor □ Broca's
transcortical sensory □ Wernicke's
conduction

Fig. 3. Transcortical motor aphasia. (*Adapted from* Perkin GD. Mosby's color atlas and text of neurology. St. Louis (MO): Mosby; 1998. p. 104; with permission.)

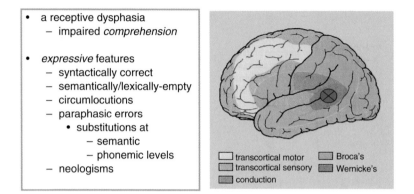

Fig. 4. Wernicke's aphasia. (*Adapted from* Perkin GD. Mosby's color atlas and text of neurology. St. Louis (MO): Mosby; 1998. p. 104; with permission.)

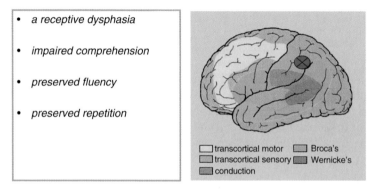

Fig. 5. Transcortical sensory aphasia: receptive aphasia, impaired comprehension, preserved fluency, preserved repetition. (*Adapted from* Perkin GD. Mosby's color atlas and text of neurology. St. Louis (MO): Mosby; 1998. p. 104; with permission.)

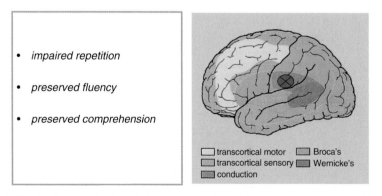

Fig. 6. Conduction aphasia: impaired repetition; preserved fluency; preserved comprehension. (*Adapted from* Perkin GD. Mosby's color atlas and text of neurology. St. Louis (MO): Mosby; 1998. p. 104; with permission.)

| dysphasia | fluency | repetition | compre-hension | naming |
|---|---|---|---|---|
| transcortical motor | X | ✓ | ✓ | X |
| Broca | X | X | ✓ | X |
| conduction | ✓ | X | ✓ | X |
| Wernicke | ✓ | X | X | X |
| transcortical sensory | ✓ | ✓ | X | X |
| global | X | X | X | X |

key: **expressive dysphasias**
receptive dysphasias

Fig. 7. Dysphasias.

There are few standardized assessment procedures for paralinguistic communication. The Profile of Nonverbal Sensitivity [19] can be administered by a neuropsychologist. This assessment can be useful for informing rehabilitation planning and tracking progress in patients with nonverbal learning disorders (eg, Asperger's syndrome).

## Memory

### Conceptual foundations

Memory is a complex and intrinsically multidimensional phenomenon [20]. For example, working memory comprises a complicated coordination of attention, memory, and executive operations (Fig. 8).

It is important to distinguish between memory processes and memory systems. Diagnostically informative assessment requires a methodical

Table 6
Paralinguistic communication

| Paralinguistic domain | Modality | Assessment task examples |
|---|---|---|
| Prosody | Receptive | Have patient rate emotional valence of utterances said out of patient's field-of-view |
|  | Expressive | Assess amplitude and semantic congruence of expressive linguistic prosody |
| Facial expression | Receptive | Have patient rate emotional valence of facial expressions |
|  | Expressive | Ask patient to make facial expressions concordant with various emotional valences |

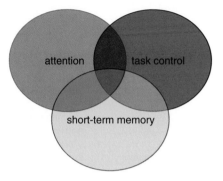

Fig. 8. Working memory.

approach informed by this distinction. Memory processes are outlined in Box 7; memory systems are outlined in Table 7.

*Assessment*

Memory assessment is difficult and extremely vulnerable to confounding executive and affective influences. Many complaints of memory impairment actually represent memory epiphenomena secondary to other cognitive or affective dysfunction. Secondary memory dysfunction often is mediated by attentional deficits that impair robust memory formation and are misinterpreted by patients as poor memory retrieval. For example, it is well known that depression-related cognitive impairment (previously termed pseudodementia) can involve memory dysfunction that is reversible with treatment of the affective disturbance (although the pathophysiology of depression-related cognitive impairment is more complicated than conventional

---

**Box 7. Memory processes**

*Memory formation*
  Registration
  Evaluation for relevance
  Encoding
  Consolidation
  Storage

*Memory retrieval*
  Euphony
  Recognition
  Free recall

Table 7
Memory systems

| Memory system | | | Function | Temporal dynamic |
|---|---|---|---|---|
| Echoic memory | | | Facilitates registration (?) | $\leq$5-s perceptual echo |
| Short-term memory | | | Relatively passive on-line maintenance | Seconds to minutes |
| Working memory | | | Active on-line maintenance | Seconds to minutes |
| Long-term memory | Explicit/declarative (conscious or preconscious) | Semantic | Factual knowledge | Minutes to years |
| | Implicit (nonconscious) | Episodic | Event memory | |
| | | Procedural (praxicon) | Skilled motor tasks | |
| | | Classic conditioning | Stimulus association | |
| | | Emotional | Emotional memory | |

attributions to motivational and attentional effects suggested). Memory assessment procedures are summarized in Table 8.

Neuropsychologic testing should be performed when ceiling effects preclude detection of dys/amnesias for high-functioning patients, to clarify memory dysfunction as primary or secondary, and to track patient

Table 8
Memory assessment procedures

| Clinical setting | Memory system | Assessment task | Comments |
|---|---|---|---|
| Emergency room/ bedside/clinic/ office | Registration | Repeat item set | Vary number/complexity according to clinical context |
| | Short-term memory | 7 $\pm$ 2-item set delayed recall | Vary semantic categories and emotional valence |
| | | 3 words–3 shapes test [21] | Combines lexical and visual assessment |
| | | Narrative task | Assess number of recalled elements, intrusions |
| | | Hidden object task | Hide objects in room |
| | Long-term memory | Current events | Vary number/complexity according to clinical context |
| | | Serial presidents or equivalent | Vary according to education level |
| | | Personal biography | Corroborate with informants |
| Neuropsychologic testing | California Verbal Learning Task (CVLT) | | |
| | Rey-Osterrieth Complex Figure Test | | |

Table 9
Dys/amnesia categorization

| Amnestic type | | Features | | |
|---|---|---|---|---|
| By temporal nature of memory loss | Anterograde | Impaired ability to form new memories | | |
| | Retrograde | Loss of old memories | No temporal gradient | |
| | | | Temporal gradient | Recent > distant |
| | | | | Distant > recent |
| By temporal nature of amnestic onset | Anterograde | Impaired memory function after pathogenic event | | |
| | Retrograde | Impaired memory function before pathogenic event | | |

performance quantitatively over time. Memory disorders are characterized according to features outlined in Table 9.

Dys/amnesia syndromes are outlined in Tables 10 and 11.

### Visuospatial processing function

#### Conceptual foundations

Visuospatial function involves a complex mixture of perceptual, attentional, and associational processing. The functional neuroanatomy of visual processing is organized classically according to ventral and dorsal streams. The dorsal stream, composed of occipital-parietal association regions, subserves localization (the "where" function). The ventral stream, composed of occipital-temporal association regions, subserves identification (the "what" function). Visual-spatial processing features warranting neuropsychiatric assessment are summarized in Box 8.

#### Assessment

Visuospatial function assessment procedures are outlined in Table 12.

Visuospatial syndromes are summarized in Table 13.

### Body representation

#### Conceptual foundations

Body representation involves a complex mixture of somatotopic, proprioceptive, and visuomotor integration. Levels of information integrated to subserve body representation include vestibular, kinesthetic, tactile, and visual. Consequently, body representation dysfunction can be mediated by multiple potential mechanisms.

#### Assessment

Disorders of body representation are summarized in Table 14.

Table 10
Dys/amnestic syndromes: amnesias

| Subtypes | | Hypothesized lesion site | Clinical features |
|---|---|---|---|
| Transient global amnesia (TGA) | | Unknown | Anterograde dys/ amnesia; typically resolves within 24 hours |
| Primary neuro- degenerative | Mild cognitive impairment (MCI) – amnestic type | Variable | Anterograde dys/ amnesia |
| | Alzheimer's disease | Hippocampal, entorhinal | Anterograde amnesia, temporally graded retrograde amnesia |
| | Dementia with Lewy body (DLB) | Variable | Anterograde amnesia, temporally graded retrograde dys/ amnesia |
| | Fronto-temporal lobar dementia (FTLD) | Varying permutations of frontal/temporal cortex | Variable dys/ amnesias |
| Stroke | Anterior communicating artery aneurysm | Basal forebrain, striatum | Variable dys/ amnesias |
| | Thalamic arteries | Thalamus | |
| | Posterior cerebral artery | Inferior/medial temporal cortex | |
| Anoxia | | Hippocampus (CA1 region) | Variable dys/ amnesias |
| Nutritional | Wernicke-Korsakoff syndrome | Thalamic nuclei | Anterograde dys/ amnesia, confabulation |
| | | Mamillary bodies | |
| Neoplastic | Paraneoplastic limbic encephalitis | Medial temporal cortex | Variable dys/ amnesias, multiple associated features |
| Infectious | Herpes simplex encephalitis (HSE) | Anterior temporal cortex | Anterograde dys/ amnesia, laterality determines linguistic vs. non-linguistic predominance |
| | Creutzfeldt-Jacob Disease (CJD) | Diffuse cortical | Variable dys/ amnesias, multiple associated features |

Table 11
Para-amnesias

| re-duplicative para-amnesia | Unknown | Delusional duplication of objects/places/people |
|---|---|---|
| Capgras syndrome | Affect–memory association disconnection? | Delusional belief that people of emotional significance are imposters |
| Fregoli syndrome | Affect–memory association dysfunction | Delusional belief that a person recurrently reappears as others |

---

**Box 8. Visual-spatial processing parameters**

Bilateral visual integration
Localization (where)
Percept analysis (what)
    Detail (parts)
    Synthesis (whole)
    Pattern recognition

---

Table 12
Visuospatial assessment

| Clinical setting | Assessment task |
|---|---|
| Emergency room/bedside | Left–right orientation<br>Line bisection<br>Geometric shape copying<br>Clock drawing |
| Clinic/office | Navigation<br>Visual cancellation tasks |
| Neuropsychologic testing | Hooper Visual Organization Task<br>Benton judgment of line orientation task<br>Block design (WAIS-III) |

*Abbreviation:* WAIS, Weschler Adult Intelligence Scale.

## Praxis

### Conceptual foundations

Praxis is the act of translating intent into action. Praxis requires two fundamental types of knowledge: (1) conceptual ("what to do"), and (2) performance ("how to do it"). Praxis can be analogized crudely to sports, with the conceptual component corresponding to the coach's knowledge and the performance component corresponding to the additional skill possessed by an athlete.

The construct of praxicon, a motor equivalent of lexicon, has been developed to aid conceptualization of praxis and its dysfunction. The praxicon

Table 13
Visuospatial syndromes

| Deficit level | Deficit | | | Neuroanatomy |
|---|---|---|---|---|
| Perceptual | Ocular impairment | | | Retinal, prechiasmal |
| | Visual field cut | | | Chiasmal, retrochiasmal |
| | Achromatopsia | | | inferno-medial calcarine |
| | Cortical blindness | | | Bilateral occipital |
| Visual attention/ awareness | Visual neglect | | | Nondominant parietal |
| Bilateral integration | Extinction to double simultaneous stimulation | | | Nondominant parietal |
| Percept integration | Simultanagnosia | | | Nondominant parietal |
| Percept recognition | Words | | Alexia | Dominant occipito-temporal-parietal |
| | Faces | | Prosopagnosia | Fusiform gyrus (fusiform facial area?) |
| | Object | | Object agnosia | |
| Oculo-motor integration | Oculo-motor dyspraxia | | Impaired voluntary saccades | Parieto-occipital |
| | Balint syndrome | optic ataxia | Impaired visual-guided reaching | Intraparietal sulcus (Brodmann areas 5, 7) |
| | | Ocular dyspraxia | Impaired voluntary saccades | Parieto-occipital |
| | | Simultanagnosia | Impaired simultaneous percept integration | Parieto-occipital |

is composed of neural representations of programs for motor tasks. Like the lexicon, programs are layered in their level of function. Higher-order programs code for the temporo-spatial patterns of learned skilled movements, whereas lower-order programs determine actual motor innervation patterns. The functional neuroanatomy of praxis is summarized in Table 15 and Fig. 9.

*Assessment*

In assessing dyspraxia, it is important to perform an adequate elementary neurologic screening examination to ensure the absence of primary motor, sensory, or praxis-unrelated cognitive dysfunction that can secondarily cause dyspraxias or confound praxis assessment. It is also important to test each side and limb independently. Criteria that should be used when

Table 14
Disorders of body representation

| Body representation dysfunction | Definition | Defect | Neuroanatomy |
|---|---|---|---|
| Hemi-body neglect | Unawareness of half of body | Unawareness of half of body | Usually nondominant parietal |
| Auto-/somato-topagnosia Finger agnosia All other | Inability to recognize body parts/locations | Inability to link preserved spatial orientation on body to conceptual representation of body schema | Interparietal sulcus, Brodmann areas 5, 7 |
| Body part phantoms | Hallucinatory perception of sensory input from amputated limb | Impaired sensory adaptation | Unknown |
| Gerstmann syndrome | Left–right disorientation Finger agnosia Dyslexia Dyscalculia | Unknown | Dominant parietal lobe |

Table 15
Functional neuroanatomy of praxis

| Functional component | Neuroanatomy |
|---|---|
| Temporo-spatial patterns of learned skilled movements (higher-order programs) | Dominant parietal lobe |
| Motor innervatory patterns (lower-order programs) | Premotor cortex Supplementary motor area |
| Semantic motor association | Dominant parietal lobe |
| Visual-motor association | Occipito-parietal association |
| Interhemispheric connectivity | Corpus callosum |

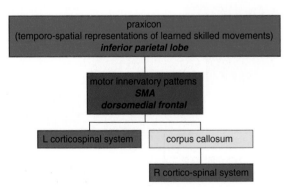

Fig. 9. Functional neuroanatomy of dyspraxia.

Table 16
Praxis assessment procedures

| Graduated examination tasks | Examples | Difficulty |
|---|---|---|
| Pantomime to verbal instruction | "Show me how you brush your teeth." | |
| Imitate examiner action | Model pantomime action for patient | |
| Actual object utilization: | | |
|     Transitive | "Show me how you would work this key." | |
|     Intransitive | "Show me how you wave goodbye." | |

evaluating dexterity include speed, precision, sequencing, and capacity for simultaneous independent movements. Praxis assessment is summarized in Table 16 and Figs. 10 through 12.

Dyspraxia syndrome classification is summarized in Table 17.

## Agnosias

### Conceptual foundations

Agnosias, a term originally introduced by Freud, represent a set of disorders sharing the clinical feature of impaired recognition of sensory stimuli. Agnosias represent a disturbance of higher-order sensory processing. The core neuropsychologic deficit seems to be a disturbance of integrative awareness causing impaired ability to recognize the nature or meaning of sensory stimuli and is typically sensory modality–specific. There are two basic categories of agnosias. Apperceptive agnosia involves impaired generation of the minimal integrated percept necessary for meaningful recognition, yielding an inadequate or defective minimal object recognition unit. Apperceptive agnosia therefore represents a defect before percept–meaning association. Associative agnosia involves postperceptual recognition dysfunction—a defect in associating a correctly perceived

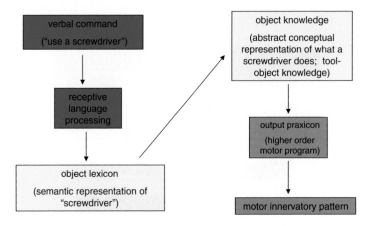

Fig. 10. Dyspraxia to auditory verbal command.

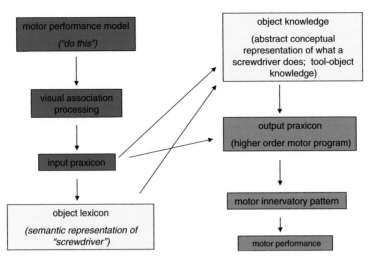

Fig. 11. Dyspraxia to pantomime demonstration command.

percept with its meaning. Visual agnosias are the most common subtype of agnosia. Patients are unable to recognize images or visually presented objects. Astereoagnosia is agnosia for tactually presented objects.

Agnosia subtypes are summarized in Tables 18 and 19.

*Assessment*

Agnosia assessment requires a neuropsychologically sophisticated approach. Figs. 13 through 16 summarize agnosia assessment strategies:

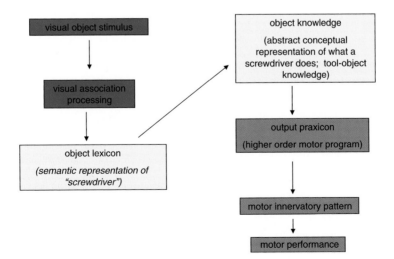

Fig. 12. Dyspraxia to object cue command.

Table 17
Dyspraxias

| Apraxia type | | Definition | Neuroanatomy |
|---|---|---|---|
| General | Limb-kinetic | Impaired dexterity of distal limb movements | Contralateral cortico-spinal system Premotor/supplementary motor area |
| | Ideomotor | Impaired ability to perform learned movement; use of body part as tool | Supplementary motor area, inferior parietal, callosal |
| | Ideational/ conceptual | Impaired ability to perform multistep motor act | Temporo-parietal junction |
| Specific | Conduction | Impaired motor imitation (ie, akin to conduction aphasia) | Unknown |
| | Constructional | Disturbance of visuo-constructive ability | Nondominant > dominant parietal |
| | Dressing | Multiple potential mechanisms Visuospatial integration Object recognition Praxis Body representation | Multiple potential sites |

Table 18
Visual agnosias

| Type | Stimulus category | Subtype | Clinical distinction | Functional neuroanatomy |
|---|---|---|---|---|
| Visual object agnosia | Objects | Apperceptive | Cannot match/draw | Bilateral occipito-parietal |
| | | Associative | Can match/draw | Bilateral occipito-temporal |
| Simultanagnosia | Multiple objects/ object features | Dorsal/ apperceptive | Cannot perceive multiple objects simultaneously | Bilateral occipito-parietal |
| | | Ventral/ associative | Cannot recognize multiple objects simultaneously | Dominant fusiform |
| Prosopagnosia | Faces | Apperceptive | Cannot match faces | Bilateral fusiform |
| | | Associative | Can match faces | Bilateral anterior medial temporal |
| Color agnosia | Colors | Apperceptive | Cannot perform nonverbal color tasks | Visuo-linguistic disconnection (eg, posterior corpus callosum) |
| | | Associative | Can perform nonverbal color tasks | Dominant occipito-parietal |

Table 19
Auditory agnosias

| Type | Stimulus category | Subtype | Clinical distinction | Functional neuroanatomy |
|------|-------------------|---------|----------------------|-------------------------|
| Pure word deafness | Speech | Apperceptive/ pre-phonemic | Cannot match phonemes | Bilateral Heschl Wernicke disconnection |
| | | Associative/ phonemic | Can match phonemes | Perisylvian |
| Nonverbal sound agnosia | Nonverbal sounds | Apperceptive | Cannot match sounds | Unclear |
| | | Associative | Can match sounds | Unclear |
| Sensory dysmusia | Musical sounds | | | Nondominant > dominant |

## Executive function

### Conceptual foundations

Executive performance constitutes a diverse set of cognitive functions that can be subdivided into three overarching domains: (1) "go," (2) "no-go," and (3) "how-to-go," summarized in Table 20. (A detailed discussion of executive function is presented elsewhere in this volume.)

Because of the traditional localization of executive operations to the frontal lobes, the terms frontal and executive function are often used interchangeably. Contemporary neuropsychiatric investigative techniques, however, have demonstrated that many executive functions previously assumed to be exclusively prefrontal are in fact subserved by distributed neural networks.

Inhibitory control constitutes an especially crucial component of behavioral regulation. Successful adaptation requires that both mentation and behavior be modulated by a context-appropriate balance of agency and inhibition. Inhibitory control is a multidomain executive function critical for flexible interaction with changing task demands and is thereby an essential component of cognitive, emotional, and motor regulation.

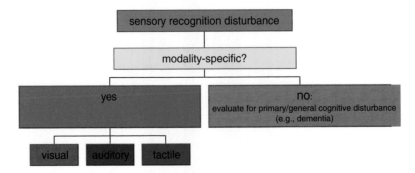

Fig. 13. Agnosia: general differential diagnostic algorithm.

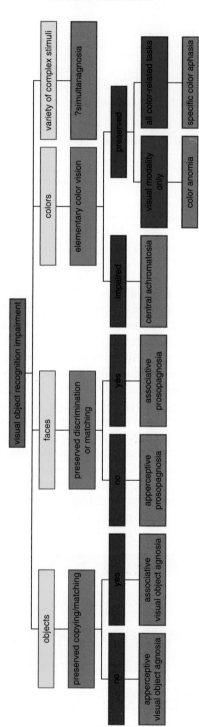

Fig. 14. Visual agnosia: differential diagnostic algorithm.

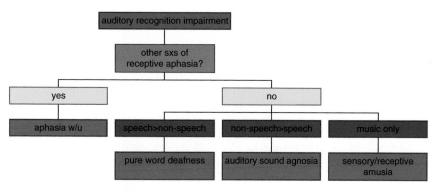

Fig. 15. Auditory agnosia: differential diagnostic algorithm.

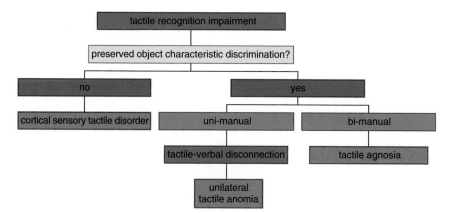

Fig. 16. Tactile agnosia: differential diagnostic algorithm.

Table 20
Executive operations

| Executive function | | |
|---|---|---|
| Global | Specific | Principal neuroanatomy |
| Go | Initiative/agency | Anterior cingulate |
| No-go | Inhibitory control | Orbito-frontal cortex |
| How-to-go | Task control operations | Dorso-lateral prefrontal cortex |
| | Set acquisition | |
| | Set maintenance | |
| | Set shifting | |
| | Conflict detection | Anterior cingulate |
| | Conflict resolution | Anterior cingulate, lateral PFC, OFC |

Inhibitory control is susceptible to impairment in a variety of neuro-developmental [22], neurodegenerative [23], primary psychiatric [24], and acquired [25] processes. Inhibitory control thereby constitutes a fundamental assessment target (especially in forensic contexts).

*Assessment*

Procedures for assessing executive function are outlined in Table 21.
Although many executive functions have extrafrontal neuroanatomic components, nosologic classification of many dysexecutive syndromes remains "frontal." Executive syndromes are summarized in Table 22.

*Interhemispheric integration*

Deficits of interhemispheric integration are prototypic examples of disconnection syndromes involving structural or functional disturbance of

Table 21
Executive assessment

| Clinical setting | Assessment procedure | Domain assayed | Potential deficits |
| --- | --- | --- | --- |
| Emergency room/ bedside | Go/no-go | Agency | Abulia |
| | | Inhibitory control | Impulsivity |
| | | Task operation control | Disinhibition Perseveration |
| | Ramparts, loops copying | Task operation control | Perseveration |
| | | Inhibitory control | |
| | Clock drawing | Task operation control | Impaired organization |
| | | Abstraction (Visuospatial function) | Concreteness (Neglect) |
| Office/clinic | Sequential finger movements | Premotor function | Poor sequencing |
| | Reciprocal motor/Luria alternating tasks | Task operation control | Perseveration |
| | | Inhibitory function | Missing components |
| | Unimanual task Bimanual task | | |
| | Continuous performance tasks | Set maintenance | Loss of set |
| | Set-shifting tasks | Flexibility | Impaired task control |
| | | Working memory Task operation control | Perseveration |
| | Multi-item free recall tasks | Search strategy | Impaired free recall |
| | Proverb interpretation Judgment questions | Abstraction | Concreteness |
| Neuropsychologic testing (examples) | Stroop tasks | Inhibitory control | Disinhibition |
| | Wisconsin Card Sort Task | Set shifting | Perseveration |

Table 22
Executive syndromes

| Syndrome | Functional neuroanatomy | Features |
|---|---|---|
| Abulic-akinetic | Medial PFC (AC) dysfunction | Hypo/akinetic |
| | | Impaired initiation |
| | | Impaired persistence |
| | | Decreased responsivity to environmental cues |
| | | Blunted affect |
| | | Apathetic/abulic comportment |
| | | Depression-mimic |
| Disinhibition syndrome | OFC dysfunction | Inhibitory failure |
| | | Perseveration |
| Dysexecutive syndrome | DLPFC dysfunction | Loss of set (task goal) |
| | | Reduced response repertoire |
| | | Reduced generativity |
| | | Decreased response flexibility |
| | | Impaired error monitoring |
| | | Inefficient learning |
| | | Poor free recall/top-down retrieval (better recognition) |
| Environmental dependency | ? Release of parietal exploratory behavior because of absence of frontal inhibition | Stimulus-boundedness |
| | | Utilization behavior |
| Frontal-striatal | | Cognitive flexibility |
| | | Reward |
| | | Punishment |
| Frontal white matter | | Slowed processing speed |

the corpus callosum. Because a task rarely tests function based in solely one hemisphere, assessment of callosal function is essentially a component of the majority of cognitive/behavioral assays. Tasks specifically evaluating callosal function explicitly test for interhemispheric coordination. One simple task involves having the patient place the fingers of one hand in various configurations and then, with eyes closed, reproducing these configurations using the other hand. In the absence of global signs of cerebral dysfunction (eg, as in advanced Alzheimer's disease), impaired performance suggests interhemispheric disconnection.

*Thought processes*

Disturbance of thought process can be a component of many neuropsychiatric disease states. Table 23 summarizes the features of thought process assessment, disturbances in thought processes, and examples of disease states.

Table 23
Thought process assessment

| Criteria | Abnormality | Examples of disease states |
|----------|-------------|----------------------------|
| Coherence | Incoherence | Delirium/encephalopathy |
| | Loosening of associations | Schizophrenia |
| Linearity | Tangentiality | FTLD |
| | Circumstantiality | Asperger's syndrome |
| | Circumlocution | Dysnomia |
| Flow | Blocking | Major depression, FTLD, schizophrenia |
| | Flight-of-ideas | Mania |

## Thought content

Disturbances of thought content can be a feature of many neuropsychiatric disease states. Table 24 summarizes the parameters of thought content assessment and gives examples of pathologic features.

## Perceptual disturbances

Perceptual disturbances represent gross dysfunction at the level of percept generation such that the percept submitted for higher-order processing contains stimulus-independent features (therefore, these disturbances are distinct from visual processing impairments discussed previously). Disturbances can be positive or negative. Positive perceptual disturbances include illusions and hallucinations of all sensory modalities. Negative disturbances (eg, scotoma) involve select sensory loss secondary to central processes. Perceptual abnormalities should be assessed by direct inquiry as well as by observation for signs of internal stimuli. Perceptual disturbances can be a component of multiple primary and secondary neuropsychiatric disease states. Table 25 summarizes perceptual disturbance states.

Table 24
Thought content assessment

| Criteria | Abnormality | | Examples of disease states |
|----------|-------------|---|----------------------------|
| Abundance | Paucity | | FTLD |
| Reality testing | Delusionality | Paranoia | Schizophrenia |
| | | Grandeur | Mania |
| | | Erotic | Erotomania |
| | | Somatic | Depression |
| Abstraction | Concreteness | | Schizophrenia |
| Meaningfulness | Ganser syndrome | | Encephalopathy |
| Veridicality | Confabulation | | Korsakoff syndrome |
| Violence potential | Suicidality | | Depression |

Table 25
Perceptual disturbances

| Modality | Examples of disease states | Features |
|---|---|---|
| Auditory | Schizophrenia | Variable hallucinations |
| Visual | | |
|   positive | Classic migraine | Fortifications |
| | Charles Bonnet syndrome | Variable hallucinations |
| | | Associated perceptual acuity impairment |
| | Peduncular hallucinosis | Formed hallucinations (often magical figures) |
| | Lewy body disease | Associated cognitive impairment and parkinsonism |
|   negative | Migraine | Visual scotoma |
| Olfactory | Temporal lobe epilepsy | Often malodorous hallucinations |
| Gustatory | Temporal lobe epilepsy | Variable hallucinations |
| Tactile | Alcohol withdrawal | Formication |

## Affect

### Conceptual foundations

Affective disturbances can represent a primary psychiatric syndrome (eg, major depression, bipolar disorder) or constitute a component of a multidomain neuropsychiatric disease state. Almost any primary or secondary disturbance of the central nervous system can manifest with emotional features. Assessment of mood and affective regulation is therefore an essential component of neuropsychiatric assessment.

Although emotional function has long been localized to limbic structures, neural substrates of emotion, emotional–cognitive integration, and socio-emotional regulation are complex and remain under intense study. Fig. 17 summarizes well-documented emotional circuitry.

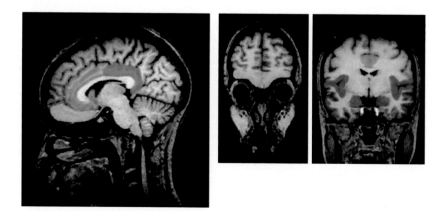

Fig. 17. Functional neuroanatomy of emotion. (*From* Dolan RJ. Emotion, cognition and behavior. Science 2002;298:1191–4; with permission.)

*Assessment*

By nature, the assessment of affective function is less structured than the assessment of cognitive performance. Important features of affective function assessment are summarized in Table 26.

*Speech*

Speech disturbances are complex to analyze. It is crucial to distinguish speech components to identify pathology accurately. These components are summarized in Table 27.

*Mixed syndromes*

Certain neuropsychiatric syndromes are intrinsically multidomain and so defy category-specific classification.

For example, Gerstmann syndrome consists of left–right disorientation, finger agnosia, dysgraphia, and dyscalculia. Most commonly attributable to a dominant parietal lobe dysfunction, when all components are present the syndrome reliably localizes to the dominant angular gyrus. Screening for Gerstmann syndrome should be performed on all patients presenting with any one of the four component features. Other multidomain neuropsychiatric syndromes are discussed throughout this volume.

Anosagnosias are marked by absence of recognition of a deficit. The most common form of deficit unawareness is anosognosia for hemiplegia, a phenomenologic admixture of hemi-body neglect and deficit agnosia. The functional neuroanatomy usually localizes to the nondominant parietal lobe. Visual anosognosias are a common form of anosognosia. Normal

Table 26
Affective assessment features

| Affective feature | Abnormalities | Examples of syndromes |
| --- | --- | --- |
| Emotional valence | Elevated | Mania |
| Context-appropriateness | Inappropriate | Schizophrenia |
| Reactivity | Blunted | FTLD |
| Range | Restricted | Depression |
| Stability | Lability | Pseudobulbar affect |

Table 27
Speech components

| Component | Abnormality | Examples of disease state |
| --- | --- | --- |
| Linguistic | Dysphasia | Cortical stroke |
| | Dysnomia | Alzheimer's disease |
| Rate | Pressured | Mania |
| Production | Dysarthria | Bulbar pathology |
| | Tachyphemia | Parkinson's disease |
| | Stuttering | Congenital speech disturbance |

forms of visual anosognosia include unawareness of a physiologic blind spot. Acquired forms include unawareness of acquired scotomas (which can be adaptive) and unawareness of acquired hemianopias. A particularly striking form of anosognosia is Anton's syndrome, which involves absence of awareness of blindness, usually cortical. The functional neuroanatomy typically involves occipito-parietal areas with or without involvement of occipito-temporal visual association areas (in addition to bilateral occipital regions if blindness is cortical).

## Psychodynamics

Although not conventionally conceptualized as a neuropsychiatric domain, psychodynamics provides crucial context for assessment of essentially all neuropsychiatric phenomenology above stupor. Psychodynamics can substantially influence the content of patient presentation involving cognitive, affective, and comportmental domains. Even the most "hardware-related" neuropsychiatric pathology rarely exists within a psychodynamic vacuum. Consequently, neuropsychiatric assessment conducted without a psychodynamically informed perspective risks missing critical diagnostic data.

## Elementary neurologic examination

Because many primary and secondary neuropsychiatric disease states have associated elementary neurologic signs, a quality general neurologic examination is an important component of comprehensive neuropsychiatric assessment. Because of the frequent association of neuropsychiatric phenomenology with movement disorders, a quality motor examination is particularly essential. Table 28 outlines key components.

## Diagnostic investigations

The scope of neuropsychiatric assessment dictates a wide assortment of potentially relevant diagnostic test procedures. The selection of diagnostic tests should be informed by findings from neuropsychiatric history and examination. Screening tests can be employed strategically to guide subsequent investigations to balance sensitivity, specificity, invasive risk, and cost control optimally. Box 9 outlines an inventory of potentially useful neuropsychiatric diagnostic tests. The rapidly expanding applications of neuroimaging in neuropsychiatry are discussed in detail elsewhere in this volume.

## Somatoform and factitious disorders, malingering

Assessment of patients presenting with signs and symptoms that do not match known pathophysiologic syndromes represents a special challenge.

Table 28
Screening neurologic examination inventory (including relevant general medical)

| Examination sets | | | | Sample abnormalities |
| --- | --- | --- | --- | --- |
| General medical | Vital signs | Blood pressure | | Orthostasis |
| | | Temperature | | Fever |
| | Cardiovascular | Heart rhythm | | Atrial fibrillation |
| | | Carotids | | Bruits |
| | | Peripheral vascular integrity | | Atherosclerosis |
| | Dermatolologic | | | Café au lait spots, rashes (eg, erythema chronicum migrans) |
| | Muscular-skeletal | Muscle bulk | | Wasting |
| Elementary neurologic | Head | Developmental abnormalities trauma signs | | Fetal alcohol syndrome |
| | | | | Battle's signs |
| | | | | Raccoon's eyes |
| | | Eyes | Sclerae | Icterus |
| | | | Fundi | Hypertensive retinopathy, papilledema |
| | | Ears | | Tympanic membrane pathology |
| | Neck | | | Nuchal rigidity |
| | | | | Mass |
| | Cranial nerves | I/olfactory | | Anosmia |
| | | II/optic | | Optic neuritis |
| | | III/oculomotor | | Papillary asymmetry, ptosis ophthalmoplegia |
| | | IV/trochlear | | Ophthalmoplegia |
| | | V/trigeminal | | Neuralgia, numbness |
| | | VI/abducens | | Ophthalmoplegia |
| | | VII/facial | | Facial asymmetry |
| | | VIII/vestibule-cochlear | | Vertigo |
| | | IX/glossopharyngeal | | Impaired gag |
| | | X/vagus | | Asymmetric palate |
| | | XI/accessory | | Asymmetric trapezius power |
| | | XII/hypoglossal | | Asymmetric tongue protrusion |
| | Motor | Power | | Paresis |
| | | Muscle tone | | Dystonias |
| | | | | Cogwheel rigidity |
| | | | | Lead pipe rigidity |
| | | | | Waxy flexibility (eg, as in catatonia) |
| | | Movement amount | | Hypokinesia, hyperkinesia |
| | | Movement speed | | Bradykinesia |

Table 28 (*continued*)

| Examination sets | | | Sample abnormalities |
|---|---|---|---|
| | Psychomotor tone | | Akathisia |
| | Adventitial movements | Resting | Tremors |
| | | | Dyskinesias |
| | | | Choreoathetoid movements, clonus |
| | | | Fasciculations |
| | | | Convulsive activity |
| | | Postural | Tremors, titubation |
| Coordination | | | Intention tremor |
| | | | Dystaxia |
| | | | Dysdiadochokinesis |
| Station | | | Positive Romberg |
| Gait | | | Dystaxia |
| Deep tendon reflexes | | | Hyper-reflexia |
| Babinski reflexes | | | Extensor |
| Frontal release signs | | | Myerson's sign |
| | | | Snout |
| | | | Routing |
| | | | Grasp |
| | | | Palmo-mental |
| Frontal eye fields function | | | Ipsilateral gaze preference |
| | | | Contralateral gaze paresis |
| | | | Impaired contralateral smooth pursuit |
| | | | Inefficient contralateral visual search |
| Neurologic soft signs | | | Impaired smooth pursuit |
| | | | Mirror movements |
| | | | Synkinesis |
| | | | Asymmetric dyscoordination |

First, because neuropsychiatric pathology can be complexly protean, definitive declaration that a clinical sign or symptom is psychogenic should be a diagnosis of exclusion [26]. Indeed, many patients with clinical syndromes deemed hysteric have later been determined to have "valid" disease [27]. Second, the terminology used to describe such disorders can be controversial, because terms can be subtly (eg, functional) or not so subtly (eg, hysteric, embellished, overlay) conflated with examiner bias. Part of the problem is discipline-dependent terminological inconsistency. Table 29 summarizes relevant terminology from *DSM-IV*.

**Box 9. Neuropsychiatric diagnostic test inventory**

*Blood*
  Complete blood count
  Electrolytes
  Kidney function tests
  Liver function tests
  Prothrombin time, partial thromboplastin time, fibrinogen
  Erythrocyte sedimentation rate
  C-reactive protein
  Serum drug levels
  Antinuclear antibodies
  $B_{12}$/folate levels
  Homocysteine, methylmalonic acid
  Cu, ceruloplasmin
  Lyme antibody, rapid plasma reagin, HIV
  Heavy metal screen
  ApoE4 allele
  Aβ42 peptide, Tau protein, PS-1
  High-density trinucleotide repeat

*Cerebrospinal fluid*
  Protein
  Cytology
  α-Fetoprotein/viral/fungal/VDRL/Lyme screens
  Aβ42 peptide, Tau protein
  Protein 14-3-3
  Cysticercosis antibody

*Urine*
  Urinalysis, catecholamines, porphyrin

*Biopsy*
  Nerve
  Brain
  Muscle

*Ophthalmologic*
  Slit lamp (eg, Kayser-Fleischer rings)

*Electrophysiologic*
  Electroencephalogram
  Polysomnography (sleep study)
  Electromyogram
  Nerve conduction velocity

*Radiologic*
  Structural neuroimaging
    CT
    MRI
  Functional neuroimaging
    Single-proton emission computed tomography
    Positron emission tomography

Table 29
Psychogenic syndrome diagnostic classification

| Disorder | | Criteria (abridged) |
|---|---|---|
| Somatoform disorders | Conversion | ≥ 1 voluntary motor and/or sensory symptom(s) |
| | | No conscious intent/exaggeration |
| | | Temporal concordance of symptom with an underlying psychologic conflict |
| | Hypochondriasis | Preoccupation with having a serious disease despite adequate medical evaluation |
| | | ? based on misinterpretation of bodily symptoms |
| | Somatization disorder | Must have all of following: |
| | | ≥ 4 pain symptoms |
| | | ≥ 2 gastrointestinal symptoms |
| | | ≥ 1 sexual symptom(s) |
| | | ≥ 1 neurologic symptom(s) |
| | Pain disorder | Pain in non-neuroanatomic distribution or without detectable structural/functional basis |
| Factitious disorders | Munchausen's syndrome | Intentional expression/generation/fabrication of sign/symptom |
| | | No overt external incentive |
| | | Internal/dynamic motivation (eg, assumption of sick role) |
| Malingering | | Intentional production of sign/symptom |
| | | External incentive |

Because neuropsychiatry encompasses the entirety of behavioral phenomena, even the most factitious of clinical signs warrants serious investigation and conceptualization, even if solely psychodynamically based. For such clinical states, once it has been reasonably satisfied that a syndrome does not represent known neuropathophysiology, the authors generally prefer the descriptor psychogenic, because it is neutral regarding intent, maintaining the principle of diagnostic conservatism in neuropsychiatric assessment. A variety of methods can be applied to disentangle these complicated cases; the reader is encouraged to consult suggested references [28–30].

## Summary

Neuropsychiatric examination is an interdisciplinary approach to diagnostic assessment of mental and brain diseases. When performed in a skillful way, with a conceptually grounded structure, neuropsychiatric assessment offers the potential for comprehensive diagnostic insight, thereby facilitating optimally informed treatment planning.

## Suggested reading

Borod J, editor. Neuropsychology of emotion. New York: Oxford University Press; 2000.
Cummings JL, Mega MS. Neuropsychiatry and behavioral neuroscience. New York: Oxford University Press; 2003.

Feinberg TE, Farah MJ, editors. Behavioral neurology and neuropsychology. New York: McGraw Hill; 2003.

Schiffer RB, Rao SM, Fogel BS. Neuropsychiatry. Philadelphia: Lippincott; 2003.

Lezak MD, Howieson DB, Loring DW. Neuropsychological assessment. New York: Oxford University Press; 2004.

Mesulam MM. Principles of behavioral and cognitive neurology. New York: Oxford University Press; 2000.

Strub RL, Black FW. The mental status examination in neurology. Philadelphia: F.A. Davis Co.; 2000.

# References

[1] Martin J. The integration of neurology, psychiatry, and neuroscience in the 21st century. Am J Psychiatry 2002;159(5):695–704.

[2] Kosik KS. Beyond phrenology at last. Nat Rev Neurosci 2003;4(3):234–9.

[3] Price BH, Adams R, Coyle J. Neurology and psychiatry: closing the great divide. Neurology 2000;54:8–14.

[4] Kandel ER. A new intellectual framework for psychiatry. Am J Psychiatry 1998;155(4): 457–69.

[5] Gorman J. Neuropsychiatry: now more than ever. CNS Spectr 2001;6(12):947.

[6] Diagnostic and statistical manual of mental disorders. 4th edtion. Washington (DC): American Psychiatric Association Press; 1994.

[7] Peterson RC, Stevens JC, Ganguli M, et al. Practice parameter: early detection of dementia: mild cognitive impairment (an evidence-based review). Neurology 2001;56: 1133–42.

[8] Knopman DS, DeKosky ST, Cummings JL, et al. Practice parameter: diagnoses of dementia (an evidence based review). Neurology 2001;56:1143–53.

[9] Folstein MF, Folstein S, McHugh PR. Mini-mental state: a practical method for grading the cognitive state of patients for the clinician. J Psychiatr Res 1975;12(3):189.

[10] Cummings JL, Mega M, Gray K, et al. The neuropsychiatric inventory: comprehensive assessment of psychopathology in dementia. Neurology 1994;44(12):2308–14.

[11] Royall DR, Mahurin RK, Gray KF. Bedside assessment of executive cognitive impairment: the executive interview. J Am Geriatr Soc 1992;40(2):1221–6.

[12] Hughes CP, Berg L, Danziger WL, et al. A new clinical scale for the staging of dementia. Br J Psychol 1982;140:566–72.

[13] Hofer SM, Piccinin AM, Hershey D. Analysis of structure and discriminative power of the Mattis Dementia Rating Scale. J Clin Psychol 1996;52(4):395–409.

[14] Zeman A. Consciousness. Brain 2001;124(7):1263–89.

[15] Oldfield RC. The assessment and analysis of handedness: the Edinburgh inventory. Neuropsychologia 1971;9(1):97–113.

[16] Knecht S, Drager B, Deppe M, et al. Handedness and hemispheric language dominance in healthy humans. Brain 2000;123:2512–8.

[17] Peters M. How sensitive are handedness prevalence figures to differences in questionnaire classification procedures? Brain Cogn 1992;18:208–15.

[18] Pujol J, Deus J, Losilla JM, et al. Cerebral lateralization of language in normal left-handed people studies by functional MRI. Neurology 1999;52(5):1038–43.

[19] Rosenthal R, Hall J, Archer D, et al. The PONS test manual. New York: Irvington Publishers; 1979.

[20] Budson AE, Price BH. Memory dysfunction. N Engl J Med 2005;352(7):692–9.

[21] Weintraub S. Neuropsychological assessment of mental state. In: Mesulam M-M, editor. Principles of behavioral neurology. New York: Oxford University Press; 2000. p. 121–73.

[22] Casey BJ, Trainor R, Orendi JL, et al. A developmental functional MRI study of prefrontal activation during performance of a go/no-go task. J Cogn Neurosci 1997;9:835–47.
[23] Shulman KI. Disinhibition syndromes, secondary mania and bipolar disorder in old age. J Affect Disord 1997;46(3):175–82.
[24] Stein DJ, Hollander E, Liebowitz MR. Neurobiology of impulsivity and the impulse control disorders. J Neuropsychiatr 1993;5:9–17.
[25] Damasio AR. A neural basis for sociopathy. Arch Gen Psychiatry 2000;57:128–30.
[26] Orr-Andrawes A. The case of Anna O: a neuropsychiatric perspective. J Am Psychoanal Assoc 1985;35(2):387–419.
[27] Gould R, Miller BL, Goldberg MA, et al. The validity of hysterical signs and symptoms. J Nerv Ment Dis 1986;174(10):593–7.
[28] Keane JR. Neuro-ophthalmic signs and symptoms of hysteria. Neurology 1982;32:757–62.
[29] Deuschl G, Koster B, Lucking CH, et al. Diagnostic and pathophysiologic aspects of psychogenic tremors. Mov Disord 1998;13(2):294–302.
[30] Lesser RP. Psychogenic seizures. Neurology 1996;46:1499–507.

ELSEVIER
SAUNDERS

PSYCHIATRIC
CLINICS
OF NORTH AMERICA

Psychiatr Clin N Am 28 (2005) 549–566

# Neuroimaging in Neuropsychiatry

## Daniel F. Broderick, MD

*Mayo Clinic College of Medicine, Mayo Clinic, 4500 San Pablo Road,
Jacksonville, FL 32224, USA*

### Neuroimaging of neuropsychiatry

The neuroimaging of neuropsychiatric disorders continues to evolve as the field of neuroradiology progresses. New imaging techniques and modalities move from the research realm into the clinical world, increasing the imaging options for the clinician. Until quite recently, imaging of the psychiatric patient was characterized by and essentially limited to structural imaging techniques including CT and MRI, which provide anatomic images with excellent spatial and contrast resolution, and perfusion imaging techniques such as single-photon emission computed tomography (SPECT), which examines regional cerebral blood flow of an injected radiopharmaceutical agent [1]. With advances in neuroimaging techniques, radiographic evaluation of the psychiatric patient now encompasses additional, more sophisticated modalities, including functional MRI (fMRI), MR spectroscopy, and positron emission tomography (PET), which complement the structural and existing functional techniques [2]. These modalities allow noninvasive in vivo examination of the human brain, contributing significantly to the understanding of the pathophysiology of neuropsychiatric disorders.

This article reviews the basics of current neuroimaging techniques available to the practicing psychiatrist. These techniques include modalities clearly within the clinical realm as well as those that are primarily research tools. Structural and functional imaging techniques are addressed separately. Basic acquisition techniques of CT, MRI, fMRI, MR spectroscopy, and PET are provided. Although technical details are kept to a minimum, essential parameters are discussed, and the interested reader is directed to more detailed reviews as appropriate. Basic interpretations of each modality are also provided. Rather than providing a systematic review of research findings of neuropsychiatric disorders that have been investigated with

---

*E-mail address:* broderick.daniel.f@mayo.edu

0193-953X/05/$ - see front matter © 2005 Elsevier Inc. All rights reserved.
doi:10.1016/j.psc.2005.05.007        *psych.theclinics.com*

neuroimaging, the discussion of imaging techniques is framed within the context of applications to neuropsychiatry.

It is hoped that this information will familiarize the nonimager with these sophisticated and powerful imaging techniques and will provide insight regarding the appropriate selection and application of these modalities to benefit the neuropsychiatric patient.

## Structural neuroimaging

### CT and MRI

CT and MRI are powerful techniques that provide exquisite anatomic images of the brain with excellent contrast and spatial resolution. Both can be used to evaluate for intracranial mass lesions, hemorrhage, and other pathologies and can demonstrate focal or regional brain atrophy. There are important differences between the two, including the generation of the images, specific advantages and disadvantages, and particular clinical indications of each technique.

To generate an image, CT uses ionizing radiation, a highly collimated X-ray beam that passes through the patient's head and then is recorded by CT detectors. The image produced depends on the degree of X-ray attenuation. Dense bone attenuates more of the X-ray beam than less dense tissue, such as air; the density of soft tissues lies between that of bone and air. Dense structures (like bone and acute blood) appear brighter or whiter on CT than less dense tissue (like air, cerebrospinal fluid, or fat), which appear darker or blacker (Fig. 1). Iodinated contrast material increases the attenuation of vessels and structures lacking an intact blood–brain barrier and appears white (Fig. 2). The degree of attenuation of a given tissue is measured in

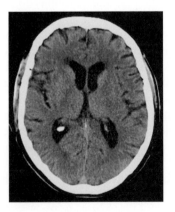

Fig. 1. Unenhanced axial CT image. The calvarium appears white, the cerebrospinal fluid appears black, and the gray matter is relatively "more white" (of greater attenuation) than the white matter.

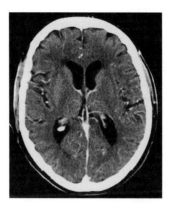

Fig. 2. Enhanced axial CT image demonstrating normal enhancement of cerebral arteries and veins.

Hounsfield units (HU), named after Sir Godfrey Hounsfield who developed CT for clinical use. The scale of attenuation ranges from +1000 HU for bone to −1000 HU for air. Similarly, the appearance of different tissues on CT ranges between white and black (Table 1). CT is relatively less expensive, quicker, and more available than MRI. CT is more sensitive than MRI in detecting acute hemorrhage and calcification and is superior in the depiction of bony architecture. CT remains the study of choice for evaluating the acute trauma patient, the uncooperative patient, suspected acute subarachnoid hemorrhage, and any acute neurologic emergency. There are essentially no contraindications for obtaining a CT scan. Although radiation exposure to the fetus from a head CT is low [3], a female patient should always inform the radiologist or technologist if there is a chance that she could be pregnant; alternative imaging tests, including MRI, may be chosen to reduce or eliminate radiation exposure to the fetus [4]. The risk of severe allergic reaction to iodinated contrast material is low. A relative disadvantage is that, practically, CT imaging is limited to the axial or transverse plane. Also, evaluation of the posterior fossa and brainstem may be degraded significantly by artifact from dense bone. Cwinn and Grahovac [5] provide an excellent discussion of basic CT physics and the use of CT head scans in the emergency patient.

The physical principles of MRI are much too complex to address in this article, but it is important to realize that MRI uses no ionizing radiation and uses a completely different mechanism to generate an image than CT. Rather than X-ray beam attenuation, MRI involves a complex interaction between external magnetic fields and tissues within the patient. One can think simplistically of MRI in terms of energy exchange between an external magnetic field and certain atomic nuclei. When a radiofrequency (RF) pulse is applied and then switched off, the tissue absorbs and then re-emits the energy. The energy is measured as an RF signal; translation of this information can

Table 1
CT attenuation values and appearance of central nervous system tissues

| Tissue | Attenuation (HU) | Appearance |
|---|---|---|
| Bone | +1000 | very white |
| Calcification | +140–200 | white |
| Acute blood | +56–76 | white |
| Gray matter | +32–41 | White relative to white matter |
| White matter | +23–34 | Gray relative to gray matter |
| Cerebrospinal fluid (water) | 0 | gray-black |
| Fat | −30–−100 | black |
| Air | −1000 | very black |

produce an anatomic image. The appearance of the image depends on multiple factors, including specific intrinsic tissue properties (such as T1 and T2 relaxation times and proton density) and particular imaging techniques and parameters (including conventional spin-echo, fast spin-echo, or gradient-echo sequences, echo planar imaging, and different repetition times [TR], echo times [TE], and flip angles). Very simply, on a T1-weighted image (short TR, short TE) (Fig. 3), tissue with short T1 relaxation time (eg, fat) appears bright; long-T1 tissue (eg, water) is dark. On a T2-weighted image (long TR, long TE) (Fig. 4), tissue with short T2 relaxation time (fat) is dark; long-T2 tissue (water) is bright (Table 2). Balanced or proton density sequences essentially have been replaced by fluid attenuation inversion recovery (FLAIR) sequences, which provide T2-weighted contrast with dark cerebrospinal fluid (Fig. 5). Intravenous contrast material shortens the T1 relaxation time, resulting in increased T1 signal intensity of venous structures and those with

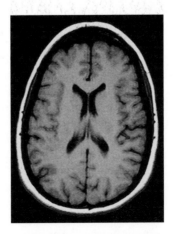

Fig. 3. Unenhanced axial T1-weighted MR image. The scalp fat appears bright or white, the cerebrospinal fluid appears dark or black, and the white matter appears white relative to the gray matter.

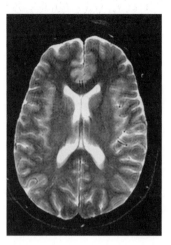

Fig. 4. Unenhanced axial T2-weighted MR image. The scalp fat appears dark, the cerebrospinal fluid appears white, and the white matter is dark relative to the gray matter.

an altered or absent blood–brain barrier (Fig. 6). Like contrast-enhanced CT, enhanced MRI complements the unenhanced examination and often increases the sensitivity and specificity of the examination in the detection of disease. MRI can be performed in any imaging plane (axial, sagittal, coronal, or oblique). It is relatively more expensive, takes longer to perform, and is less available than CT. Still, MRI is the initial study of choice in the evaluation of most intracranial processes because of its superior inherent tissue contrast and multiplanar imaging capabilities. MRI is more sensitive than CT in the evaluation of white matter disease, including multiple sclerosis, and in the screening of patients for suspected intracranial metastases. MRI is superior to CT in the differentiation of gray matter and in both cortical and subcortical regions. Contraindications for MRI include cardiac pacemakers, non–MRI-compatible aneurysm clips, neurostimulators, cochlear implants, and other

Table 2
MRI signal intensities of central nervous system tissues

| Tissue | T1-weighted sequence | T2-weighted sequence |
| --- | --- | --- |
| Bone | very dark | very dark |
| Calcification | very dark | very dark |
| Acute blood (oxyhemoglobin) | isointense | hyperintense |
| Subacute blood (intracellular methemoglobin) | very bright | dark |
| Chronic blood (hemosiderin) | very dark | very dark |
| Gray matter | isointense | bright |
| White matter | bright | isointense |
| Cerebrospinal fluid (water) | dark | bright |
| Fat | bright | intermediate |
| Air | very dark | very dark |

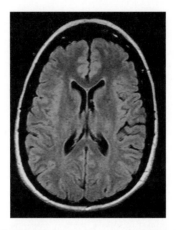

Fig. 5. Unenhanced axial FLAIR MR image. Note that the brain has a T2 appearance (white matter dark, relative to the gray matter), whereas the cerebrospinal fluid is dark.

metallic or electronic devices within the body [4]. Claustrophobia and acoustic noise are potential problems with MRI. For a more comprehensive discussion of MRI physics and techniques, the reader is directed to Sanders [6].

Structural images of the brain provided by CT and MRI can provide useful information in the evaluation of the psychiatric patient. MRI, with its superior depiction of cerebral white matter, has proved useful in investigating the possible role of oligodendroglial dysfunction in myelin maintenance and repair and the associated alteration in neuronal connectivity thought to be a central abnormality in schizophrenia. White matter hyperintensities have been seen in schizophrenic patients; white matter hyperintensities are

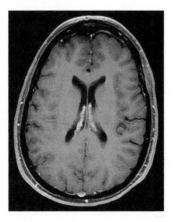

Fig. 6. Enhanced axial T1-weighted MR image demonstrating normal enhancement of the choroid plexus in the lateral ventricles, sagittal sinus, and cortical veins. The scalp fat appears dark because of the fat-saturation technique.

significantly more common in subjects who have late-life schizophrenia-like symptoms than in with age-matched controls. Also, decreases in both global and regional cerebral white matter have been seen; reductions in white matter volume in the prefrontal cortical region have been associated with negative symptoms [7].

Volumetric imaging of the brain can be performed with both CT and MRI and provides more quantitative assessment of regional atrophy in certain psychiatric disorders. A recent MRI study using high-resolution volumetric analysis comparing patients who had Huntington's disease with normal control subjects demonstrated extensive subcortical gray matter atrophy (particularly in the caudate nucleus and putamen), as well as significantly reduced cortical gray matter volume, consistent with previous findings. Novel findings from this study include significantly reduced volume of cerebellar gray and white matter, extensive reduction of cerebral white matter, and increased volume of abnormal cerebral white matter, suggesting that both the cerebellum and cerebral white matter integrity may be significant in the symptomatology of Huntington's disease [8]. An MRI study of patients who have Huntington's disease compared with age-matched healthy controls employing volumetric, diffusion-weighting, and magnetization transfer techniques has shown smaller caudate, putamen, and whole-brain volumes in patients who have Huntington's disease. An accompanying increase in the apparent diffusion coefficient values was seen on diffusion-weighted images in these regions as well as in the cerebral periventricular white matter, suggesting tissue damage at these sites. These imaging findings show correlation with disease severity [9]. The understanding of the pathophysiology of neurodegenerative central nervous system conditions such as Huntington's disease will continue to be advanced by such structural imaging techniques, allowing earlier diagnosis and serving as measures to monitor disease progression and treatment response.

Volumetric MRI is also useful in the study of patients who have schizophrenia. A recent study of 39 schizophrenic patients studied with high-resolution whole-brain morphometry contradicted the supposition that the enlargement of the lateral cerebral ventricles seen in schizophrenia reflects diffuse brain atrophy. Rather, this study showed an association of larger ventricles with regionally specific decreases of brain parenchyma in both paraventricular and remote areas, including the thalamus, putamen, and superior temporal gyrus [10]. A similar study found reduction in volume of the mediodorsal and pulvinar nuclei of the thalamus in schizophrenia [11]. Results of both studies point to the possible role that the thalamus may have in schizophrenia.

Diffusion tensor imaging is a variation of MRI able to study brain tissue microstructure and examine white matter tracts. Although this tool is still in its infancy, it may improve the understanding of neural connectivity and how specific regions of the brain interconnect, with specific applications to neuropsychiatric disorders including dementia, schizophrenia, and addictions [12]. For example, results of a recent study suggest abnormal patterns on diffusion tensor imaging linking declarative-episodic verbal memory deficits to the left uncinate fasciculus and deficits in executive function to the left cingulate bundle in patients who have schizophrenia [13].

## Functional neuroimaging

### Functional MRI

fMRI complements the excellent spatial and contrast resolution of the brain provided by structural MRI. Although fMRI identifies the regions of the brain that are active in response to a task, the technique does not actually identify the neuronal firing. Rather, by coupling changes in local cerebral blood flow with neural activation, fMRI allows noninvasive evaluation and localization of motor, sensory, and cognitive deficits or symptoms. Because fMRI can be performed at the same time as the structural MRI study, functional activity can be mapped onto high-resolution anatomic brain images.

Although it is possible to study cerebral blood volume with fMRI using the injection of contrast material, the fMRI technique most frequently employed in the evaluation of the neuropsychiatric patient takes advantage of the changes in signal intensity associated with variations in the level of cerebral blood oxygenation. Called blood oxygen level–dependent contrast, this technique is noninvasive and does not require the injection of exogenous contrast material. Neural activation is followed by increased cerebral blood flow to the activated region. An increased number of red blood cells carrying oxyhemoglobin flow into the particular activated region. The supply of oxyhemoglobin exceeds the neuronal demand, resulting in a net decrease in the local concentration of deoxyhemoglobin. Oxyhemoglobin is diamagnetic, and deoxyhemoglobin is paramagnetic. The significance for the imager is that the increased signal intensity seen on fMRI in the activated brain actually is caused by the loss of decreased signal intensity associated with the paramagnetic deoxyhemoglobin.

Regardless of the mechanism, fMRI allows the study of brain activity without use of either ionizing radiation or the injection of radiopharmaceuticals needed in SPECT and PET. FMRI can be performed on most clinical MR systems (1.5 T) with conventional hardware, although the increased signal/noise ratio (SNR) and the increased imaging speed of the higher-field-strength magnets (3 T) are distinct advantages of those systems. The advantage of increased SNR can be appreciated when one realizes that the changes in signal intensity associated with variations in the level of blood oxygenation are extremely small. Still, one can perform single-case fMRI studies on individual patients, rather than averaging data from several studies. Because of the rapid image acquisition possible with fMRI, repetitive studies also can be performed on the same patient at one sitting.

The temporal and spatial resolution of fMRI are better than those of PET or SPECT.

The fMRI technique is very sensitive to motion, and minor patient movement can make it difficult to identify neural activation. Limiting head motion is essential for obtaining high-quality images. Like other MR techniques, patient claustrophobia may be an issue.

A variety of task paradigms can be used with fMRI. Typically, baseline images are acquired with the patient at rest. Then the patient performs a specific task, and another set of images is acquired. Various motor, sensory, and cognitive paradigms can be employed, and visual and auditory stimuli can be presented. In each case, increased signal intensity associated with changes in blood oxygenation in the activated cortex can be visualized. For a more detailed explanation of the principles, techniques, and applications of fMRI, the reader is referred to Chong and colleagues [14].

A significant current use of fMRI is preoperative brain mapping, especially the mapping of the eloquent cortex in patients being considered for neurosurgery [15]. The technique also holds great promise in the evaluation of psychiatric and neurodegenerative conditions. Functional imaging can be of great help in testing hypotheses of disease etiology. For example, frontal lobe dysfunction is thought to be of fundamental importance in schizophrenia. The term hypofrontality describes a failure of task-induced frontal cerebral response [16]. Hypofrontality has been shown on fMRI studies of neuroleptic-naive schizophrenic patients during Wisconsin Card Sorting Test; specifically, reduced activation was seen in the right frontal lobe, left temporal lobe, and left cerebellum, findings consistent with prior PET and SPECT studies [17]. Enhanced prefrontal function on fMRI with verbal working memory experiments was demonstrated in schizophrenia patients after 6 weeks of treatment with an atypical antipsychotic agent [18]. Functional imaging may also provide useful information in the evaluation of patients who have dementia, providing a means for earlier diagnosis, for differentiation among various dementias, and for monitoring drug response. For example, fMRI was used to investigate the memory-associated activation of the medial temporal lobe in nondemented elderly patients who had mild cognitive impairment. The individuals who progressed to Alzheimer's disease within 2.5 years showed greater medial temporal lobe activation at initial fMRI, suggesting that this finding may serve as a marker for impending clinical decline [19]. Future fMRI research will certainly include investigation of other conditions in which abnormal brain function can be observed before visible structural alterations.

## MR spectroscopy

MR spectroscopy is a noninvasive technique with broad applications in neuropsychiatry that relies on the same basic principles used by nuclear MR but provides unique metabolic and biochemical information not available with MRI. MR spectroscopy allows noninvasive interrogation of the chemical environment of tissues, providing relative quantification of particular compounds and their constituents in certain regions of the brain. The complex physical principles behind MR spectroscopy cannot be addressed adequately in this article, but there are excellent more comprehensive reviews of basic MR spectroscopy techniques [20–22].

The nuclei studied with MR spectroscopy include proton [$^1$H], phosphorus [$^{31}$P], carbon [$^{13}$C], lithium [$^7$Li], fluorine [$^{19}$F], and sodium [$^{23}$Na]. The most current MR spectroscopy involves $^1$H (proton MR spectroscopy), which can distinguish certain metabolites including N-acetyl aspartate (NAA), creatine and phosphocreatine, and choline-containing phospholipids. NAA is the largest peak seen on MR spectroscopy and is considered a marker on neuronal integrity. It is depleted in most conditions that replace or damage neurons. Creatine and phosphocreatine serve as useful internal references, because they are relatively constant metabolites in the brain, even in disease states. Choline reflects total choline brain stores and is associated with cell membrane synthesis and degradation; choline elevation suggests membrane turnover and often is seen with acute demyelination and cerebral neoplasms [23].

With MR spectroscopy, a spectrum associated with a particular region of interest is generated. A spectrum is simply a plot of peaks at different frequencies. Each peak is characterized by its resonant frequency and its height. Each metabolite in the spectrum is identified by its characteristic resonant frequency or location; the location is expressed in units of parts per million, plotted on the x-axis from right to left. The height of the peak (or area under the peak) yields the relative concentration of the metabolite.

Two main pulse sequences used in MR spectroscopy: stimulated echo acquisition method (STEAM) and point-resolved spectroscopy. Each has distinctive advantages and disadvantages. STEAM uses a shorter TE, has better water suppression, and is better able to identify more metabolites. These metabolites are often of interest to the psychiatrist and include myoinositol, glutamate, glutamine, and γ-aminobutyric acid (GABA). For example, myoinositol has been suggested as a marker for Alzheimer's disease, with increased myoinositol and decreased NAA seen in patients who have Alzheimer's disease [23]. Point-resolved spectroscopy uses a longer TE and has relatively greater SNR. The longer TE, however, results in loss of signal from most brain compounds, allowing the detection of only four metabolites: NAA, creatinine, choline-containing phospholipids, and lactate. Still, this technique may be adequate if one is interested in NAA and creatinine. For example, significantly lower NAA/creatine ratios were seen in ill Gulf War veterans than in healthy control subjects, confirming reduction of functioning neuronal mass in the basal ganglia and brainstem [24]. Appropriate selection of the particular pulse sequence is influenced by the metabolites of interest. If the referring clinician is especially interested in a metabolite such as myoinositol or GABA, this information should be relayed to the radiologist so that the STEAM technique is used.

A unique application of MR spectroscopy in the psychiatric patient is the in vivo measurement of psychoactive drugs in the human brain, specifically the quantification of brain lithium and fluorinated drugs, which include most of the serotonin-specific reuptake inhibitors. Lithium is used for the treatment of bipolar disorders, with poor correlation between serum and brain lithium levels. A certain percentage of patients who have therapeutic serum lithium levels experience a relapse of symptoms, and serious toxicity can result from modest elevations of serum levels. [7]Li-MR spectroscopy can provide a noninvasive measurement of brain lithium in patients. Similarly, [19]F-MR spectroscopy may be useful in providing an in vivo means of measuring fluorinated drugs and their metabolites in the brain [25].

Another neuropsychiatric application of MR spectroscopy is the in vivo measurement of brain GABA levels. Abnormal GABA levels have been measured in several neuropsychiatric conditions, including epilepsy, anxiety disorders, major depression, and drug addiction. In disorders with abnormally low GABA levels, treatment may include medications that block the reuptake or degradation of GABA [26].

Results of an MR spectroscopy study of nine autistic children found lower NAA levels in the cerebellum, consistent with neuropathic reports of decreased numbers of Purkinje cells and granule cells in the cerebellar cortex of autistic patients. Also, lactate was detected in the frontal cortex of one autistic child; lactate is not detectable in normal brain on MR spectroscopy. Plasma lactate levels were also significantly higher in the autistic group. These findings are consistent with altered energy metabolism in some children, which may have therapeutic implications [27]. Although the study was small, the results suggest further evaluation of autistic individuals may be warranted.

[1]H-MR spectroscopy of patients who had parkinsonism showed significant correlation between the severity of various diseases causing parkinsonism and the NAA/creatinine ratios in the both the putamen and the frontal lobe. Significant correlation was also seen between the impairment of executive function and frontal lobe NAA/creatinine ratio. These findings suggest that MR spectroscopy may be helpful in the diagnosis and monitoring of patients who have parkinsonism syndromes [28].

Future directions include MR spectroscopy with higher-field-strength magnets. Performing MR spectroscopy with 3T magnets will provide increased sensitivity, better SNR, and improved spatial resolution. Metabolite peaks can be detected and measured more precisely. The study of GABA with [1]H-MR spectroscopy would certainly benefit from higher magnetic field [27]. Detection of GABA will also be improved with [13]C-MR spectroscopy, in which injected [13]C-labeled glucose is incorporated into glutamate and then into GABA [27]. The increased SNR available with higher-field-strength systems would facilitate [31]P-MR spectroscopy, which may be of benefit in the study of membrane phospholipid metabolism in patients who have schizophrenia [29] and the study of high-energy phosphate metabolism in the frontal lobes of patients who have panic disorder [30].

### Positron emission tomography

Emission tomography includes PET and SPECT. Both nuclear imaging techniques involve the injection of certain short-lived radiopharmaceuticals and the detection of particular emitted radiation by gamma scintillation cameras. In SPECT, gamma rays are detected as the primary decay product. In PET, emitted positrons collide with electrons, annihilating both particles. Two 511-kEv gamma rays are produced 180° apart. For the event to be recorded, nearly simultaneous detection on opposite sides of the patient is required. The information originating in different regions of the brain is processed to create a three-dimensional image. SPECT tracers are more limited than PET tracers in the types of brain activity that can be studied. SPECT tracers have longer half-lives than PET agents and do not require an onsite cyclotron for production. With the greater temporal and spatial resolution of PET compared with SPECT, the development of newer PET tracers, and the increasingly greater availability and affordability of PET, PET will probably be the imaging study of choice for emission tomography studies of the brain. This article therefore focuses solely on PET and its applications in neuropsychiatry. The reader is directed to Hartshorne [31] for a more comprehensive discussion of the performance of PET in the central nervous system.

PET has wide applications in the study of brain disorders, cardiac disease, and oncology [32]. Radionuclides used in PET include Carbon 11 [$^{11}$C], Nitrogen 13 [$^{13}$N], Oxygen 15 [$^{15}$O] and Fluorine 18 [$^{18}$F]. Clinically, the most widely used PET radionuclide is $^{18}$F, which has a longer half-life than $^{11}$C, $^{13}$N, or $^{15}$O and is a label for the glucose analogue fluoro-2-deoxy-D-glucose (FDG). [$^{18}$F]-FDG-PET is especially valuable in the study of brain function because the rate of glucose metabolism increases in regions of brain activity. Regional cerebral metabolism has been studied in various neurodegenerative and psychiatric conditions, stroke, and trauma with [$^{18}$F]-FDG-PET [33]. PET also allows noninvasive study of cerebral blood flow and volume, oxygen metabolism, and drug concentrations in particular brain regions. For example, PET studies with $^{11}$C tracers can provide valuable information in the study of neuroreceptor mapping and for psychotropic drug development [34].

PET/CT fusion is a relatively new technique that allows the nearly synchronous acquisition of images and precise coregistration of the functional (PET) and anatomic (CT) data sets. Potential advantages of the combined technique also include better-quality PET images because of more accurate attenuation correction and shorter imaging times [32,35]. Studies comparing standard PET with PET/CT in patients who have head and neck cancer demonstrated that the combined technique provided improved anatomic localization of abnormalities identified on PET, resulting in improved diagnostic accuracy and a reduced number of equivocal PET findings. These findings led to a change in patient care in 12 of the 68 patients studied [36]. It is reasonable to assume that the improved anatomic localization PET/CT findings will have similar positive applications for the neuropsychiatric patient.

Coregistration of PET images with MRI images has also proved useful. A recent [18F]-FDG-PET study of glucose metabolism within specific thalamic subdivisions of schizophrenic patients co-registered the PET and axial T1-weighted MRI images of 41 unmedicated schizophrenic patients compared with 60 matched control subjects. In the schizophrenic patients, glucose metabolism in the mediodorsal nucleus and the centromedian nucleus was significantly lower and glucose metabolism in the pulvinar was significantly higher than in controls. Lower glucose metabolism in the mediodorsal nucleus was associated with more negative symptoms, whereas lower glucose metabolism in the pulvinar was associated with more hallucinations and more positive symptoms. The demonstration of abnormal glucose metabolism in distinct thalamic regions with specific cortical connections and the association of these abnormalities with clinical symptoms furthers the understanding of schizophrenia [37].

PET has proved to be important in the evaluation of patients who have neurodegenerative disorders, especially in aiding with the difficult diagnosis of Alzheimer's disease. [18F]-FDG-PET demonstrates bilateral temporoparietal hypometabolism in patients who have probable and definite Alzheimer's disease [38]. Frontotemporal deficits are seen on PET scans of patients who have frontotemporal dementia (Fig. 7) [39]. [18F]-FDG-PET studies may allow earlier and more definite diagnosis of Alzheimer's disease, aiding in the differentiation of patients who have various types of dementia. [40]. Recently developed molecular imaging agents include [18F]-FDDNP, a PET ligand that can determine the localization and load of neurofibrillary tangles and beta-amyloid plaques in the brains of living patients who have Alzheimer's disease; specifically, greater accumulation of the ligand was seen in the temporal lobes of nine patients who had Alzheimer's compared with seven controls [41]. Another agent that targets beta-amyloid deposits, [11C]PIB, which is a thioflavin-T analogue, localized in the frontal and temporoparietal regions of nine patients who had "mild" Alzheimer's disease compared with five healthy controls. [11C]PIB is now in clinical trials in Sweden [42]. These agents certainly hold promise in the development of effective drug therapy, in aiding early diagnosis, and in monitoring a patient's progress.

The study of the central serotonin system in mood disorders has been greatly advanced with PET imaging and the development of particular

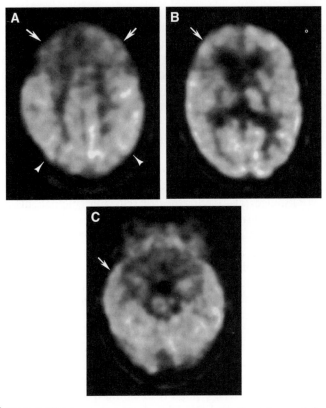

Fig. 7. [$^{18}$ F]-FDG-PET image in a 70-year-old woman with frontotemporal dementia. (*A*)
Normal metabolic activity is seen within both parietal lobes (*arrowheads*). (*A, B*) FDG-PET
shows prominent diminished FDG uptake in both frontal lobes, more marked on the right
(*arrows*). (*C*) Diminished FDG uptake is seen to a lesser degree within the temporal lobes and is
more marked on the right (*arrow*).

ligands. Alterations of brain serotonin (5-HT) transmission, especially
changes in availability of the presynaptically located serotonin transporter
(SERT), have been implicated in the pathophysiology of depression [43].
[$^{11}$C](+)McN5652 is a selective PET radioligand for imaging the human 5-
HT transporter site, which allows the in vivo detection of cerebral SERT
availability. Serotonin transporter binding is a marker of the level of
intrasynaptic serotonin. Decreased transporter binding indicates fewer
serotonin nerve terminals or less intrasynaptic serotonin; either condition
results in reduced serotonin function [34]. Thirteen antidepressant-naive
or -free patients who had either major depressive disorder or bipolar disorder and 21 healthy controls were recently studied with [$^{11}$C](+)McN5652
PET. Thalamic SERT availability was significantly increased in the patient
group, especially in those who had major mood disorder, compared with
controls; no difference between the two groups was found in midbrain

SERT availability [44] This finding suggests an altered integration of the serotonergic neurons in patients who have mood disorders and possibly a thalamic role in mood disorder pathophysiology. Another recent $[^{11}C](+)$McN5652 PET study reported significantly greater ligand binding to the 5-HT transporter sites in the left frontal region and right cingulate region of four drug-free depressed patients compared with healthy controls [45]. These findings suggest increased 5-HT transporter sites in the frontal and cingulated cortex of depressed patients and support the hypothesis that alterations in 5-HT transporter sites may be significant in the pathophysiology and treatment of depression and mood disorders. PET and SPECT studies using SERT tracers have also investigated other psychiatric disorders, including obsessive-compulsive disorder, schizophrenia, and drug abuse, and neurologic diseases such as Parkinson's and Wilson's disease [43]. Further PET studies will continue to expand the understanding of the role of the serotonergic and other neurotransmitter systems in the pathophysiology of neuropsychiatric disorders.

PET also has an important role in epilepsy. $[^{18}F]$-FDG-PET has been useful in the localization of the epileptic focus, because seizure foci are seen as areas of hypermetabolism ictally and hypometabolism interictally [33]. Imaging has been especially helpful in evaluating patients who have refractory temporal lobe epilepsy being considered for surgery. Single hypometabolic foci can be seen on interictal PET studies in 55% to 80% of patients who have focal electroencephalographic abnormalities [33]. In seizures caused by foci in the medial and inferior aspects of the frontal lobes, PET has been shown to be superior to electroencephalography in the accurate localization of the seizure focus [33]. Foci of hypometabolism on $[^{18}F]$-FDG-PET studies have been seen in patients who have temporal lobe epilepsy and no evidence of hippocampal sclerosis on MRI [46]. PET may also be a useful tool in the general epilepsy population, in the exclusion of pathology in patients who have nonepileptic seizures, in primary generalized epilepsies, and in the identification of patients previously thought not to be surgical candidates [47]. Finally, SPECT may still be useful in the evaluation of the seizure patient. SPECT with $[^{123}I]$-iododexetimide (IDEX) can depict tracer uptake by muscarinic acetylcholine receptors, which are thought to play an important role in the generation of seizures. A recent study showed that IDEX SPECT was superior to the interictal PET in localizing seizures in patients who have temporal lobe epilepsy and suggested that the 6-hour IDEX SPECT scan is a viable alternative to $[^{18}F]$-FDG-PET imaging in localizing seizure foci in these patients [48].

Future applications of PET imaging in neuropsychiatry seem almost limitless in areas of scientific interest and of clinical importance. The use of coregistered or fused anatomic images with PET data will continue to bridge the gap between structural and functional imaging. The continued development of additional PET ligands will allow further in vivo molecular imaging of the brain.

## Summary

Once limited to structural imaging modalities such as CT and MRI, radiographic evaluation of the psychiatric patient now includes more sophisticated functional techniques such as fMRI, MR spectroscopy, and PET. With the increased sensitivity that these new tools bring comes greater complexity. As new imaging techniques continue to transition from research to clinical application, the imaging options and associated complexity will increase. Consultation with neuroradiology colleagues will allow the practicing psychiatrist to evaluate their patients optimally. These techniques will continue to provide insight into the pathophysiology, etiology, diagnosis, treatment, and prognosis of these patients.

## References

[1] Weight D, Bigler E. Neuroimaging in psychiatry. Psychiatr Clin North Am 1998;21(4): 725–59.

[2] Gupta A, Elheis M, Pansari K. Imaging in psychiatric illnesses. Int J Clin Pract 2004;58(9): 850–8.

[3] Parry R, Glaze S, Archer B. Typical patient radiation doses in diagnostic radiology. Radiographics 1999;19:1289–302.

[4] Shellock F, Crues J. MR procedures: biologic effects, safety, and patient care. Radiology 2004;232(3):635–52.

[5] Cwinn A, Grahovac S. Emergency CT scans of the head: a practical atlas. St. Louis (MO): Mosby-Year Book; 1998.

[6] Sanders J. Computed tomography and magnetic resonance imaging. In: Orrison WW Jr, editor. Neuroimaging. Philadelphia: WB Saunders; 1998. p. 12–36.

[7] Davis K, Stewart D, Friedman J, et al. White matter changes in schizophrenia. Arch Gen Psychiatry 2003;60:443–56.

[8] Fennema-Notestine C, Archibald S, Jacobson M, et al. In vivo evidence of cerebellar atrophy and cerebral white matter loss in Huntington disease. Neurology 2004;63:989–95.

[9] Mascalchi M, Lolli F, Della Nave R, et al. Huntington disease: volumetric, diffusion-weighted, and magnetization transfer MR imaging of brain. Neuroradiology 2004;232: 867–73.

[10] Gaser C, Nenadic I, Buchsbaum B, et al. Ventricular enlargement in schizophrenia related to volume reduction of the thalamus, striatum, and superior temporal cortex. Am J Psychiatry 2004;161(1):154–6.

[11] Byne W, Buchsbaum M, Kemether E, et al. Magnetic resonance imaging of the thalamic mediodorsal nucleus and pulvinar in schizophrenia and schizotypal personality disorder. Arch Gen Psychiatry 2001;58:133–40.

[12] Taylor W, Hsu E, Ranga Rama Krishnan K, et al. Diffusion tensor imaging: background, potential, and utility in psychiatric research. Biol Psychiatry 2004;55:201–7.

[13] Nestor P, Kubicki M, Gurrera R, et al. Neuropsychological correlates of diffusion tensor imaging in schizophrenia. Neuropsychology 2004;18(4):629–37.

[14] Chong B, Sanders J, Jones G. Functional magnetic resonance imaging. In: Orrison WW Jr, editor. Neuroimaging. Philadelphia: WB Saunders; 1998. p. 60–86.

[15] Moritz C, Haughton V. Functional MR imaging: paradigms for clinical preoperative mapping. Magn Reson Imaging Clin N Am 2003;11(4):529–42.

[16] Honey G, Bullmore E. Functional neuroimaging and schizophrenia. Psychiatry 2002;1(1): 26–9.

[17] Woodruff P, Wright I, Bullmore E, et al. Auditory hallucinations and the temporal cortical response to speech in schizophrenia: a functional magnetic resonance imaging study. Am J Psychiatry 1997;154(12):1676–82.

[18] Honey G, Bullmore E, Soni W, et al. Differences in frontal cortical activation by a working memory task after substitution of risperidone for typical antipsychotic drugs in patients with schizophrenia. PNAS 1999;96(23):13432–7.

[19] Dickerson B, Salat D, Bates J, et al. Medial temporal lobe function and structure in mild cognitive impairment. Ann Neurol 2004;56(1):7–9.

[20] Passe T, Charles H, Rajagopalan P, et al. Nuclear magnetic resonance spectroscopy: a review of neuropsychiatric applications. Prog Neuropsychopharmacol Biol Psychiatry 1995;19(4): 541–63.

[21] Castillo M, Kwock L, Mukherji S. Clinical applications of proton MR spectroscopy. AJNR Am J Neuroradiol 1996;17:1–15.

[22] Miller B. A review of chemical issues in 1H NMR spectroscopy: N-Acetyl-L-aspartate, creatine and coline. NMR Biomed 1991;4:47–52.

[23] Miller B, Moats R, Shonk T, et al. Alzheimer disease: depiction of increased cerebral myo-inositol with proton MR spectroscopy. Radiology 1993;187(2):433–7.

[24] Haley R, Marshall W, McDonald G, et al. Brain abnormalities in Gulf War syndrome: evaluation with $^1$H MR spectroscopy. Neuroradiology 2000;215:807–17.

[25] Lyoo K, Renshaw P. Magnetic resonance spectroscopy: current and future applications in psychiatric research. Biol Psychiatry 2002;51:195–207.

[26] Chang L, Cloak C, Ernst T. Magnetic resonance spectroscopy studies of GABA in neuropsychiatric disorders. J Clin Psychiatry 2003;64(Suppl 3):7–14.

[27] Chugangi D, Sundram B, Behen M, et al. Evidence of altered energy metabolism in autistic children. Prog Neuropsychopharmacol Biol Psychiatry 1999;23:635–41.

[28] Abe K, Terakawa H, Takanashi M, et al. Proton magnetic resonance spectroscopy of patients with parkinsonism. Brain Res Bull 2000;52(6):589–95.

[29] Stanley J, Williamson P, Drost D, et al. An in vivo study of the prefrontal cortex of schizophrenic patients at different stages of illness via phosphorus magnetic resonance spectroscopy. Arch Gen Psychiatry 1995;52:399–406.

[30] Shioiri T, Kato T, Murashita J, et al. High-energy phosphate metabolism in the frontal lobes of patients with panic disorder detected by phase-encoded $^{31}$P-MRS. Biol Psychiatry 1996; 40:785–93.

[31] Hartshorne M. Computed tomography and magnetic resonance imaging. In: Orrison WW Jr, editor. Neuroimaging. Philadelphia: WB Saunders; 1998. p. 87–122.

[32] Rohren E, Turkington T, Coleman R. Clinical applications of PET in oncology. Radiology 2004;231:305–32.

[33] Newberg A, Alavi A, Reivich M. Determination of regional cerebral function with FDG-PET imaging in neuropsychiatric disorders. Semin Nucl Med 2002;32(1):13–34.

[34] Parsey R, Mann J. Applications of positron emission tomography in psychiatry. Semin Nucl Med 2003;33(2):129–35.

[35] Kapoor V, McCook B, Torok F. An introduction to PET-CT imaging. Radiographics 2004; 24:523–43.

[36] Schöder H, Henry W, Yeung D, Gonen M, et al. Head and neck cancer: clinical usefulness and accuracy of PET/CT image fusion. Radiology 2004;231:65–72.

[37] Hazlett E, Buchsbaum M, Kemether E, et al. Abnormal glucose metabolism in the mediodorsal nucleus of the thalamus in schizophrenia. Am J Psychiatry 2004;161: 305–14.

[38] Salmon E, Sadzot B, Maquet P, et al. Differential diagnosis of Alzheimer's disease with PET. J Nucl Med 1994;35(3):391–8.

[39] Duara R, Barker W, Luis CA. Frontotemporal dementia and Alzheimer's disease. differential diagnosis. Dement Geriatr Cogn Disord 1999;10(Suppl 1):37–42.

[40] Goto I, Taniwaki T, Hosokawa S, et al. Positron emission tomographic (PET) studies in dementia. J Neurol Sci 1993;114(1):1–6.

[41] Shoghi-Jadid K, Small GW, Agdeppa E, et al. Localization of neurofibrillary tangles and beta-amyloid plaques in the brains of living patients with Alzheimer's disease. Am J Geriatr Psychiatry 2002;10(1):24–35.

[42] Helmuth L. Long-awaited technique spots Alzheimer's toxin. Science 2002;297(5582):752–3.

[43] Hesse S, Barthel H, Schwarz J, et al. Advances in in vivo imaging of serotonergic neurons in neuropsychiatric disorders. Neurosci and Biobehav Rev 2004;28:547–63.

[44] Ichimiya T, Suhara T, Sudo Y, et al. Serotonin transporter binding in patients with mood disorders: a PET study with [$^{11}$C](+)McN5652. Biol Psychiatry 2002;51:715–22.

[45] Reivich M, Amsterdam J, Brunswick D, et al. PET brain imaging with [$^{11}$C](+)McN5652 shows increased serotonin transporter availability in major depression. J Affect Disord 2004; 82:321–7.

[46] Carne R, O'Brien T, Kilpatrick C, et al. MRI-negative PET-positive temporal lobe epilepsy: a distinct surgically remediable syndrome. Brain 2004;127(10):2276–85.

[47] Swartz B, Brown C, Mandelkern M, et al. The use of 2-deoxy-2-[18F]fluoro-D-glucose (FDG-PET) positron emission tomography in the routine diagnosis of epilepsy. Mol Imaging Biol 2002;4(3):245–52.

[48] Mohamed A, Eberl S, Fulham M, et al. Sequential [123]I-iododexetimide scans in temporal lobe epilepsy: comparison with neuroimaging scans (MR imaging and [18]F-FDG PET imaging). Eur J Nucl Mol Imaging 2005;32(2):180–5.

ELSEVIER
SAUNDERS

Psychiatr Clin N Am 28 (2005) 567–580

PSYCHIATRIC
CLINICS
OF NORTH AMERICA

# Neuropsychologic Assessment of Frontal Lobe Dysfunction

Elkhonon Goldberg, PhD*, Dmitri Bougakov, PhD

*Department of Neurology, New York University School of Medicine, 315 West 57th Street, Suite 401, New York, NY 10019, USA*

Neuropsychology, a relatively recently developed discipline, is concerned with the relationship between brain structures and their functions and how this relationship is affected in brain pathology. Neuropsychologic testing consists of a wide range of quantitative procedures allowing assessment of the presence and extent of cognitive and behavioral disturbances in a number of medical conditions. Neuropsychologic assessment is central to the diagnosis of neurologic, psychiatric, neurodevelopmental, and neurogeriatric conditions and to the planning of rehabilitation and vocational training, competency determination, treatment planning, and determination of need for assisted living.

Neuropsychologic testing is used in assessing cognitive changes associated with cerebrovascular disorder, traumatic brain injury, seizures, Alzheimer's disease, Huntington disease, schizophrenia, depression, dementia, and many other medical conditions. It also may be helpful in determining side effects of various medications on cognition.

Neuropsychologic assessment is particularly important in the diagnosis of regional brain dysfunction, including the dysfunction the frontal lobes, and in the assessment of the somewhat more broadly defined executive functions in a wide range of clinical populations.

## The nature of executive control

Traditionally, the concept of executive control was linked inextricably to the function of the frontal lobes. The groundwork for elucidating the nature of executive control was laid by Alexander Luria [1] as early as 1966. Luria

This work was supported by East-West Science and Education Foundation.
* Corresponding author.
*E-mail address:* egneurocog@aol.com (E. Goldberg).

proposed the existence of a system in charge of intentionality, the formulation of goals and plans of action subordinate to the goals, the identification of goal-appropriate cognitive routines, the sequential access to these routines, the temporally ordered transition from one routine to another, and the editorial evaluation of the outcome of actions.

Subsequently, two broad types of cognitive operations linked to the executive control system figured most prominently in the literature. The first is the organism's ability to guide its behavior by internal representations [2]—formulating plans and then guiding behavior according to these plans. The second is an organism's ability to guide its behavior by internal representations and also to "switch gears" when something unanticipated happens [3]. To deal with such transitions effectively, a particular ability is needed—mental flexibility, that is, the capacity to respond rapidly to unanticipated environmental contingencies. Sometimes this capacity is referred to as the ability to shift cognitive set.

More recently, Fuster [4] enlarged on the premise originally developed by Luria by suggesting that the so-called "executive systems" can be considered functionally homogeneous in the sense that they are in charge of actions, both external and internal (eg, logical reasoning). Fuster emphasized that the function of executive control is not unique to humans. The uniqueness of this system in humans is the extent to which humans are capable of integrating factors such as time, informational novelty, complexity, and possibly ambiguity.

Currently, an ever-increasing body of research is being dedicated to the study of the nature of executive control. Unfortunately, the main thrust of many such investigations has been reductive in character, and insight into the nature of executive control has been limited. Numerous attempts have been made to show that the key to the nature of executive control lies along the lines of such distinctions as sensory modalities and submodalities, linguistic versus nonlinguistic, object versus spatial ("what" versus "where"), and so forth.

This approach has gained particular prominence in the investigation of one aspect of executive functions, working memory. In the study of working memory, two main lines of scientific inquiry can be clearly discerned: one guided by a premise of domain specificity, and the other guided by the premise of process specificity. According to the domain specificity theory, different regions of the brain process different types of information (eg, spatial information versus object information) [2,5]. This theory is an extension of the object-versus-spatial ("what"-versus-"where") visual processing streams found in posterior cortices [6]. According to the process specificity theory, which draws on earlier human lesion studies [7], different regions of the brain are responsible for maintaining and manipulating information [8,9]. In the study of the long-term memory processes, Tulving's [10,11] hemispheric encoding–retrieval asymmetry stands out. According to this theory, episodic encoding results in greater left than right hemispheric activation, and episodic retrieval results in greater right than left hemispheric activation. More specifically, left prefrontal cortical regions are differentially more involved in retrieval of information from semantic memory and in simultaneously encoding novel aspects of the retrieved information into episodic memory. Right prefrontal cortical regions, on the other hand, are differentially more involved in retrieval of episodic memory [12].

Fuster [4] refers to this conceptual approach as neural "balkanization." This line of investigation may be useful for heuristic purposes and probably represents a sensible way to conduct well-controlled experiments. In the attempt to reduce the nature of executive control to modality- and process-specific subparts, one might come to a point at which it becomes necessary to invent a new subsystem for each new finding. Unless research is guided by a comprehensive unified theory of executive control that transcends the more specialized lines of inquiry, the actual picture of executive control may prove to be difficult, if not impossible, to construct.

More recently, the contribution of additional neuroanatomic structures to executive control has become apparent. These structures include the anterior cingulate cortex, basal ganglia, possibly the dorsomedial thalamic nucleus and cerebellum, and the ventral mesencephalon. Therefore, interchangeable use of the terms executive control and frontal lobe functions should be discouraged. To this extent, the concept of executive control remains a multifactorial and not a unitary construct. As a minimum, it includes the following components: goal-setting, cognitive tool selection, cognitive switching and mental flexibility, evaluating outcome, and adapting the current plan of execution appropriately.

## Neuropsychologic measures of executive control

To the extent that current understanding of the nature of executive control is not a unitary construct, it would be impossible to design a single test to measure it. There are, however, a number of neuropsychologic tests that provide an adequate measure of specific aspects of executive control. Among them, the family of Tower tests, the Wisconsin Card Sorting Test, and the family of Stroop tests [13] stand out.

### Tower tests

Tower tests comprise a whole family of somewhat similar tests, among which the towers of London [14], Hanoi, and Toronto [13] are most frequently used. The Tower tests measure the ability to plan. The subjects are required to build a tower or a pyramid according to a specified arrangement of pieces. The solution to the puzzle must be found in the fewest number of moves possible under such constraints as using only one hand, moving only one piece at a time, and not placing a larger piece on top of a smaller piece.

## The Wisconsin Card Sorting Test

The Wisconsin Card Sorting Test, originally developed by Grant and Berg [15], permits the assessment of mental flexibility, the ability to use feedback to shift cognitive sets, and goal-directed behavior [13]. Normed for individuals aged 6.5 through 89 years, the test challenges the ability to develop and maintain an appropriate problem-solving strategy across changing stimulus conditions to achieve a future goal. The four stimulus cards incorporate three stimulus parameters (color, form, and number). Respondents are required to sort the cards according to different principles during the test.

## Stroop tests

The family of Stroop tests [16,17] measures freedom from distractibility, selective attention, ability to resolve response conflict, and response inhibition. These tests are based on the phenomenon that it takes longer to name colors than to read words and even longer to name the color of the ink in which a color name is printed when they are different [17,18]. Patients with frontal lesions have been shown to perform worse on this test than patients with posterior lesions [19]. A typical version of a Stroop test might consist of three trials: word reading, color naming, and interference trial in which the first two are a baseline measure and the third is a critical measure. On an interference trial, respondents are required to name the color of the ink in which a color name is printed when they are different.

## Executive control batteries

Among the several batteries of executive control evaluation that exist, the Delis-Kaplan Executive Function System (D-KEFS) [20] and the Executive Control Battery (ECB) [21] stand out.

## The Delis-Kaplan Executive Function System

The D-KEFS is comprised of nine specific tests. These tests are mostly an updated version of commonly used stand-alone tests of executive function with better standardization and quantitative error scoring. The D-KEFS is normed for ages 8 through 89 years. The authors provide more exhaustive norms than the stand-alone tests. In the D-KEFS, the subtests were lengthened to avoid ceiling and floor effects. A number of quantitative measurements were designed to allow a wide variety of scores to be generated. No allowance, however, is made for composite score calculation.

The nine independent tests are

1. The Trail Making Test, which has five subtests: Visual Scanning, Number Sequencing, Letter Sequencing, Number-Letter Switching, and Motor Speed.
2. The Verbal Fluency Test, in which the subject says as many words starting with letters F, A, and S as possible in 1 minute and also says as many words as possible that belong to a category of animals, boys' names, and switching between the categories of fruits and furniture.
3. Design Fluency, which involves drawing as many different designs as possible in 1 minute using four straight lines to connect five dots.
4. The Color-Word Interference Test, which is a modification of the Stroop test, with the color, word, and interference conditions; unique to this version of the Stroop test is the interference/switching condition, in which the person must perform the interference task, except for the words that have a box drawn around them and must be read.
5. The Sorting Test, which consists of six cardboard tokens with a word written on each. The subject must sort these into two groups of three items according to some principle, explain the principle, then sort them a different way, to produce as many different sorts as possible. There is also a category recognition condition. This test measures abstract reasoning and mental flexibility.
6. The Twenty Questions Test, which resembles the familiar game of the same name and measures abstraction, strategy, and mental flexibility.
7. Word Context Test, which involves inferring the meaning of a nonsense word based on clues and measures the ability to infer and integrate information.
8. The Tower Test, which involves moving five concentric rings among three different pegs according to rules. It measures planning abilities.
9. The Proverb Test involves interpreting common and uncommon proverbs and measures the ability to think abstractly. It includes a recognition condition.

## The Executive Control Battery

The ECB [21] is a neuropsychologic battery designed to document the presence and the extent of certain qualitative features of executive dyscontrol. The battery is based on approaches and procedures developed and used by Alexander Luria and Elkhonon Goldberg while studying patients with focal prefrontal lesions. It is useful to think of the ECB as a battery of tests to detect pathognomic signs. The battery combines the advantages of qualitative and quantitative measurement. It preserves the qualitative type of error analysis inherent in the Lurian tradition of neuropsychology while adding the methodologic advantages of quantitative analysis.

The ECB was designed to elicit the various qualitative manifestations of the executive dyscontrol syndrome (ie, perseverations, echopraxia, field-dependent behavior, inertia, stereotypies, and so forth) through standard, quantitative procedures. Various qualitative types of deficits are identified, and their magnitude is quantified. The battery therefore combines the advantages of qualitative and quantitative, psychometric approaches. It enables the investigator to elicit and score errors in a standardized and quantitative fashion.

The ECB consists of four subtests, each known to be particularly capable of eliciting the features of the executive dyscontrol syndrome. These subtests are the Graphical Sequence test, the Competing Programs test, the Manual Postures test, and the Manual Sequences test.

### The Graphical Sequence Test

The Graphical Sequence Test involves drawing graphical sequences in accordance with verbal commands under time constraint. This test was designed to elicit various kinds of perseverations and various behavioral stereotypies. It allows the following four types of perseverations to be elicited: hyperkinetic motor perseverations, perseveration of elements, perseveration of features, and perseveration of activities.

### The Competing Programs Test

The Competing Programs Test, designed to elicit various types of echopraxia, behavioral stereotypies, and disinhibition, requires the respondent to execute various commands whose physical characteristics are in conflict with appropriate responses. The two types of sequences employed are the conflict visual version and the "go/no-go" version.

### The Manual Postures Test

The Manual Postures Test involves imitations by the respondent of various asymmetric static manual postures (unimanual and bimanual) produced by the examiner who is facing the patient. The task assesses the patient's ability to relate egocentric and allocentric spaces. The test allows the eliciting of various types of echopraxia and mirroring.

### The Motor Sequences Test

The Motor Sequences Test requires rapid alternation of both simple and complex unimanual and bimanual motor sequences. The six types of sequences are (1) unimanual two-stage movement, (2) unimanual two-stage movement reversal, (3) unimanual three-stage movement, (4) bimanual (reciprocal) coordination—distal, (5) bimanual (reciprocal) coordination—proximal, and (6) bimanual (reciprocal) coordination—mixed. The test allows the eliciting of various types of motor perseverations, stereotypies, and other deficits of sequential motor organization.

## Actor-centered nature of executive control

In a typical neuropsychologic test, one possible response is correct and others are incorrect. The determination of what is correct and what is incorrect is inherent in the test design and does not require any knowledge of the patient making the choice. To this extent, a typical neuropsychologic test is deterministic and veridical. A rigid structure of the test minimizes its ability to identify the executive control deficit in a clinical evaluation. A new generation of tests is needed to measure actor-centered rather than veridical decision-making. Because the prefrontal cortex is particularly critical for actor-centered decision making, such innovative experimental procedures are required to characterize the contribution of the prefrontal cortex to cognition.

Actor-centered and veridical decision making are based on different mechanisms. Veridical decision making is based on the identification of the correct response, which is intrinsic to the external situation and is actor-independent, whereas actor-centered decision making is guided by the actor's priorities. The actor-centered, as opposed to veridical, decision-making process involves relating individual priorities to the parameters of the external situation. For example, a person deciding what to order in a restaurant is faced with an ambiguous situation. After weighing individual priorities, the person usually makes the choice quickly but not randomly. These priorities characterize the actor, not only the contents of the menu. Once the priorities have been ranked, the situation has been disambiguated, and the rest of the decision-making process is veridical. It is reduced to finding items that are appropriate to the situation, a decision that is independent of any of the individual's characteristics as the agent of action. For instance, someone with little money and with no credit cards may decide to look for the most reasonably priced entrée. By contrast, a wealthy person eager to impress a date will choose the most expensive item.

In real life, veridical decision making is subordinate to actor-centered decision making. The individual's best response cannot be inferred from the properties of the external situation alone, because the choice of such a response depends on the subject's needs and the subject's perception of those needs.

The frontal lobes are central to the formation of plans and the organism's ability to guide its behavior by internal representation [22]. The frontal lobes are linked uniquely to intentionality, and to elucidate the functions of the prefrontal lobes, one must study the neural substrates of intentionality. In turn, to study intentionality, one must deal with ambiguity and cognitive relativity.

Nauta [23] emphasized that the prefrontal cortex plays a unique role in integrating neural inputs from the organism's external and internal environments. This integrative role of the prefrontal lobes is essential to actor-centered behavior and intentionality. By extension, the study of the functions of the frontal lobes requires a particular type of cognitive tasks measuring actor-centered decision-making.

Even cognitive tasks that have been traditionally accepted as the frontal lobe tasks (eg, the Wisconsin Card Sorting Test, Category Test, or Stroop Test) are quite limited in their ability to elucidate the functions of the frontal lobes, because they are veridical, rather than actor-centered. Because the frontal lobes are particularly critical for actor-centered decision making, innovative experimental procedures are required to characterize the contribution of the prefrontal cortex to actor-centered decision making. Currently, few tests capable of examining adaptive decision making and its impairment exist in clinical neuropsychology.

Two tests, the Cognitive Bias Task (CBT) and the Iowa Gambling Test, are among the first steps in this direction.

*The Cognitive Bias Task*

The CBT [24] consists of stimuli characterized along five dimensions: color (red/blue), shape (circle/square), number (one/two), size (large/small), and contour (outline/filled with a homogenous color). Thirty-two different stimuli can be constructed. Any two stimuli can be compared according to the number of dimensions that they share. A similarity index ranging between 5 and 0 can be computed.

The unique feature of the CBT is that it requires the subject to make a selection based on preference, rather than on any of the external stimulus characteristics or constraints. Earlier work demonstrated that CBT is sensitive to the effects of prefrontal lesions, as long as the choice of response is ambiguous and up to the subject; once the ambiguity is removed, the effects of the prefrontal lesion disappear [24].

A trial consists of the presentation of three stimuli: a target and two choices vertically aligned. The subjects are instructed to look at the target card then select the one of the two choices that they like better. In all trials, the similarity indices between the target and each of the two choices are never equal; thus the subject must make a choice that is either more similar to or different from the target. There are 60 independent trials. The similarity indices are summed across trials to generate a cumulative score ranging from 80 to 220. A low cumulative score indicates that the subject consistently chose the more different choice relative to the target. A high cumulative score indicates that the subject consistently responded by choosing the more similar choice relative to the target. A middle-range score indicates that the subject's choices are either unrelated to the target or that the subject makes a relatively equal number of similar and different choices. Both high and low cumulative scores imply guidance by the properties of the target and reflect context-dependent response preference. Middle-range scores imply context-independent response (not using the target as a context) or the preference to produce an inconsistent response pattern. Two control tasks are used. The format is the same, but instead of selecting the card they "like better," the subjects are asked to choose the card that is more similar to or more different from the target card.

The original study introducing the CBT [24] reported a robust effect of frontal lobe lesions in the ambiguous condition, when the subjects respond according to their own preferences. The effect disappears when the task is disambiguated and becomes veridical. The role played by the prefrontal cortex in the CBT is clearly not in computing the veridical aspects of the task but in deciding how the inherently ambiguous task should be constrained. By introducing ambiguity and using preference as the basis for cognitive task design, the sensitivity of the task to frontal lobe function is significantly enhanced.

In addition, the CBT was instrumental in elucidating hemispheric and gender differences in the functional organization of the frontal lobes and showing a relationship between handedness and the functional organization of the frontal lobes [24]. In an earlier study [25], the CBT was able to show robust lateralization of frontal lobe functions in males. By contrast, The Wisconsin Card Sorting Test failed to reveal such lateralization. These differences suggest that the functional differences between the left and right prefrontal systems can be best understood in terms of actor-centered, rather than veridical, aspects of decision making.

In conclusion, findings generated by the CBT in patients with focal frontal lesions highlight strong gender and hemispheric differences in the functional specialization of the frontal lobes, which are more robust than the differences elicited with the commonly used veridical tasks, such as the Wisconsin Card Sorting Test.

*The Iowa Gambling Test*

The Iowa Gambling Test [26] was developed to assess decision-making impairment in patients with damage to the ventro-medial prefrontal cortex. This test essentially simulates gambling with varied cost-versus-payoff ratios. The ventro-medial prefrontal cortex region of the brain controls aspects of decision making. Bechara and colleagues [27] noted that one factor that was strongly associated with a poor score on the Iowa Gambling Test was the inability to maintain employment, which is one of the hallmarks of decision-making impairment in patients with damage to the ventro-medial prefrontal cortex. Additionally, Bechara and colleagues [27] report that behaviors of substance-dependent individuals are similar to behaviors seen in patients with damaged ventro-medial prefrontal cortices. This observation provides additional insight as to the underlying nature of substance-abuse disorders.

The CBT and the Iowa Gambling Test are among the first attempts to develop measures of nonveridical decision making. It is hoped that a new generation of neuropsychologic tests will emerge, designed to assess various aspects of adaptive decision making.

## Working memory and its assessment

Historically there are has been a great deal of controversy regarding the role of the frontal lobes in memory. During the last few decades, the work by Patricia Goldman-Rakic [2] and Joaquin Fuster [4] helped to clarify the role of the frontal lobes in memory and introduced the concept of working memory. The construct of working memory, like many other influential concepts, has been somewhat overused. Sometimes it is used interchangeably with the construct of short-term memory. Common sense tells us that if these two constructs represent the same underlying cognitive structure, then having two separate constructs is redundant and unnecessary. The authors, however, believe that the construct of working memory has a place in the field of cognitive neuroscience as a unique concept. What is unique to the concept of working memory is its actor-centered nature: the assessment by the working memory of "what needs to be memorized."

Memory is among the most extensively studied aspects of the mind. In a typical memory study, a subject is asked to memorize a list of words or view a series of pictures of faces and then recall or recognize the material under various conditions. In most memory tests, a subject is instructed explicitly by an examiner to memorize certain information and then recall it. The decision as to what to recall rests with the examiner, not with the subject. In most real-life situations, people store and recall information for solving a problem at hand. Furthermore, certain memories are accessed and retrieved not in response to an external command but in response to an internally generated need. Instead of being told what to recall, people must decide for themselves which information is useful in the context of ongoing activities at the moment.

In real-life situations, memory recall involves making a decision as to the type of information that is useful at the moment and then selecting this information out of the total fund of knowledge available. Furthermore, when necessary, people often make a smooth, instantaneous switch from one selection to another. Most of the time, such decisions, selections, and transitions are made automatically and effortlessly. These decisions are anything but trivial, however: they require complex neural computations that are performed by the frontal lobes. Different stages of solving a problem may require different types of information. Therefore, the frontal lobes must constantly and rapidly decide which information is required at which stage of decision making and bring new engrams into play while letting go of the old ones. Memory based on such an ever-changing selection process and guided by the frontal lobes is called working memory.

In real life, recall processes involve working memory and the frontal lobes, but most procedures used in memory research and clinical settings do not. In the typical memory experiment, the examiner makes the decision about what to remember, and the role of the frontal lobes is removed.

Working memory (in its proper definition) is among most vulnerable aspects of cognition, and it suffers in a wide range of neurologic and psychiatric conditions. Often overlooked, working memory frequently suffers in early dementias. Unfortunately, at present, neuropsychologic measures that directly assess the working memory as an actor-centered construct are scarce. One of the indirect measures of working memory is the semantic clustering index of The California Verbal Learning Test [28]. This index provides a measure of the extent to which an individual is capable of independently coming up with a strategy that facilitates the learning of items that at a first glance are seemingly unrelated and overwhelming in quantity.

## Clinical conditions requiring the assessment of executive functions

The prefrontal cortex is afflicted in a wide range of conditions [29,30]. Historically, it was thought that to find prefrontal dysfunction one has to look for focal frontal lesions. The findings of the last few decades make it clear that the frontal lobes are particularly vulnerable in numerous nonfocal conditions. Today, schizophrenia is regarded as substantially involving the frontal lobes [31,32]. Traumatic brain injury often produces frontal lobe syndrome accompanied by pronounced hypofrontality (reduction in the frontal cerebral activation relative to other regions of the cortex) [33]. Frontal lobe dysfunction in traumatic brain injury is caused by either direct frontal injury or injury that disrupts the reticular–frontal connection.

The role of prefrontal dysfunction in attention deficit disorder has been emphasized by Barkley [34]. Executive functions are also vulnerable in dementia and in depression.

A frontal lobe lesion is not necessary for a frontal lobe syndrome. In many conditions functional neuroimaging and neuropsychologic studies show evidence of frontal lobe dysfunction, but there is no evidence of structural damage to the frontal lobes. These conditions are characterized by frontal lobe dysfunction in the absence of morphologic damage to the frontal lobes. The existence of these conditions suggests that the threshold for functional breakdown of the frontal cortex is lower than that of other parts of neocortex.

Because of the high prevalence of frontal lobe dysfunction in a wide range of conditions, it is important to include tests of executive functioning in any comprehensive neuropsychologic evaluation. Because of the heterogeneous nature of executive control, various aspects of executive functioning can be impaired. Therefore, it is often prudent to administer a number of different neuropsychologic tests of executive functions.

Following is a more detailed discussion of some of the nonfocal conditions characterized by frontal lobe dysfunction.

It would be an overstatement to talk about unique neuropsychologic profiles of most neuropsychiatric conditions, nor is it advisable to make a psychiatric diagnosis solely on the basis of neuropsychologic data. Nonetheless, several useful diagnostic considerations should be kept in mind. For instance, cognitive impairment in schizophrenia usually is dominated by executive deficit. Although the presence of executive deficit is nonspecific and by itself should not lead to the diagnosis of schizophrenia, its absence may be sufficient grounds for questioning this diagnosis.

In depression, both executive deficit and memory impairment are often present. Depression also tends to affect those functions traditionally associated with the right hemisphere (ie, processing of and memory for nonrepresentational visuospatial information). By contrast, functions commonly associated with the posterior aspect of the left hemisphere (eg, language, ideational praxis, and processing of meaningful visuospatial information) are usually spared in depression. This consideration may be particularly valuable in distinguishing between depression and dementia, a diagnostic dilemma commonly arising in the context of geriatric psychiatry. The presence of significant anomia (naming deficit), associative agnosia (deficit of recognizing common objects), or dressing apraxia immediately raises the possibility of dementia, because, none of these findings is usually caused by depression alone.

A neuropsychologic diagnosis never should be made in a piecemeal, test-by-test basis. Instead, the whole profile of performance on a number of tests should be considered. Therefore, a referral made by a psychiatrist for a neuropsychologic evaluation should specify the diagnostic or/and treatment question, rather than specify a menu of specific tests.

## Summary

Given the pervasive nature of executive deficit, assessment of executive functions is of crucial importance in neuropsychiatry, child and adolescent psychiatry, geriatric psychiatry, and other related areas. A number of neuropsychologic tests of executive function commonly are used in assessing several clinical disorders, including but not limited to traumatic brain injury, schizophrenia, depression, attention deficit disorder/attention deficit hyperactivity disorder, and dementia. Because the concept of executive control in its current form constitutes an overarching construct, a construct that is based on the cognitive symptoms of the frontal lobe disorder caused by many disparate underlying conditions, no single measure of executive function can adequately tap the construct in its entirety. Therefore, it is necessary to administer several tests of executive function, each assessing a particular aspect of the executive function. An appropriate combination of such neuropsychologic tests and batteries, including the Wisconsin Card Sorting Test, Tower test, Stroop test, the D-KEFS, and the

ECB, provides an adequate but relatively crude mechanism for assessing executive systems dysfunction. Neuroscientists continue to refine their understanding of the nature of executive control, and additional innovative procedures that reflect state-of-the-art insights of cognitive neuroscience have been introduced recently. Among a few first steps in that direction are nonveridical, actor-centered procedures such as the CBT and the Iowa Gambling Test.

## References

[1] Luria AR. Higher cortical functions in man. New York: Basic Books; 1966.
[2] Goldman-Rakic PS. Circuitry of primate prefrontal cortex and regulation of behavior by representational memory. In: Plum F, editor. Handbook of physiology: nervous system, higher functions of the brain (part 1), vol. 5. 5th edition. Bethesda (MD): American Physiological Association; 1987. p. 373–417.
[3] Milner B. Some cognitive effects of frontal lobe lesion in man. Philos Trans R Soc Lond B Biol Sci 1982;298:211–26.
[4] Fuster J. The prefrontal cortex: anatomy, physiology, and neuropsychology of the frontal lobe. 3rd edition. Philadelphia: Lippincott-Raven; 1997.
[5] Goldman-Rakic PS. The prefrontal landscape: implications of functional architecture for understanding human mentation and the central executive. In: Roberts AC, Robbins TW, Weiskrantz L, editors. The prefrontal cortex: executive and cognitive functions. Oxford (UK): Oxford University Press; 1998. p. 87–102.
[6] Mishkin M, Ungerleider LG, Macko KA. Object vision and spatial vision: two cortical pathways. Trends Neurosci 1983;6:414–7.
[7] Petrides M, Milner B. Deficits on subject-ordered tasks after frontal- and temporal-lobe lesions in man. Neuropsychologia 1982;20(3):249–62.
[8] Petrides M. Frontal lobes and working memory: evidence from investigations of the effects of cortical excision in nonhuman primates. In: Boller F, Grafman J, editors. Handbook of neuropsychology, vol. 9. Amsterdam: Elsevier; 1994. p. 59–82.
[9] Petrides M. Impairments on nonspatial self-ordered and externally ordered working memory tasks after lesions of the mid-dorsal part of the lateral frontal cortex in the monkey. J Neurosci 1995;15(1 Pt 1):359–75.
[10] Tulving E, Kapur S, Craik FI, et al. Hemispheric encoding/retrieval asymmetry in episodic memory: positron emission tomography findings. Proc Natl Acad Sci U S A 1994;91(6): 2016–20.
[11] Tulving E, Markowitsch HJ, Kapur S, et al. Novelty encoding networks in the human brain: positron emission tomography data. Neuroreport 1994;5(18):2525–8.
[12] Fletcher PC, Henson RN. Frontal lobes and human memory: insights from functional neuroimaging. Brain 2001;124(Pt 5):849–81.
[13] Lezak MD. Neuropsychological assessment. 4th edition. New York: Oxford University Press; 2004.
[14] Shallice T. Specific impairments of planning. Philos Trans R Soc Lond B Biol Sci 1982; 298(1089):199–209.
[15] Grant DA, Berg EA. A behavioral analysis of degree of reinforcement and ease of shifting to new responses in a Weigl-type card-sorting problem. J Exp Psychol 1948;38:404–11.
[16] Stroop JR. Studies of interference in serial verbal reactions. J Exp Psychol 1935;18:643–62.
[17] Jensen AR, Rohwer WD Jr. The Stroop color-word test: a review. Acta Psychol (Amst) 1966; 25(1):36–93.
[18] Dyer FN, Severance LJ. Stroop interference with successive presentations of separate incongruent words and colors. J Exp Psychol 1973;98(2):438–9.

[19] Stuss DT, Floden D, Alexander MP, et al. Stroop performance in focal lesion patients: dissociation of processes and frontal lobe lesion location. Neuropsychologia 2001;39(8): 771–86.

[20] Delis D, Kaplan E, Kramer J. Delis-Kaplan Executive Function Scale. San Antonio (TX): Psychological Corporation; 2001.

[21] Goldberg E, Podell K, Bilder R, et al. The executive control battery. Sydney (Australia): Psych Press; 2000.

[22] Goldberg E, Bilder RM. The frontal lobes and hierarchical organization of cognitive control. In: Perecman E, editor. The frontal lobes revisited. New York: IRBN Press; 1987. p. 159–87.

[23] Nauta WJ. The problem of the frontal lobe: a reinterpretation. J Psychiatr Res 1971;8(3): 167–87.

[24] Goldberg E, Harner R, Lovell M, et al. Cognitive bias, functional cortical geometry, and the frontal lobes: laterality, sex, and handedness. J Cogn Neurosci 1994;6(3):276–96.

[25] Podell K, Lovell M, Zimmerman M, Goldberg E. The Cognitive Bias Task and lateralized frontal lobe functions in males. J Neuropsychiatry Clin Neurosci 1995;7(4):491–501.

[26] Bechara A, Damasio AR, Damasio H, et al. Insensitivity to future consequences following damage to human prefrontal cortex. Cognition 1994;50(1–3):7–15.

[27] Bechara A, Dolan S, Denburg N, et al. Decision-making deficits, linked to a dysfunctional ventromedial prefrontal cortex, revealed in alcohol and stimulant abusers. Neuropsychologia 2001;39(4):376–89.

[28] Delis D, Kaplan E, Kramer J, et al. California Verbal Learning Test—Second Edition (CVLT-II). San Antonio (TX): Psychological Corporation; 2000.

[29] Goldberg E. The frontal lobes in neurological and psychiatric conditions [introduction]. Neuropsychiatry Neuropsychol Behav Neurol 1992;5(4):231–2.

[30] Goldberg E, Bougakov D. Novel approaches to the diagnosis and treatment of frontal lobe dysfunction. In: Christensen A-L, Uzzel BP, editors. International handbook of neuropsychological rehabilitation. New York: Kluwer Academic/Plenum Publishers; 2000. p. 93–112.

[31] Ingvar DH, Franzen G. Abnormalities of cerebral blood flow distribution in patients with chronic schizophrenia. Acta Psychiatr Scand 1974;50(4):425–62.

[32] Franzen G, Ingvar DH. Absence of activation in frontal structures during psychological testing of chronic schizophrenics. J Neurol Neurosurg Psychiatry 1975;38(10):1027–32.

[33] Deutsch G, Eisenberg HM. Frontal blood flow changes in recovery from coma. J Cereb Blood Flow Metab 1987;7(1):29–34.

[34] Barkley RA. ADHD and the nature of self-control. New York: The Guilford Press; 1997.

ELSEVIER
SAUNDERS

Psychiatr Clin N Am 28 (2005) 581–597

PSYCHIATRIC
CLINICS
OF NORTH AMERICA

# Disorders of Memory

## John A. Lucas, PhD, ABPP/ABCN

*Department of Psychiatry and Psychology, Mayo Clinic, 4500 San Pablo Road, Jacksonville, FL 32224, USA*

Memory reflects the ability to maintain information within a searchable, internal storage system so that it can be accessed and used later. Perhaps more than for any other cognitive construct, the understanding of normal and disordered memory has advanced greatly in recent decades. Once believed to be a unitary construct, memory has been shown through medical observation and neuropsychologic studies to be characterized instead by a number of unique and dissociable dimensions with distinct underlying neuroanatomic substrates. This article reviews some of the common classifications of memory constructs, the basic underlying neuronal bases of learning and memory, and the contributions of distinct brain systems to normal and disordered memory functioning.

## Conceptual divisions of memory

Human memory is a complex cognitive process that manifests in multiple parallel pathways. These manifestations can be fractionated along a number of different dimensions reflecting different underlying processing demands or features of the information to be remembered. For example, one can characterize memory by the amount of time that elapses between presentation and recall of information (eg, immediate versus delayed recall), by the nature of the information that is remembered (eg, knowledge-based facts versus personal experiences), or by the means by which information is remembered (eg, free recall or recognition), among others. Some of the more common conceptual divisions of memory are reviewed in this section.

---

*E-mail address:* jlucas@mayo.edu

*Short- and long-term memory*

It has long been observed that some memories are brief in duration whereas others endure long after the experience leaves conscious awareness [1]. The ability to recall material immediately after it is presented is known as short-term memory (STM), whereas the ability to remember information later is known as long-term memory (LTM).

STM is of limited capacity, with the ability to hold only an average of seven pieces of information at any one time [2,3]. This information can remain available to conscious recall for several minutes but will be lost or replaced by new information if not sustained by active rehearsal. For example, when one looks up a telephone number in a directory, the information remains in STM as one briefly looks away from the directory and dials the number. If the telephone is across the room, one can maintain the number in STM by rehearsing it continuously until it is dialed. Soon after dialing, however, the number is usually forgotten.

In contrast, LTM has an extraordinarily large capacity, with the potential to hold information indefinitely without the need for continued rehearsal [3]. One can, for example, recall one's own telephone number, as well as myriad other facts, past experiences, and personal information, without needing to reference external resources or actively rehearse the information.

The clinical significance of the distinction between STM and LTM has been well documented in patients who have amnesic disorders [4–8]. Perhaps the most famous medical case study of disordered memory was of patient H.M., a man with medically intractable epilepsy who became densely amnesic after tissue from both temporal lobes including the hippocampus was removed to control his seizures [6]. After his surgery, H.M. could accurately repeat back information immediately following presentation, but once he was distracted by another task, he could not recall the information that was originally presented. He could recall information, events, and people that he had encountered or learned before his surgery, but he could not learn new information that he encountered following his surgery. Together, these observations provided evidence for the fractionation of the processes and brain systems required for STM, the creation of new LTM, and the ability to retain and access old LTM.

*Encoding, retention, and retrieval*

Information processing models reveal evidence of three distinct processes involved in memory: encoding, retention, and retrieval of information [9]. Encoding is the process by which information is acquired and transformed into a stored mental representation. Retention refers to the process by which the encoded information is maintained over time in the absence of active rehearsal. Of course, encoding and retaining information is of little value if the information cannot be sought out and brought back into consciousness when needed (ie, retrieved).

The encoding process allows the storage of considerably more information than would normally could held in STM alone. Although the precise mechanisms involved in memory encoding remain poorly understood, one theory [10] suggests that as information is processed by the brain, various features of the information (eg, visual perceptual, semantic, and others) are analyzed, manipulated, reorganized, and coded in such a way that they become functionally associated with each other.

As one might expect, information that is poorly or incompletely encoded typically is poorly retained and is lost to future recall. Even if memories are normally encoded and retained, however, one might experience poor recall because of difficulties accessing the stored information. To distinguish between failures of recall caused by poor encoding/retention versus poor retrieval, neuropsychologists typically examine the relationship between free recall and recognition performances on formal memory tests. Free recall requires the subject to search memory actively to find and access information, placing maximum demands on retrieval processes. These demands are diminished when the subject is provided multiple choices and asked to recognize the correct information. A primary retrieval deficit is surmised if recognition memory is intact in the presence of impaired free recall. In contrast, if both recall and recognition are equally poor, an encoding/retention deficit is likely.

## Anterograde and retrograde memory

The terms anterograde and retrograde refer to the ability to recall information consciously and deliberately before or after a given point in time or sentinel event. Specifically, anterograde memory is the ability to form new memories from a given time forward, whereas retrograde memory is the ability to remember information or events that occurred before a specific event or moment in time. For example, patients who suffer acquired brain injuries in motor vehicle accidents may not recall the events leading up to the accident (ie, a retrograde deficit) or the events that occurred immediately following the accident (ie, an anterograde deficit) caused by disruption of the mechanisms required for reliable memory encoding. The length of anterograde and retrograde amnesia following a head injury is often correlated with the extent of brain damage sustained [11]. Anterograde and retrograde memory deficits are dissociable and often differ in length, with anterograde deficits typically spanning a longer time frame than retrograde deficits. It is also common for anterograde deficits to occur in the absence of retrograde amnesia. The reverse pattern, however, is rare. Isolated retrograde impairments, including loss of past memories, personal history, and personal identity, typically are psychologic rather than neurologic in origin [12].

*Recent and remote memory*

Retrograde memory is commonly divided into two temporal components, recent versus remote. Recent memory typically refers to information acquired shortly (ie, days to weeks) before a specified time or event, whereas remote memory refers to information about events or experiences that occurred months to years in the more distant past.

Patients who have retrograde memory impairments often demonstrate a temporal gradient in which memory for more recent events is disrupted more than memory for remote events. Such is the case in amnesic disorders such as alcoholic Korsakoff syndrome. In a classic study of a prominent scientist with this disorder, Butters and Cermak [13] used the patient's own autobiography to test his memory for past life events. His most accurate memories were for events that occurred early in his life, with progressively worse memory for events in subsequent decades and no memory for significant life events that occurred within the decade immediately before his disease onset.

*Declarative versus nondeclarative memory*

Declarative memory (or explicit memory) refers to the acquisition of facts, experiences, and information about events [14,15]. It is memory that is directly accessible to conscious awareness and thus can be "declared." In contrast, nondeclarative memory (also called implicit memory) refers to various forms of memory that are not directly accessible to consciousness [14,16,17]. These memories include skill and habit learning, classical conditioning, priming, and other circumstances in which memory is expressed through performance rather than through conscious recollection. Most clinical memory disorders involve disruption of declarative memories, so this discussion focuses on declarative memory.

*Episodic memory*

Episodic memory is a subtype of declarative memory that refers to information linked to a particular place and time. To remember such information, the spatial and temporal context must be retrieved also. Recalling events from one's last birthday or what one ate for dinner last night are examples of episodic memory, because in each case the appropriate time and place of the events must be accessed to recall the target information correctly.

*Semantic memory*

Semantic memory is a second type of declarative memory that refers to one's general knowledge of facts or information that is not linked to a particular temporal or spatial context. For example, recalling one's birth date or the meaning of the word "dinner" can be achieved without processing where or when such information was originally learned.

## Neurobiologic bases of memory

Most scientists view memory as a special case of neuronal plasticity, a phenomenon by which neurons can change their structure or function in a lasting way. Although several competing hypotheses regarding the nature and mechanism of this change have been advanced over the years, it is now widely accepted that neuronal changes associated with new learning and memory reflect modifications in neuronal connectivity and efficiency at the level of the synapse [18].

### Memory as change of synaptic structure and efficacy

A synapse is a functional juxtaposition of two or more neurons (Fig. 1). When a neuron is stimulated to a sufficient degree, neurotransmitters are

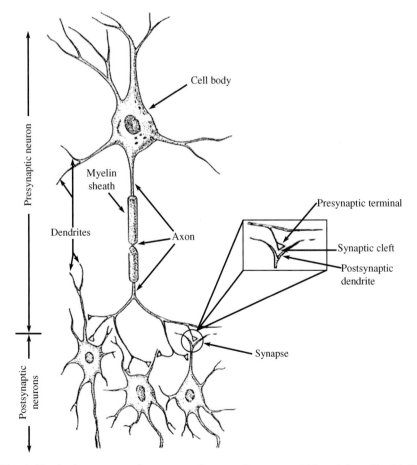

Fig. 1. The basic structure of neurons and neuronal synapses. (*Adapted from* Kandel E, Schwartz JH, Jessell TM, editors. Principles of neural science. 3rd edition. The McGraw-Hill Companies; 1993; with permission.)

released from the axon terminal into the microscopic space that separates it from neighboring neurons. The presence of neurotransmitters within this region produces characteristic changes in the membranes of adjacent neurons. Memories are believed to be the result of structural and functional changes of neuronal activity and synaptic transmission in response to experience.

### Neuronal processes underlying short-term memory

A neuron's function can be modified by intense activity, such as high-frequency stimulation by a presynaptic neuron. Such activity increases the responsiveness and efficiency of postsynaptic membranes, with some neurons being capable of increased responsiveness lasting from several minutes to more than an hour after active stimulation has ceased. This temporary increase in synaptic effectiveness is known as posttetanic potentiation (PTP) and reflects one possible way that newly presented information may be remembered [19]. PTP may cause neurons activated during learning to remain active for a brief time after learning has ceased, thus allowing a trace of that information to remain available for recall.

Another proposed mechanism by which neuronal activity may be maintained for a brief period is by means of a feedback loop. Excitatory input entering a closed loop could be maintained after active input ceases if neurons within that loop are excitatory (Fig. 2). Such neuronal feedback systems are known as reverberatory circuits [14,20].

The time that elapses before information in STM degrades is believed to be a function of PTP strength or the level of neuronal excitement in reverberatory circuits. More intense changes in these neuronal dynamics

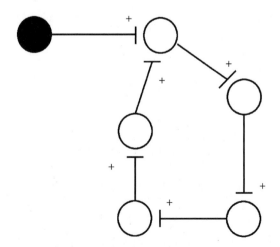

Fig. 2. A reverberatory neuronal circuit. Excitatory input to a neuron within the circuit (*unfilled circles*) yields prolonged activation even after input from outside the circuit (*filled circle*) ceases.

typically are associated with more persistent memory, whereas weaker changes are associated with more rapid forgetting.

## Neuronal processes underlying long-term memory

The ability to encode information into a more permanent long-term storage system is believed to be a function of long-term potentiation (LTP). LTP is similar to PTP, in that high-intensity stimulation increases the effectiveness of the neuronal synapse. LTP is more powerful and enduring than PTP, however, and cannot be produced by activation of only a single presynaptic neuron in a single pathway. Instead, a minimum number of inputs must be present to produce an effect.

When neurons in the brain's memory consolidation centers are activated by LTP, enzymes in the neuronal membrane are released and form a chemical messenger known as cyclic adenosine monophosphate (cAMP). This messenger activates specific proteins, including cAMP-response element binding protein, which promotes a synaptic growth process that strengthens the functional relationships among active neurons. These neuronal changes are believed to provide the biologic substrate for consolidation of information into LTM [21–23].

## Neuroanatomic correlates of memory

In mammals, the first neurons observed to demonstrate LTP were found in the structures of the medial temporal lobe of the brain, including the hippocampus and surrounding regions. Other brain regions identified as important to declarative memory include the medial diencephalon, basal forebrain, prefrontal cortex, subcortical nuclei, and cerebral white matter pathways.

### Medial temporal lobes

The temporal lobe is a large brain region with several anatomically distinct areas. The structures in the medial aspect of the temporal lobes, including the hippocampus, its surrounding cortex, and the amygdala, are most important for memory (Figs. 3 and 4).

### Hippocampus and related structures

The human hippocampus and associated cortices are located bilaterally in the cerebral hemispheres, forming a ridge that extends along the temporal horn of each lateral ventricle. As illustrated in Fig. 4, these structures are convoluted, with several distinct regions defined by differences in cellular structure and organization. Recent studies indicate that projections from area CA1 of the hippocampus to the subiculum and prefrontal cortex can

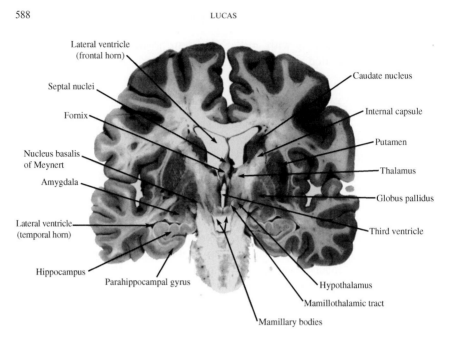

Fig. 3. Coronal section of the brain showing the relative locations of selected medial temporal lobe, diencephalic, and basal forebrain structures important to memory functioning. (*Adapted from* DeArmond SJ, Fusco MM, Dewey MM. Structure of the human brain: a photographic atlas. 3rd edition. New York: Oxford University Press; 1989; with permission.)

express several forms of neuronal plasticity and probably play an important role in consolidating information into LTM [24–26].

*Amygdala*

The amygdala is a collection of nuclei and specialized cortical areas in the dorsomedial portion of the temporal lobe (Fig. 3). It plays an important role in emotional and autonomic behaviors and has substantial interconnections with brain regions involved in memory consolidation (eg, hippocampal formation, thalamus, hypothalamus, prefrontal cortex, basal forebrain). Studies of nonhuman primates suggest that damage to the amygdala itself does not impair the ability to learn new information, provided the information is neutral in emotional valence [27–29]. In contrast, the ability to learn a conditioned fear response is highly dependent upon the amygdala and is absent in animals with lesions to this brain region [30,31].

*Medial diencephalon*

The diencephalon is a region of several important nuclei located at the top of the brainstem. The regions important to memory functioning include portions of the thalamus and hypothalamus (Fig. 3). In particular, patients who have injuries involving the midline structures of these regions

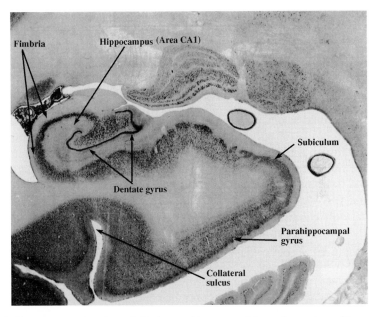

Fig. 4. Transverse section through the human hippocampal formation and parahippocampal gyrus, including area CA1 of the hippocampus proper. (*Adapted from* DeArmond SJ, Fusco MM, Dewey MM. Structure of the human brain: a photographic atlas. 3rd edition. New York: Oxford University Press; 1989; with permission.)

demonstrate severe anterograde amnesia and often demonstrate a temporally graded retrograde amnesia. The structures most often implicated in diencephalic amnesia include the dorsomedial nucleus of the thalamus, the mamillary bodies of the hypothalamus, and the white matter (mamillothalamic) tract connecting these structures [32–35]. Some animal studies have shown that the internal medullary lamina of the thalamus is also important to memory [36,37].

*Basal forebrain*

The basal forebrain is located superior to the optic chiasm and includes the medial septal nuclei, nucleus accumbens, anterior hypothalamus, diagonal band of Broca, nucleus basalis of Meynert, and part of the prefrontal cortex. The septal nuclei and nucleus basalis of Meynert (Fig. 3), in particular, have extensive connections to and from the hippocampal formation, amygdala, and neocortex and are believed to be important to memory functioning [38,39]. In monkeys, combined lesions to the nucleus basalis of Meynert, medial septal nuclei, and diagonal band of Broca result in significant memory impairment. No significant impairment is noted, however, if each structure is lesioned separately, suggesting that extensive damage to the basal forebrain may be necessary to produce memory impairment. Basal forebrain neurons are rich in the neurotransmitter acetylcholine, which is important to memory functioning. [40] Most investigators believe that input from this region plays a role in modulating memory processes that occur in other brain systems [14,41].

### The prefrontal cortex

The prefrontal cortex plays an important role in directing the attentional and organizational resources needed to encode and retrieve information. In addition, disruption of prefrontal systems is associated with characteristic memory impairments, including source memory deficits and impaired temporal ordering [42,43]. Source memory and temporal ordering refer to the ability to recall the spatial and temporal contexts within which information was originally acquired. Thus, episodic memory is affected to a greater degree than semantic memory. For example, when given two successive word lists to learn, patients who have prefrontal cortex damage may be able to recall the words but have difficulty indicating the list from which each word originated.

### Subcortical nuclei and white matter

The ability to search and retrieve information from LTM is a function of subcortical nuclei and white matter systems. These observations come primarily from studies of patients who have basal ganglia diseases, such as Parkinson's disease and Huntington's disease, or white matter disorders, such as diffuse ischemic cerebrovascular disease and multiple sclerosis. Damage to subcortical nuclei or white matter is associated with slowed information processing, inefficient learning, and poor free recall. Recognition memory, however, is usually equivalent to that of neurologically normal individuals, suggesting a deficit in retrieval processes rather than in retention of information [44–48].

### A neuroanatomic model of long-term memory processing

Although the precise mechanisms by which information is encoded, stored, and retrieved from LTM remain unclear, most investigators believe that declarative memory systems work together to encode and store new memories. Once information is processed by the neocortex, it is sent along parallel pathways to the hippocampal cortices and medial diencephalon for memory processing. The stimulus features are indexed to the cortical sites where they were originally processed, and associations are created to link various stimulus features together. Inputs from the basal forebrain and prefrontal cortex to these regions stamp the newly learned information with temporal and spatial information, and the constituent features of the memory representation are then distributed throughout the brain's neocortex. In this model, no single location contains the complete record of any given memory; therefore, the ability to remember a given experience or piece of information requires the activation of enough subcomponent constituent features to reconstruct the memory [49]. This model is known as the constructive memory theory of information processing.

## Memory disorders in clinical populations

Disordered memory can be observed in a number of patient populations as well as with normal human aging. A brief overview of these memory profiles reveals how different components of learning and memory can be disrupted or spared selectively.

### Normal aging

Older adults commonly complain that their memory is no longer reliable, and studies confirm a strong negative relationship between age and performance on tests of learning and memory [50]. Memory problems associated with normal aging tend to reflect a generalized decrease in the efficiency by which information is processed and retrieved [51]. STM is typically well preserved unless there is high demand placed on processing resources. For example, older and younger individuals perform essentially equally when asked to repeat strings of digits read aloud by an examiner. Older subjects, however, have greater difficulty than younger subjects in manipulating the information being held in STM (eg, arranging the digits in order or repeating the string of digits back in reverse order). With regard to LTM, age-related impairments in free recall of stories and word lists are evident by age 50 years [52]. When structure is provided by the use of recognition testing or cueing, however, the age differences diminish, suggesting greater impairment of retrieval processes than of encoding or retention [53,54].

### Alzheimer's disease and mild cognitive impairment

Anterograde episodic memory impairment is often one of the first observable symptoms in patients who have Alzheimer's disease [55]. In the earliest stages, patients may demonstrate memory impairment in isolation of any other cognitive or behavioral changes, a condition known as mild cognitive impairment (MCI) [56]. Memory difficulties in MCI and Alzheimer's disease begin insidiously and progress gradually over time. Although it often can be difficult to distinguish the memory changes of normal aging from MCI or early Alzheimer's disease on casual observation, the pattern of memory test results on formal neuropsychologic studies can often assist in early diagnosis. Specifically, patients who have MCI and Alzheimer's disease typically demonstrate poor retention and rapid forgetting of newly learned information [56–59], which differs from the inefficient retrieval difficulties associated with normal aging.

Patients who have amnestic MCI and Alzheimer's disease typically demonstrate hippocampal atrophy on brain imaging studies [60,61] and significant deficiencies in the neurotransmitter acetylcholine [40]. Although currently there is no cure for Alzheimer's disease, several therapies have demonstrated success in slowing disease progression by making acetylcholine more available to brain cells or by reducing neuronal apoptosis through regulation of brain glutamate levels.

### Subcortical and white matter diseases

Patients who have subcortical degenerative diseases or white matter disorders often display similar memory profiles. Early disease stages are characterized by poor delayed free recall, often at the same level of impairment as seen in patients who have Alzheimer's disease of similar disease staging/severity. Patients who have subcortical or white matter disease, however, typically demonstrate significantly better recognition memory than seen in patients who have Alzheimer's disease, suggesting that the primary mechanism of memory failure lies in deficient retrieval [44,45,62]. As disease progresses, however, evidence of encoding and retention deficits also can be observed in subcortical and white matter disorders [63].

### Frontal lobe dementia

Patients who have disorders that preferentially affect the frontal lobes often demonstrate characteristic changes in behavior and memory. Changes in personality and adaptive behaviors are common and typically are characterized by difficulties modulating or regulating thoughts and actions. Patients may be disinhibited and behave inappropriately, or they may be passive and abulic. When memory deficits appear, they typically occur within the context of poor planning, organization, attention, and mental flexibility [64]. Ability to sustain attention is disturbed, and learning strategies are inefficient [32]; however, there is no evidence of rapid forgetting of information, as is seen in Alzheimer-type dementia [65]. Source memory problems, as described earlier, are common when prefrontal regions are affected.

### Amnesic Korsakoff syndrome

Amnesic Korsakoff syndrome is caused by damage to medial diencephalic structures, including the dorsomedial nucleus of the thalamus and mammillary bodies, resulting from severe thiamine deficiency, most often related to excessive alcohol consumption. Patients who have amnesic Korsakoff syndrome demonstrate largely normal intelligence and STM ability, but their ability to encode new information into LTM is severely impaired [4]. Patients demonstrate equally poor free recall and recognition [66] and at times "recall" information that was never presented, a phenomenon known as confabulation [4,67]. Many patients who have amnesic Korsakoff syndrome also present with a severe, temporally graded retrograde amnesia, as described earlier [13,68,69].

## Depression

Patients who have clinical depression frequently have impaired attention and STM, often secondary to vegetative signs (eg, poor sleep) and distraction associated with dysphoric preoccupation and obsessive thinking [70]. They do not adopt active, efficient encoding strategies [71], and they tend to put forth minimal effort, often giving up easily on tasks. Although initial learning is usually below normal, patients who have clinical depression typically recall much of what they initially learned when assessed after a delay interval. Memory also often improves to nearly normal with recognition testing [72].

## Medication-related memory deficits

Several commonly used classes of prescription medications may disrupt memory functioning, especially in elderly patients. Katzman and colleagues [73] reported that medication-induced cognitive dysfunction was the most common form of reversible dementia in the elderly. Moreover, the incidence of medication-related cognitive difficulties increases steadily with the number of medications the patient is taking [74]. A complete review of all the medications that can impair memory functioning is beyond the scope of this article. Discussion is therefore limited to two medication classes most commonly associated with memory impairment: long-acting benzodiazepine and anticholinergic agents.

## Benzodiazepine

One of the most pronounced cognitive effects of benzodiazepine use is impaired ability to learn new information [75–77]. Patients taking high dosages of benzodiazepine for long periods perform poorly on tasks requiring sustained attention and report improved concentration after discontinuation of the medication [78,79]. The ability to recall information that has been learned previously does not seem to be disrupted by benzodiazepine use. The mechanism by which benzodiazepine affects memory encoding remains unclear. The depressant effect of the medication on the central nervous system probably contributes to this impairment; however, many believe that benzodiazepine action extends beyond the sedating effects of the medication.

*Anticholinergics*

Direct anticholinergic agents such as atropine and scopolamine cause significant memory impairment, as do a number of other commonly used medications with anticholinergic side effects. These drugs include most heterocyclic antidepressants (eg, imipramine, amitriptyline), over-the-counter sleep and cold preparations containing antihistamines, some antiparkinsoninan medications (eg, benztropine), and some neuroleptics (eg, phenothiazines). Anticholinergic agents produce an imbalance in the cholinergic and adrenergic pathways of the reticular activating system, thereby disrupting arousal and attentional capabilities [74]. At higher doses, anticholinergics can cause memory impairment and acute confusional episodes, especially in the elderly. Fortunately, alternative medications with minimal anticholinergic effects are available.

## Summary

The understanding of the neuroanatomic substrates and cognitive processes underlying memory functioning has improved dramatically during the past several decades. Animal studies and observations of patients who have brain diseases show that memory is not a unitary factor but instead can be parsed into overlapping but dissociable constructs; that encoding, retention, and retrieval processes depend on the integrity of several distinct brain regions; and that the creation of new memories depends on structural and functional changes within the neuronal systems of those brain regions. Much remains to be learned, however, regarding the specific biologic, genetic, and information-processing mechanisms underlying many features of this complex cognitive construct. As this knowledge base grows, new and improved pharmacologic and behavioral treatments for patients who have memory disorders may be realized.

## References

[1] James W. Principles of psychology. New York: Holt; 1890.
[2] Miller GA. The magical number seven: plus or minus two. Some limits on our capacity for processing information. Psychol Rev 1956;9:81–97.
[3] Lezak MD. Neuropsychological assessment. 2nd edition. Oxford (UK): Oxford University Press; 1983.
[4] Butters N, Cermak LS. Alcoholic Korsakoff's syndrome. New York: Academic Press; 1980.
[5] Milner B, Corkin S, Teuber HL. Further analysis of the hippocampal amnesic syndrome: a 14-year follow-up study of H.M. Neuropsychologia 1968;6:215–34.
[6] Scoville WB, Milner B. Loss of recent memory after bilateral hippocampal lesions. J Neurol Neurosurg Psychiatry 1957;20:11–21.
[7] Squire LR, Moore RY. Dorsal thalamic lesions in a noted case of chronic memory dysfunction. Ann Neurol 1979;6:503–6.
[8] Teuber HL, Milner B, Baughan HG. Persistent anterograde amnesia after stab wound of the basal brain. Neuropsychologia 1968;6:267–82.

[9] Klatzky RL. Human memory: structures and processes. 2nd edition. San Francisco (CA): Freeman; 1980.

[10] Verfaille M, Cermak LS. Neuropsychological issues in amnesia. In: Martinez JL, Kesner RB, editors. Learning and memory: a biological view. San Diego (CA): Academic Press; 1991. p. 467–97.

[11] Lucas JA, Addeo R. Traumatic brain injury and post-concussive syndrome. In: Snyder PJ, Nussbaum PD, editors. Clinical neuropsychology: a pocket handbook for assessment. 2nd edition. Washington (DC): American Psychological Association, in press.

[12] Kopelman MD. Amnesia: organic and psychogenic. Br J Psychiatry 1987;150:428–42.

[13] Butters N, Cermak LS. A case study of the forgetting of autobiographical knowledge: implications for the study of retrograde amnesia. In: Rubin D, editor. Autobiographical memory. New York: Cambridge University Press; 1986. p. 253–72.

[14] Squire LR. Memory and brain. Oxford (UK): Oxford University Press; 1987.

[15] Tulving E. Elements of episodic memory. Oxford (UK): Clarendon Press; 1983.

[16] Schacter DL, Chiu C-YP, Ochsner KN. Implicit memory: a selective review. Annu Rev Neurosci 1993;16:159–82.

[17] Heindel WC, Salmon DP, Shults CW, et al. Neuropsychological evidence for multiple implicit memory systems: a comparison of Alzheimer's, Parkinson's and Huntington's disease patients. J Neurosci 1989;9:582–7.

[18] Rose SPR. The biochemistry of memory. Essays Biochem 1991;26:1–12.

[19] Kandel E. Transmitter release. In: Kandel E, Schwartz JH, Jessell TM, editors. Principles of neural science. 3rd edition. Norwalk (CT): Appleton & Lange; 1991. p. 194–212.

[20] Hebb DO. The organization of behavior. New York: Wiley; 1949.

[21] Abel T, Kandel E. Positive and negative regulatory mechanisms that mediate long-term memory storage. Brain Res Rev 1998;26:360–78.

[22] Scott R, Bourtchuladze R, Gossweiler S, et al. CREB and the discovery of cognitive enhancers. J Mol Neurosci 2002;19:171–7.

[23] Nguyen PV, Woo NH. Regulation of hippocampal synaptic plasticity by cyclic-AMP-dependent protein kinases. Prog Neurobiol 2003;71:401–37.

[24] Laroche S, Davis S, Jay TM. Plasticity at hippocampal to prefrontal cortex synapses: dual roles in working memory and consolidation. Hippocampus 2000;10:438–46.

[25] O'Mara SM, Commins S, Anderson M. Synaptic plasticity in the hippocampal area CA1-subiculum projection: implications for theories of memory. Hippocampus 2000;10:447–56.

[26] Mehta MR. Cooperative LTP can map memory sequences to dendritic branches. Trends Neurosci 2004;27:69–72.

[27] Squire LR, Zola-Morgan S. The medial temporal lobe memory system. Science 1991;253: 1380–6.

[28] Mahut HS, Zola-Morgan S, Moss M. Hippocampal resections impair associative learning and recognition in the monkey. J Neurosci 1982;2:1214–29.

[29] Zola-Morgan S, Squire LR. Memory impairment in monkeys following lesions of the hippocampus. Behav Neurosci 1986;100:155–60.

[30] Davis M. Pharmacological and anatomical analysis of fear conditioning using the fear-potentiated startle paradigm. Behav Neurosci 1986;100:814–24.

[31] Kesner RP. Learning and memory in rats with an emphasis on the role of the amygdala. In: Aggleton J, editor. The amygdala. New York: Wiley; 1992. p. 379–400.

[32] Mayes A, Meudell P, Mann D, et al. Location of lesions in Korsakoff's syndrome: neuropsychological and neuropathological data on two patients. Cortex 1988;24:367–88.

[33] Cramon Dv, Hebel N, Schuri U. A contribution to the anatomical basis of thalamic amnesia. Brain 1985;108:993–1008.

[34] Graff-Radford NR, Tranel D, Van Hoesen GW, et al. Diencephalic amnesia. Brain 1990; 113:1–25.

[35] Squire LR, Amaral DG, Zola-Morgan S, et al. Description of brain injury in amnesic patient N.A. based on magnetic resonance imaging. Exp Neurol 1989;105:23–35.

[36] Mair RG, Lancourse DM. Radio-frequency lesions of thalamus produce delayed non-matching to sample impairments comparable to pyrithiamine-induced encephalopathy in rats. Behav Neurosci 1992;106:634–45.

[37] Mair RG, Robinson JK, Koger SM, et al. Delayed non-matching to sample is impaired by extensive, but not by limited lesions of the thalamus in the rat. Behav Neurosci 1992;106: 646–56.

[38] Zola-Morgan S, Squire LR. Neuroanatomy of memory. Annu Rev Neurosci 1993;16: 547–63.

[39] Mesulam MM, Mufson EJ, Levey AI, et al. Cholinergic innervation of cortex by the basal forebrain: cytochemistry and cortical connections of the septal area, diagonal band nuclei, nucleus basalis (substantia innominata), and hypothalamus in the rhesus monkey. J Comp Neurol 1983;214:170–97.

[40] Auld DS, Kornecook TJ, Bastianetto S, et al. Alzheimer's disease and the basal forebrain cholinergic system: relations to beta-amyloid peptides, cognition, and treatment strategies. Prog Neurobiol 2002;68:209–45.

[41] Damasio AR, Graff-Radford NR, Eslinger PJ, et al. Amnesia following basal forebrain lesions. Arch Neurol 1985;42:263–71.

[42] Squire LR. Memory and the hippocampus: a synthesis from findings with rats, monkeys, and humans. Psychol Rev 1992;99:195–231.

[43] Paulsen JS, Butters N, Salmon DP, et al. Prism adaptation in Alzheimer's and Huntington's disease. Neuropsychology 1993;7:73–81.

[44] Heindel WC, Salmon DP, Butters N. Cognitive approaches to memory disorders of demented patients. In: Sutker PB, Adams HE, editors. Comprehensive handbook of psychopathology. 2nd edition. New York: Plenum Press; 1993.

[45] Grafman J, Rao SM, Litvan I. Disorders of memory. In: Rao SM, editor. Neurobehavioral aspects of multiple sclerosis. New York: Oxford University Press; 1990. p. 102–17.

[46] Pillon B, Deweer B, Agid Y, et al. Explicit memory in Alzheimer's, Huntington's, and Parkinson's diseases. Arch Neurol 1993;50:374–9.

[47] Vanderploeg RD, Yuspeh RL, Schinka JA. Differential episodic and semantic memory performance in Alzheimer's disease and vascular dementias. J Int Neuropsychol Soc 2001;7: 563–73.

[48] Zakharov VV, Akhutina TV, Yakhno NN. Memory impairment in Parkinson's disease. Neurosci Behav Physiol 2001;31:157–63.

[49] Schacter DL, Norman KA, Koutstaal W. The cognitive neuroscience of constructive memory. Annu Rev Psychol 1998;49:289–318.

[50] Craik FIM, Rabinowitz JC. Age differences in the acquisition and use of verbal information. In: Bouma H, Bouwhuis DG, editors. Attention and performance X. Hillsdale (NJ): Erlbaum; 1984.

[51] Craik FIM. Age differences in remembering. In: Squire LR, Butters N, editors. Neuropsychology of memory. New York: Guilford; 1984. p. 3–12.

[52] Albert MS, Duffy FH, Naeser MA. Nonlinear changes in cognition and their neurophysiologic correlates. Can J Psychol 1987;41:141–57.

[53] Craik FIM, Byrd M, Swanson JM. Patterns of memory loss in three elderly samples. Psychol Aging 1987;2:79–86.

[54] Albert MS. Cognitive function. In: Albert MS, Moss MB, editors. Geriatric neuropsychology. New York: Guilford; 1988. p. 33–53.

[55] Zec RF. Neuropsychological functioning in Alzheimer's disease. In: Parks RW, Zec RF, Wilson RS, editors. Neuropsychology of Alzheimer's disease and other dementias. New York: Oxford University Press; 1993. p. 3–80.

[56] Petersen RC, Stevens JC, Ganguli M, et al. Practice parameter: early detection of dementia. Mild cognitive impairment. Neurology 2001;56:1133–42.

[57] Ober BA, Koss E, Friedland RP, et al. Processes of verbal memory failure in Alzheimer-type dementia. Brain Cogn 1985;4:90–103.

[58] Moss MB, Albert MS, Butters N, et al. Differential patterns of memory loss among patients with Alzheimer's disease, Huntington's disease, and alcoholic Korsakoff's syndrome. Arch Neurol 1986;43:239–46.

[59] Wilson RS, Bacan LD, Fox JH, et al. Primary memory and secondary memory in dementia of the Alzheimer type. J Clin Neuropsychol 1983;5:337–44.

[60] Jack CR Jr, Petersen RC, O'Brien PC, et al. MR-based hippocampal volumetry in the diagnosis of Alzheimer's disease. Neurology 1992;42:183–8.

[61] Kantarci K, Xu Y, Shiung MM, et al. Comparative diagnostic utility of different MR modalities in mild cognitive impairment and Alzheimer's disease. Dement Geriatr Cogn Disord 2002;14:198–207.

[62] Butters N, Wolfe J, Granholm E, et al. An assessment of verbal recall, recognition and fluency abilities in patients with Huntington's disease. Cortex 1986;22:11–32.

[63] Kramer JH, Delis DC, Blusewicz MJ, et al. Verbal memory errors in Alzheimer's and Huntington's dementias. Dev Neuropsychol 1988;4:1–5.

[64] Sungaila P, Crockett DJ. Dementia and the frontal lobes. In: Parks RW, Zec RF, Wilson RS, editors. Neuropsychology of Alzheimer's disease and other dementias. Oxford (UK): Oxford University Press; 1993. p. 235–64.

[65] Shimamura AP, Janowski JS, Squire LR. What is the role of frontal damage in memory disorders? In: Levin HS, Eisenberg HM, Benton AL, editors. Frontal lobe function and dysfunction. Oxford (UK): Oxford University Press; 1991. p. 173–95.

[66] Butters N, Salmon DP, Cullum CM, et al. Differentiation of amnesic and demented patients with the Wechsler Memory Scale-Revised. Clin Neuropsychol 1988;2:133–48.

[67] Butters N, Stuss DT. Diencephalic amnesia. In: Boller F, Grafman J, editors. Handbook of neuropsychology, vol. 3. Amsterdam: Elsevier; 1989. p. 107–48.

[68] Zangwill OL. The amnesic syndrome. In: Whitty CWM, Zangwill OL, editors. Amnesia. London: Butterworths; 1966.

[69] Cermak LS. The episodic-semantic distinction in amnesia. In: Squire LR, Butters N, editors. Neuropsychology of memory. New York: Guilford Press; 1984. p. 55–62.

[70] Breslow R, Kocsis J, Belkin B. Memory deficits in depression: evidence utilizing the Wechsler Memory Scale. Percept Mot Skills 1980;51:541–2.

[71] Weingartner H, Grafman J, Boutelle W, et al. Forms of memory failure. Science 1981;221: 380–2.

[72] Caine ED. The neuropsychology of depression: the pseudodementia syndrome. In: Grant I, Adams KM, editors. Neuropsychological assessment of neuropsychiatric disorders. New York: Oxford University Press; 1986. p. 221–43.

[73] Katzman R, Lasker B, Bernstein N. Advances in the diagnosis of dementia, accuracy of diagnosis, and consequences of misdiagnosis of disorders causing dementia. Aging and the Brain 1988;32:17–62.

[74] McConnell H, Duffy J. Neuropsychiatric aspects of medical therapies. In: Coffey CE, Cummings JL, editors. Textbook of geriatric neuropsychiatry. Washington (DC): American Psychiatric Association; 1994. p. 549–74.

[75] Taylor JL, Tinklenberg JR. Cognitive impairment and benzodiazepines. In: Meltzer HY, editor. Psychopharmacology: the third generation of progress. New York: Raven; 1987. p. 1449–54.

[76] Bixler EO, Kales A, Manfredi RL, et al. Next-day memory impairment with triazolam use. Lancet 1991;337:827–31.

[77] Pomara N, Deptula D, Singh R, et al. Cognitive toxicity of benzodiazepines in the elderly. In: Salzman C, Lebowitz BD, editors. Anxiety in the elderly: treatment and research. New York: Springer; 1991. p. 175–96.

[78] Golombok S, Moodley P, Lader M. Cognitive impairment in long-term benzodiazepine users. Psychol Med 1988;18:365–74.

[79] Petursson H, Gudjonsson GH, Lader MH. Psychosomatic performance during withdrawal from long-term benzodiazepine treatment. Psychopharmacology (Berl) 1983;81:345–9.

PSYCHIATRIC
CLINICS
OF NORTH AMERICA

ELSEVIER
SAUNDERS

Psychiatr Clin N Am 28 (2005) 599–611

# The Medial Temporal-Lobe Amnesic Syndrome

## Brenda Milner, ScD

*Montreal Neurological Institute, 3801 University Street, Montreal, QC H3A 2B4, Canada*

Bekhterev [1], in 1899, provided the first hint that the medial parts of the temporal lobes might play a critical role in human memory processes. At a medical meeting in St. Petersburg, he demonstrated the brain of a patient who had shown severe memory impairment as her earliest and most striking clinical abnormality; the main pathologic finding was bilateral softening in the regions of the uncus, hippocampus, and adjoining medial temporal cortex. After this early and brief report, there came a number of more detailed clinicopathologic case studies suggesting a relationship between memory disorder and hippocampal damage [2–6], as well as descriptions of post-encephalitic amnesias believed to be associated with lesions of the hippocampus and neighboring temporal lobe structures [7]; but the most compelling evidence for a major contribution to memory processes from the hippocampal region came from the systematic study of a few patients who had become amnesic after a medial temporal-lobe resection undertaken to control epilepsy. This article provides a historical overview of this work, showing how the research evolved.

I first encountered this amnesic syndrome in a patient of Dr. Wilder Penfield's, at the Montreal Neurological Institute, in the early 1950s, where the condition manifested as an unforeseen consequence of a left temporal-lobe resection for the relief of epilepsy. In the early days of temporal-lobe surgery, Penfield usually confined surgical removal to the anterior neocortex, but this limited resection was rarely effective in controlling the patient's seizures, so that by 1950 most removals included the anterior hippocampus and parahippocampal gyrus, together with the amygdala, on the medial surface of the hemisphere, with no striking behavioral change resulting from what by then had become a routine procedure. During this early period, several patients who had undergone unilateral neocortical

---

*E-mail address:* brenda.milner@mcgill.ca

doi:10.1016/j.psc.2005.06.002

removal returned with continuing seizures, requiring completion of the temporal lobectomy. Such unilateral operations tended at most to be associated with mild material-specific memory deficits that varied with the side of the lesion (verbal from the left, nonverbal from the right) but no generalized memory disorder [8–12]. However, in one such case, a 46-year-old civil engineer (PB), this second operation, which involved only the medial structures of the left temporal lobe, was followed by a severe, persistent, and generalized impairment of recent memory, unaccompanied by other cognitive deficits. The impairment was manifested clinically as progressive anterograde amnesia, such that the events of daily life were forgotten as soon as the patient's attention shifted to a new topic. In addition, there was a retrograde amnesia covering the salient events of the preceding few months. PB's unexpected memory loss was a troubling outcome of elective surgery; in that preneuroimaging era, his remained a single, puzzling case until the following year, when another patient (FC), a 28-year-old glove cutter, exhibited a similar amnesic syndrome after a one-stage left temporal lobectomy that included the amygdala, uncus, and the anterior hippocampus and parahippocampal gyrus. In FC's case, the retrograde amnesia extended to the previous 4 years, but, as with PB, memory for events before that appeared to be normal.

Despite the severe anterograde amnesia, both these patients continued to earn their living. Their professional skills, whether for preparing blueprints or for cutting gloves, were well maintained. PB was, however, too forgetful to handle the administrative part of his former work and had to be demoted to draftsman. There had been no change in intelligence quotient (IQ) from preoperative levels, and neither patient showed any attention deficit. In fact, PB had an excellent immediate memory, and he was able to repeat nine digits forward and seven backward and to carry out complex mental arithmetic with speed and accuracy; yet, he was unable to recall or recognize test material after a lapse of 5 minutes or less if his attention was diverted [13].

To account for these two instances of memory loss after a unilateral temporal-lobe removal, Penfield and Milner hypothesized that in each case there had been a pre-existing but preoperatively unsuspected atrophic lesion in the medial temporal region of the opposite hemisphere, so that when Penfield removed a large part of the hippocampus and parahippocampal gyrus in the left hemisphere, he effectively deprived the patients of hippocampal function bilaterally. The reason we emphasized the hippocampal region was that PB had had his temporal lobectomy in two stages, 5 years apart, and it was only after the medial temporal-lobe removal that the memory loss occurred. In this case, our hypothesis was confirmed 12 years later when PB died of a pulmonary embolism and the autopsy findings revealed the presence of a long-standing right hippocampal atrophy. In contrast, on the operated (left) side, the 22 mm of remaining hippocampus appeared to be normal [14].

The preliminary report of these two cases [15] attracted the attention of Dr. William Scoville, a neurosurgeon from Hartford, CT, who contacted

Penfield to say that he had observed a similar memory disturbance in a patient (HM) in whom he had performed a bilateral medial temporal-lobe resection, also in an attempt to control epileptic seizures. As a result, I was invited to go to Hartford to study HM and Scoville's other patients who had undergone similar removals.

Scoville had designed the operation of bilateral medial temporal-lobe resection as an alternative to frontal lobotomy in the treatment of seriously ill schizophrenic patients. Because of the known connections between the medial temporal region and the orbital frontal cortex, he had hoped that this procedure would prove to be beneficial psychiatrically, while avoiding what he termed the "blunting" effects of a frontal lobotomy. As it turned out, the operation did little to alleviate the psychosis, and any memory changes went undetected until much later, when I had the opportunity to examine eight of these patients [16]. Although some patients were difficult to test, I did manage to establish the presence of anterograde amnesia in all cases in which the removal encroached on the hippocampus and parahippocampal gyrus, and there seemed to be a rough positive correlation between the extent of removal and the degree of memory impairment. No residual memory impairment was observed after removals that were limited to the uncus and amygdala, a finding consistent with those of Sawa and colleagues [17].

## Case history: insights into amnesia

Scoville had first become aware of the risk to memory in this operation in 1953, when he performed an extensive bilateral medial temporal-lobe resection on a nonpsychotic 27-year-old patient (HM) whose frequent major and minor epileptic seizures had failed to respond to near toxic doses of anticonvulsant medication [18]. This frankly experimental procedure had been proposed because HM, an assembly line worker by trade, had become unable to work or lead a normal life, and the operation did in fact control the epilepsy, despite the fact that neither electrographically nor clinically did the seizure pattern suggest an origin in the temporal lobes. Yet, this success was achieved at too high a price, because it was already apparent in the early postoperative period that HM had a major memory impairment [18]. He could no longer recognize the hospital staff, apart from Scoville, whom he had known for many years; he did not remember and could not relearn the way to the bathroom, and he seemed to retain nothing of the day-to-day happenings in the hospital. At the same time, it was discovered that he had an extensive, although patchy, retrograde amnesia, such that he did not remember the death of a favorite uncle 3 years previously, or anything of the period spent in hospital before the operation, but he did recall a few minor incidents from the previous month. His early memories were seemingly vivid and intact, his speech was normal, and his social behavior and emotional responses were entirely appropriate. There has been little change in this clinical picture over the years since the operation. HM has shown no personality change, remaining rather placid but having occasional outbursts of irritability; nor is there any intellectual loss. In fact, the Wechsler IQ of 117, which he achieved in 1962, compared favorably with the IQ of 104 reported in 1953, a finding that may be the result of the marked reduction in the number and severity of his seizures.

On my first encounter with HM, in April 1955, it was apparent that his memory disorder was the same kind as that of Penfield's two patients but more severe. All three patients reported that at any given moment "everything is clear," but that they felt as though they were constantly waking from a dream. In the intervals between tasks, HM frequently expressed anxiety about what might have gone just before and particularly about whether he had done or said anything amiss. We all tend to feel responsible for our own actions and, therefore, not to know what these actions have been must be troubling. However, in HM's case, such worries were short lived, and, as soon as a new task was presented, he showed a remarkable capacity for sustained attention. For example, I found that he could retain the number 584 for at least 15 minutes by continuous rehearsal, combining and recombining the digits according to an elaborate mnemonic scheme, although the moment his attention was diverted by a new topic, the entire event was forgotten [19,20].

HM's success in remembering a three-digit number for 15 minutes in the absence of distraction is at first sight consistent with the view of Drachman and Arbit [21] that amnesic subjects can hold a simple memorandum indefinitely provided that no interfering event claims their attention. Yet, it was already clear that for HM, verbal rehearsal played a key role in this holding process. When we switched to nonverbal memoranda, a very different picture emerged. In 1959, Konorski [22] had described a method for testing memory for single events, which was later adapted by Stepien and Sierpinski [23] for work with human subjects. This delayed paired comparison technique consists of presenting two stimuli in succession separated by a short time interval. The subject must then indicate whether the second stimulus is the same as or different from the first. To succeed, the subject must retain an accurate representation of the first stimulus to compare the second one with it. The task difficulty may be increased by lengthening the intratrial interval or by interpolating a distracting task.

Using this method, Prisko [24] (see Milner [25]) has demonstrated HM's rapid forgetting of simple perceptual material that could not be easily verbalized. The study [25] sampled five different sets of stimuli (three visual and two auditory), each set constituting a separate task. The stimuli comprised flashing lights, clicking sounds, pure tones, shades of red, and nonsense patterns. At least five values were assigned to each variable, to prevent as far as possible the use of verbal mediation to bridge the retention interval. All paired stimuli were easily distinguishable when one stimulus succeeded the other with no delay, and normal subjects rarely made errors, even with a 60-second delay and an interpolated distraction. In contrast, HM performed all tasks well at zero delay, but with increasing intratrial intervals (even without distraction), his performance deteriorated sharply, falling to the chance level at 60-seconds' delay.

In a subsequent study, Sidman and colleagues [26] have confirmed Prisko's [24] findings using an elegant delayed matching-to-sample technique that allowed the plotting of discrimination gradients to show how far the subject's choice of a matching stimulus deviated from the sample stimulus as the delay lengthened. In the nonverbal form of their task, HM was required to indicate which one of eight ellipses matched a sample ellipse. Once again, HM performed normally at zero delay, but as the interval lengthened, his performance deteriorated rapidly, until at 32 seconds, the sample no longer exerted any control over his choice. In contrast, HM had no difficulty with a verbal version of the task, which required the matching of consonant trigrams. However, as with other verbal memory tasks, he succeeded only by constant rehearsal; his lips could be seen moving throughout the delay period. These and related studies concur in showing that HM was able to register perceptual information normally but that the information ceased to be available to him within 30 to 60 seconds. Such results support the distinction between a primary memory process with a rapid decay [27,28] and an overlapping secondary process (impaired in HM) by which the long-term storage of information is achieved.

## What can the patient HM learn?

HM's failure on tasks that assess memory after a single presentation accords well with the clinical finding that he forgets from moment to moment the individual events of daily life. But this does not rule out the possibility that he might be capable of some learning, given intensive practice, or even that certain kinds of learning might take place at a normal rate. Accordingly, in 1960, I set out to explore this possibility by means of two different learning tasks, which yielded widely divergent results.

The first, a maze-learning task, required the subject to discover and remember by trial and error the one correct path through a "stepping stone" stylus maze, with the loud clicks of the error counter as a guide. This task is not difficult for most subjects, who typically achieve errorless performance within 20 trials. In contrast, HM failed to show any learning at all after 215 trials spread over 3 days, and at the end he was still having "a little argument" with himself over which way to turn at the first choice point. In retrospect, this total failure is less surprising than it seemed at the time. This maze had 28 choice points, so that, even with recourse to verbal mnemonics, it is hard to see how HM could have encompassed the entire sequence of turns within the span of immediate memory. He would inevitably, therefore, have forgotten the first part of the route by the time he reached the end. In an attempt to get around this problem, I later gave him intensive training on a shortened form of the maze that contained only six choice points and thus did not exceed his memory span. Even under these conditions, HM's learning was extraordinarily slow, requiring 155 trials before he attained the criterion of three successive errorless runs [29]. He did, however, show some partial retention of this shortened maze 2 years later [30], suggesting that the main defect is in acquisition [31] rather than in retention of what has been learned. We cannot, however, conclude that HM's retention is normal, because healthy control subjects (and many patients with unilateral temporal-lobe lesions) show nearly perfect recall of the 28 choice-point maze 1 year after having learned it.

These experimental findings parallel the slow learning of spatial relationships shown by HM in everyday life. Shortly after the operation, the family moved to a new house a few blocks away from where they had formerly lived, and it took him approximately 5 years to learn the spatial layout of the new house and to remember where objects that he used constantly (such as the lawn mower) were kept. However, once it was acquired, this knowledge was well retained [30], and he was even able to draw an accurate floor plan of the house after he had ceased to live there [32]. We do not know how such cognitive maps are represented in the brain, but presumably, they involve large populations of cells distributed widely within specialized regions of the cerebral cortex. What is impressive is to realize how slowly these regions are established when the normal medial temporal-lobe input to the cortex is absent or drastically reduced.

The second learning task on which HM was trained in 1960 involved the acquisition of a visuo-motor skill. The task of mirror drawing requires the subject to draw a line that follows the contour of a five-pointed star, always keeping within the narrow double border of that star. What makes the task difficult is that the subject cannot observe the hand or the star directly but only as reflected in a mirror. This means that at first, on reaching a point of the star, the subject tends to move in the wrong direction and thus accumulate errors, but performance improves gradually with practice over many trials until the skill is mastered. HM was given 30 trials spread over 3 days, and he achieved a normal learning curve, beginning each new session at the level he had attained at the end for the previous day's training. Yet he remained totally unaware that he had ever done the task before; this was learning without any sense of familiarity. We are now used to the idea that such dissociations are possible after a circumscribed brain lesion but witnessing this for the first time was an astonishing experience.

HM's success on the mirror drawing task and subsequently on several different motor-learning tasks [33] led to the speculation that other kinds of motor skill might be acquired independently of the medial temporal-lobe system, such as learning to skate or swim or to pronounce the words of a foreign language. Such skills tend to be acquired most easily in childhood and are remarkably stable across periods of disuse. They are built up gradually without our being able to describe just what it is that we are learning, and the attempt at introspection on this process is more likely to impair than to aid performance. It seemed reasonable to suppose that this kind of learning, later termed "procedural" by Cohen and Squire [34], would not require the participation of a conscious cognitive memory system and so would be preserved in amnesia. This generalization has held up wherever it has been tested, although the skills sampled so far have been few and of limited complexity.

The demonstration of preserved motor-skill learning in HM (and in Penfield's patients PB and FC) provided early evidence of the existence of more than one memory system, but this was only the beginning. In 1968, Warrington and Weiskrantz [35] showed that perceptual learning may also be preserved in the presence of a severe anterograde amnesia. Using a version of the Gollin Incomplete Figures task [36], they asked their patients to try to identify line drawings of common objects or animals (such as a telephone or a cat) from which most of the contour lines had been removed. This is initially quite a difficult task with the most fragmented versions of the drawings, but over successive random presentations of the series, the contours are gradually filled in, until the subject can name the item depicted. On a second presentation of the task 1 hour later, normal subjects show considerable savings, requiring fewer contour cues to name the items. On this fragmented figures task and on an analogous fragmented words task, Warrington and Weiskrantz found marked savings in their amnesic patients, with good retention 4 weeks later, although the patients did not remember doing the task previously. We subsequently replicated these findings for HM. Interestingly, his performance on first exposure to the fragmented stimuli was above the control mean, illustrating his superior perceptual abilities. On retesting 1 hour later, he reduced his error score by 48%, and he showed residual savings 4 months later, although still unaware that he had carried out the task before. This long-term effect of a prior visual experience, which I have termed "perceptual learning," is an instance of what is now known as priming [37,38], a form of learning distinct from motor skill and which, in this case, is probably mediated by higher visual cortical areas.

In 1980, Cohen and Squire [34] showed that amnesic patients could master the cognitive skill of reading mirror-reversed print as well as normal subjects do, thus further broadening the scope of what amnesic patients can remember and leading these authors to distinguish between a conscious, declarative form of memory, dependent on the medial temporal-lobe system (and thus impaired in HM), and a wide range of nondeclarative, implicit forms of memory, which are spared. These forms include not only priming but also the acquisition of habits and skills, impaired by lesions of the caudate nucleus [39,40], as well as classical conditioning, which is known to be mediated by cerebellar circuitry [41].

Up to this point in the analysis of HM's memory impairment, the important distinction made by Tulving [37] between episodic and semantic memory has been ignored. Episodic memory, as the name implies, refers to the personal, autobiographical kind of memory, with its temporal reference to past events, whereas semantic memory is exemplified in our acquired cognitive structure of the meanings of words and in the broad framework of our conceptual knowledge. Although few investigators would deny that the most salient feature of the amnesic syndrome is the loss of episodic memory (as defined here), the status of semantic memory has been [42] and remains [43] a matter for debate. Thus, it has been suggested that because HM's preoperatively acquired semantic knowledge was unaffected by the medial temporal-lobe resection, his semantic memory system was spared. This begs the question of how much new knowledge HM has in fact been able to acquire over the many years that he has been amnesic.

Some time ago, John Gabrieli, who was then a student in Corkin's laboratory at the Massachusetts Institute of Technology, began to explore this question, taking advantage of the fact that Webster's dictionary is updated every 5 years by the inclusion of words that have become current in the language since the last issue was compiled. Gabrieli [44] used a variety of experimental techniques to assess HM's knowledge of such words, and he showed that HM had learned far fewer new words than a control group of healthy subjects of the same age. Similarly, a former student of mine, Dr. Mary Lou Smith, began to explore with me in the 1980s, HM's notions of what such common objects as cars, clocks, radios, and washing machines looked like then, more than 25 years after his operation, and she found that his mental representations of these objects had not kept up with the times. Lest this ignorance be attributed to the sheltered life that HM leads, it should be pointed out that he watches television assiduously and is exposed to advertisements in magazines. HM's factual knowledge has in fact expanded with constant exposure to television, so that for example, he now has some concept of astronauts and space travel, and he believes that a famous person called Kennedy was assassinated, but such knowledge is meager and unreliable. Limited as these investigations are, they support the notion that the medial temporal-lobe structures play a role in the acquisition of semantic knowledge as well as in personal episodic memory and that in their absence such knowledge can only be acquired slowly over many repetitions, although it appears that the situation may somewhat be different in the case of young children [43].

## What is the critical lesion?

The extensive behavioral studies performed with HM, together with the findings from Montreal patients PB and FC, demonstrate the importance of the medial temporal region for human declarative memory, but the studies leave us with much to discover about the relative contributions of different structures within this region and how these structures interact with other brain areas. Attention has been drawn to the hippocampus because removals limited to the amygdala and surrounding cortex have caused no global memory impairment, but we have never claimed that the hippocampal lesion was alone responsible for the observed deficits.

It is clear now that Scoville overestimated the extent of the medial temporal-lobe removal in HM, but otherwise his description has proved remarkably accurate. The results of a subsequent magnetic resonance imaging study [45] have shown that the removal was in fact exactly as Scoville had described it, except that the resection extends only approximately 5 cm posteriorly in both hemispheres, instead of the radical 8 cm reported originally [18]. Thus, in both hemispheres, the removal included the medial temporal polar cortex, the bulk of the amygdala, the perirhinal and entorhinal cortices, and half the rostrocaudal extent of the hippocampal formation (the dentate gyrus, subiculum, and hippocampus proper). The parahippocampal cortex remained largely intact. Most importantly, the lateral temporal neocortex and the temporal stem were spared, safely attributing this impressive and enduring memory deficit to the bilateral medial temporal-lobe lesion.

Subsequent work has shown, however, that the severity of HM's memory impairment depends not only on his hippocampal damage but also on the fact that his surgery included the hippocampal region together with the perirhinal and entorhinal cortices. In this connection, it is instructive to compare the findings for HM with the results for two other amnesic patients (RB and GD) who, as a result of an ischemic event, incurred bilateral lesions limited to the CA1 region of the hippocampus [46,47]. Their memory impairment was qualitatively similar to that of HM, but quantitatively it was much milder.

## The search for an animal model

Interest in human memory processes has grown steadily over the past 30 years, and the early pioneering work with HM certainly provided much of the impetus for the growth. Yet the findings had a somewhat mixed reception at the time and for some years thereafter because of difficulty in establishing a suitable animal model for amnesia. For years we were perplexed by the seeming lack of confirmation from work with monkeys, in which, for example, animals that had undergone bilateral medial temporal-lobe resections similar to what was described in HM showed normal or nearly normal performance on visual discrimination learning tasks, even when concurrent trials on a different task were interpolated as potential distracters [48]. Such findings were troubling because they suggested either that the cross-species comparison was invalid or that the patient data had in some way been misinterpreted. What we had not considered at the time was that ostensibly similar tasks may be solved in different ways by people and monkeys and that a visual discrimination task learned by the monkey over many trials was an example of procedural learning and therefore not a good model for human amnesia. It was not until much later that the concept of multiple memory systems became accepted widely and hence that it became clearer which memory tasks were appropriate to give to experimental animals.

The first major breakthrough came in 1978 when Mishkin [49] demonstrated severe memory impairments in monkeys with bilateral medial temporal-lobe removals, similar to those of HM, when the monkeys were given a single-trial test of object-recognition memory (delayed nonmatching to sample [50,51]). This defect on a task that incorporated an intratrial delay resembled Prisko's earlier results for HM on the Konorski delayed comparison tasks [24] and thus achieved a cross-species convergence of findings. This work set the stage for further series of experimental studies designed to evaluate the relative contributions to memory of different structures within the medial temporal region [52] and their interaction with medial diencephalic structures known to play a role in human memory processes [53].

### Current issues: does the hippocampus play a role in remote memory?

Thus far this article has focused on the anterograde amnesia that is the most striking and disabling aspect of the medial temporal-lobe amnesic syndrome, but all of our patients with bilateral hippocampal lesions also have shown in varying degrees a retrograde amnesia for preoperative periods covering months or years, with the recall of more remote events and previously acquired semantic knowledge seemingly normal [19,20]. This has fostered the traditional view that the hippocampus is required for memory formation and initial consolidation of experience but that neocortical areas ultimately become responsible for memory storage and retrieval independently of the hippocampus. In contrast, the multiple trace theory contends that each autobiographical memory has a permanent trace in the hippocampus [54] and that in the absence of the hippocampus, the quality and detail of even remote memories is impoverished.

This disagreement has occasioned lively debate, but it is difficult to study remote memory in a few amnesic patients encountered postoperatively for the first time. Fortunately, thanks to modern technology, it is now possible to address the issue in healthy subjects by means of event-related functional magnetic resonance imaging. Using this technique, Maguire and Frith [55] have found both hippocampi to be active during the retrieval of autobiographical memories but with an interesting hemispheric difference. The right hippocampus showed a temporal gradient, decreasing in activity the more remote the memory retrieved, whereas no such gradient was found for the left hippocampus, suggesting an invariant involvement in recalling autobiographical events throughout the lifespan. This suggestion of lateral asymmetry adds another dimension to the unresolved question of the role of the hippocampus in the recall of remote autobiographical events. The debate continues.

## Summary

This article has attempted to show how early evidence of the existence of multiple memory systems in the brain arose from the study of a few patients with bilateral damage to the medial structures of the temporal lobe in the hippocampal region, as in the case of the now famous patient HM. Such patients exhibit a profound anterograde amnesia for the experiences of daily life, whereas previously acquired knowledge is well preserved and immediate or primary memory is intact, and other cognitive abilities, including language, perception, and reasoning also are unaffected by the lesion. Despite the seemingly global nature of HM's memory loss, it was possible to show by the appropriate choice of behavioral tasks that many implicit, procedural forms of learning were preserved, and these forms are now known to be mediated by different brain systems. The first major finding was the demonstration of normal acquisition of a motor skill by HM, although he remained unaware that he had done the task before. This finding was followed by the demonstration of preserved perceptual learning, and since then the examples of preserved learning in amnesia have multiplied. In addition, after many false starts, a convincing animal model has now been achieved, with convergent findings for human and nonhuman primates.

Although considerable progress has been made since the early 1950s, many questions remain unanswered; particularly, the distinct contributions of the various medial temporal-lobe structures to memory processes and the interaction of these structures with other brain areas need to be clarified. As in the past, the solution of such problems will call for a multidisciplinary approach.

## References

[1] von Bekhterev M. Demonstration eines Gehirns mit Zerstörung der vorderen und inneren Theile der Hirnrinde beider Schläfenlappen. Neurologisches Zeitblatt 1900;19:990–1.
[2] Grünthal E. Über das klinische Bild nach umschriebenem beiderseitigem Ausfall der Ammonshornrinde. Monatsschrift für Psychiatrie und Neurologie 1947;113:1–16.
[3] Glees P, Griffith HB. Bilateral destruction of the hippocampus (cornu ammonis) in a case of dementia. Monatsschrift für Psychiatrie und Neurologie 1952;129:193–204.
[4] Hegglin K. Über einen Fall von isolierter linkseitiger Ammonshornerweichung bei präseniler Dementz. Monatsschrift für Psychiatrie und Neurologie 1953;125:170–86.
[5] Ule G. Pathologische-anatomische Befunde bei Korsakow-Psychosen und ihre Bedeutung für die Lokalisationslehre in der Psychiatrie. Ärtzliche Wochenschrift 1958;13:6–13.
[6] Victor M, Angevine JB, Mancall GL, et al. Memory loss with lesions of hippocampal formation. Arch Neurol 1961;5:244–63.

[7] Rose FC, Symonds CP. Persistent memory defect following encephalitis. Brain 1960;83: 195–212.

[8] Kimura D. Right temporal-lobe damage. Arch Neurol 1963;8:264–71.

[9] Meyer V, Yates AJ. Intellectual changes following temporal lobectomy for psychomotor epilepsy: preliminary communication. J Neurol Neurosurg Psychiatry 1955;18:44–52.

[10] Milner B. Psychological defects produced by temporal-lobe excision. Research Publications: Association for Research in Nervous and Mental Disease 1958;36:244–57.

[11] Milner B. Laterality effects in audition. In: Mountcastle VB, editor. Interhemispheric relations and cerebral dominance. Baltimore (MD): John Hopkins Press; 1962. p. 177–95.

[12] Milner B. Visual recognition and recall after right temporal-lobe excisions in man. Neuropsychologia 1968;6:191–210.

[13] Penfield W, Milner B. Memory deficits induced by bilateral lesions in the hippocampal zone. Arch Neurol Psychiatry 1958;79:475–97.

[14] Penfield W, Mathieson G. Memory: autopsy findings and comments on the role of the hippocampus in experimental recall. Arch Neurol 1974;31:145–54.

[15] Milner B, Penfield W. The effect of hippocampal lesions on recent memory. Transactions of the American Neurological Association 1955;80:42–8.

[16] Scoville WB, Milner B. Loss of recent memory after bilateral hippocampal lesions. J Neurol Neurosurg Psychiatry 1957;20:11–21.

[17] Sawa M, Ueki Y, Arita M, et al. Preliminary report on the amygdaloidectomy on the psychotic patients, with interpretation of oral-emotional manifestation in schizophrenics. Folia Psychiatrica Neurologica Japonica 1954;7:309–29.

[18] Scoville WB. The limbic lobe in man. J Neurosurg 1954;11:64–6.

[19] Milner B. The memory defect in bilateral hippocampal lesions. Psychiatric Research Report 1959;11:43–58.

[20] Milner B. Amnesia following operation on the temporal lobes. In: Whitty CWM, Zangwill OL, editors. Amnesia. London: Butterworth; 1966. p. 109–33.

[21] Drachman DA, Arbit S. Memory and the hippocampal complex II. Is memory a multiple process? Arch Neurol 1966;15:52–61.

[22] Konorski J. A new method of physiological investigation of recent memory in animals. Bull Acad Poli Sci 1959;7:115–7.

[23] Stepien L, Sierpinski S. The effect of focal lesions of the brain upon auditory and visual recent memory in man. Journal of Neurology Neurosurgery and Psychiatry 1960;23:334–40.

[24] Prisko L. Short-term memory in focal cerebral damage [doctoral thesis]. Montreal (Canada): McGill University; 1963.

[25] Milner B. Disorders of learning and memory after temporal lobe lesions in man. Clin Neurosurg 1972;19:421–46.

[26] Sidman M, Stoddard LT, Mohr JP. Some additional quantitative observations of immediate memory in a patient with bilateral hippocampal lesions. Neuropsychologia 1968;6:245–54.

[27] James W. Principles of psychology. volume 1. New York: Rinehart and Winston; 1890. p. 85–95.

[28] Milner B. Les troubles de la mémoire accompagnant les lésions hippocampiques bilatérales. In: Physiologie de l'hippocampe, colloques internationaux. number 107. Paris: CNRS; 1962. p. 257–72.

[29] Milner B, Corkin S, Teuber H-L. Further analysis of the hippocampal amnesic syndrome: 14-year follow-up study of HM. Neuropsychologia 1968;6:215–34.

[30] Milner B. Memory and the medial temporal regions of the brain. In: Pribram KH, Broadbent DE, editors. Biology of memory. New York: Academic Press; 1970. p. 29–50.

[31] Gross GG. Effects of hippocampal lesions on memory in rats. In: Functions of the hippocampus in learning and memory. Paper presented at the Annual Meeting of the American Psychological Association. San Francisco, 1968.

[32] Corkin S. What's new with the amnesic patient HM? Nat Rev Neurosci 2002;3:153–60.

[33] Corkin S. Acquisition of motor skill after bilateral medial temporal-lobe excision. Neuropsychologia 1968;6:255–65.

[34] Cohen NJ, Squire LR. Preserved learning and retention of pattern analyzing skill in amnesia: dissociation of knowing how and knowing that. Science 1980;210:207–9.

[35] Warrington E, Weiskrantz L. New method of testing long-term retention with special reference to amnesic patients. Nature 1968;217:972–4.

[36] Gollin ES. Developmental studies of visual recognition of incomplete objects. Percept Mot Skills 1960;11:289–98.

[37] Tulving E. Episodic and semantic memory. In: Tulving E, Donaldson W, editors. Organization of memory. New York: Academic Press; 1972. p. 381–403.

[38] Schacter DL, Chiu C-YP, Ochsner KN. Implicit memory: a selective review. Annu Rev Neurosci 1993;16:159–82.

[39] Packard MG, Hirsh R, White NM. Differential effects of fornix and caudate nucleus lesions on two radial maze tasks: evidence for multiple memory systems. J Neurosci 1989;9: 1465–72.

[40] Knowlton BJ, Mangels JA, Squire LR. A neostriatal habit learning system in humans. Science 1996;273:1399–402.

[41] Thompson RF, Krupa DJ. Organization of memory traces in the mammalian brain. Annu Rev Neurosci 1994;17:519–50.

[42] Wood FB, Ebert V, Kinsbourne M. The episodic-semantic memory distinction in memory and amnesia: clinical and experimental observations. In: Cermak LS, editor. Human memory and amnesia. Hillsdale (NJ): Erlbaum; 1982. p. 167–94.

[43] Vargha-Khadem F, Gadian DG, Watkins KE, et al. Differential effects of early hippocampal pathology. Science 1997;277:376–80.

[44] Gabrieli JDE, Cohen NJ, Corkin S. The impaired learning of semantic knowledge following bilateral medial temporal-lobe resection. Brain Cogn 1988;7:157–77.

[45] Corkin S, Amaral DG, González RG, et al. HM's medial temporal lobe lesion: findings from magnetic resonance imaging. J Neurosci 1997;17:3964–79.

[46] Zola-Morgan S, Squire LR, Amaral DG. Human amnesia and the medial temporal region: enduring memory impairment following a bilateral lesion limited to field CA1 of the hippocampus. J Neurosci 1986;6:2950–67.

[47] Rempel-Clower NL, Zola SM, Squire LR, et al. Three cases of enduring memory impairment following bilateral damage limited to the hippocampal formation. J Neurosci 1996;16: 5233–55.

[48] Weiskrantz L. Comparison of amnesic states in monkey and man. In: Jarrard LE, editor. Cognitive processes of nonhuman primates. New York: Academic Press; 1971. p. 25–46.

[49] Mishkin M. Memory in monkeys severely impaired by combined but not by separate removal of amygdala and hippocampus. Nature 1978;273:297–8.

[50] Mishkin M, Delacour J. An analysis of short-term visual memory in the monkey. J Exp Psychol Anim Behav Process 1975;1:326–34.

[51] Gaffan D. Recognition impaired and association intact in the memory of monkeys after transection of the fornix. J Comp Physiol Psychol 1974;86:1100–9.

[52] Squire LR, Zola-Morgan S. The medial temporal-lobe memory system. Science 1991;253: 1380–6.

[53] Aggleton JP, Brown MW. Episodic memory, amnesia, and the hippocampal-anterior thalamic axis. Behav Brain Sci 1999;22:425–89.

[54] Nadel L. Moscovitch. Memory consolidation, retrograde amnesia and the hippocampal complex. Curr Opin Neurobiol 1997;7:217–27.

[55] Maguire EA, Frith CD. Lateral asymmetry in the hippocampal response to the remoteness of autobiographical memories. J Neurosci 2003;23:5302–7.

ELSEVIER
SAUNDERS

PSYCHIATRIC
CLINICS
OF NORTH AMERICA

Psychiatr Clin N Am 28 (2005) 613–633

# Cognition in Schizophrenia: Impairments, Determinants, and Functional Importance

## Christopher R. Bowie, PhD*, Philip D. Harvey, PhD

*Department of Psychiatry, Mount Sinai School of Medicine, 1425 Madison Avenue, 4th Floor, Box 1230, New York, NY 10029, USA*

Cognitive impairments are now recognized as one of the most ubiquitous features of schizophrenia. These impairments can be detected before the onset of symptoms that meet diagnostic criteria for schizophrenia [1], are moderate to severe in magnitude even at the time of the first break [2], and tend to persist throughout the course of the illness [3], even during episodes of remission of most other symptoms of the illness [4]. Cognitive impairments are not simply a result of other symptoms or antipsychotic treatment, because even never-medicated patients display neuropsychologic profiles similar to those with a history of antipsychotic treatment [2,5]. Moreover, with second-generation antipsychotic treatment, improvements in symptom domains seem to be relatively independent of improvements in cognitive domains [6–9], suggesting that cognitive deficits are a core feature of the illness, separable from positive and negative symptoms. In late life, a subset of patients experience a marked worsening in cognitive skills [10–12], which seems related to a concurrent decline in adaptive life skills.

Assessment of cognitive functions greatly broadens the understanding of schizophrenia. It provides windows through which investigators may look into the neural bases for schizophrenia and suggests how the patient might be expected to function when faced with real-world challenges. Although cognitive tests do not localize specific neurologic dysfunction, particularly in schizophrenia, they provide insight into dysfunctional processing systems and allow detection of relative strengths and weaknesses. Cognitive

This research was supported by a National Alliance for Research on Schizophrenia and Depression Young Investigator Award (CRB), NIMH grant # MH 63116 (PDH), and the VA VISN 3 MIRECC.

* Corresponding author.
*E-mail address:* christopher.bowie@mssm.edu (C.R. Bowie).

assessment, unlike self-reported or clinician-rated psychiatric symptoms, is based on objective performance. As a result, it can be argued that the results of cognitive testing provide valuable information on both the micro and macro levels. From an individual perspective, evaluation of functional potential can be attempted, and the success of interventions can be tracked. On a more global level, subgroups of patients can be identified based on a signature of cognitive impairments. These subgroups might share causative or course-of-illness features that allow reduction of the heterogeneity of the illness.

The recognition that cognitive dysfunction is a central feature of schizophrenia has elevated its importance for both research and treatment. One of the main incentives for understanding the signature of cognitive impairment in schizophrenia is the strong relationship between cognitive performance and functional skills and functional outcome. Cognitive impairment is one of the most functionally relevant aspects of the illness. Additionally, cognitive functioning may be a vulnerability marker. Cognitive impairments are proving to be one of the symptoms within a cluster that may eventually enhance the ability to determine who is at risk of developing a psychotic disorder. Cognitive assessment may also be used as a tool to assess the beneficial and adverse effects of treatment. For example, although conventional antipsychotic medications are not directly detrimental to cognitive functions [13], anticholinergic medications, which are often needed to treat their side effects, are known to affect several cognitive functions disadvantageously, including episodic and working memory [14]. Conversely, evidence [7–9] of consistent improvements in cognitive functioning strengthens the case for the use of atypical antipsychotic medication for the treatment of schizophrenia.

Several reports have related performance on cognitive tasks to specific brain regions or circuits. When compared with healthy subjects, schizophrenia patients typically manifest decreased activity in the frontal cortex and in the temporoparietal regions when performing cognitive tasks [15,16] and in the thalamus and anterior cingulate [17,18] during tests of sustained attention. The extensive work of Goldman-Rakic and colleagues [19,20] has tied working memory dysfunction in schizophrenia to the functioning of the dorsolateral prefrontal cortex. Recent work has clarified this relationship by demonstrating that even schizophrenia patients with good performance on working memory tasks are inefficient in their use of prefrontal networks [21].

Further validating the neural basis of cognitive deficits in schizophrenia are recent findings from genetic studies. Catechol-$O$-methyltransferase (COMT) is an enzyme that deactivates dopamine in cortical but not in subcortical regions. Several studies have demonstrated an association between COMT genotype and performance on tests of processing speed [22], verbal learning and memory [22], executive functions [23], and working memory [24]. Patients who have two valine alleles, which are associated with higher levels of COMT and greater degradation of cortical dopamine, perform more poorly. These studies provide opportunities for translational research in the genetic and neurobehavioral study of schizophrenia.

This article reviews specific domains of cognitive deficits in schizophrenia, discusses the functional implications of these deficits, and proposes new methods for assessing the relationship between cognition and functional outcome. In so doing, it briefly reviews previous studies describing some of the well-established features of impairment in cognitive ability areas and then examines the newest data that sharpen the understanding of cognitive impairment and its relevance to other aspects of the illness.

## Basic areas of impairment

Despite the widespread prevalence of cognitive impairment in schizophrenia, there is considerable controversy as to whether the deficits reflect a generalized and a global neuropsychologic impairment. Although some reports [25,26] have questioned the notion that there is a specific profile of cognitive deficits in schizophrenia, there are data suggesting that there is variability among patients in level of impairment and that there is some separability across cognitive domains in terms of the overall severity of impairment. Some of this controversy is based on the breadth of the cognitive assessments performed and the extent to which current performance is compared with information about potential decline in functioning from premorbid levels. Further, the heterogeneity in schizophrenia extends to cognitive impairment, and sampling may affect the severity of measured cognitive dysfunction. The authors define each cognitive ability area (construct), describe the degree of impairment found in studies of schizophrenia patients, and discuss correlates with symptoms and functional outcome. The degree of impairment is referenced to healthy comparison samples, to normative data groups, or to the patients' own level of functioning before the onset of illness. The authors adopt the convention that cognitive functioning is within normal limits if performance scores are within 1 SD of the normative standards, is mildly impaired if scores fall between 1 and 2 SD below the normative standards, is moderately impaired between 2 and 3 SD below the normative standards, and is severe at 3 or more SD below the normative standards.

### Attention

The construct of attention comprises several components, including detection of relevant information, maintaining focus on those stimuli, and ignoring irrelevant competing stimuli. Early descriptions of schizophrenia [27,28] recognized attentional impairments as fundamental aspects of schizophrenia long before the advent of formal neuropsychologic testing or modern experimental psychology. Perhaps more than other aspects of cognition, deficits in attention may be present before the diagnosis of a psychotic condition in individuals who are genetically vulnerable to schizophrenia [29]. These impairments may further decline slightly with the onset of frank psychosis [30]. They are detectable after diagnosis at the first episode before medication treatment [31] and tend to persist even after resolution of psychotic symptoms [32,33].

The presence and severity of attentional impairments, possibly more than some other cognitive deficits, are associated with higher severity of positive symptoms [34,35]. Greater impairments in attention have been reported to be predictive of poor treatment response [36] and to identify chronic patients who do poorly when their medication dosage is reduced [37].

Impairments in vigilance, meaning the ability to sustain effort and attention while discriminating target and nontarget stimuli, are among the most widely replicated findings in the illness and are also associated with greater deficits in social problem solving and in the ability to acquire skills in training programs [38]. Because attention is the foundation for other, higher-order cognitive skills, attentional deficits are likely to limit success in many functional domains and are thus an important feature of cognitive impairment in the illness.

*Working memory*

The ability to store and manipulate information is referred to as working memory. In a hierarchical concept of cognitive functioning, working memory is the next step in processing, following selective attention and vigilance. Information that has been detected and selected for further processing is maintained in a storage system that allows further processing. Working memory differs from episodic or long-term memory in that the stimuli are not necessarily transferred to long-term storage.

Working memory operations are complex and may be specialized for both the type of information (location, action, and object) and the modality of the information (verbal versus visual-spatial) [39]. Impairments in verbal working memory are common and frequently are severe in schizophrenia. Measurement of verbal working memory can include simple memory span as well as the ability to manipulate and reorganize information. Fleming and colleagues [40] demonstrated that schizophrenic patients showed marked impairments in recalling verbal information after distractor conditions, in which they had to produce competing verbal output. Patients typically manifest moderate to severe deficits on tasks that require storage, sequencing, and reproduction of verbal information [41,42]. Stone and colleagues [43] found that the moderate to severe impairments in verbal working memory that they detected could not be accounted for simply by deficits in attention.

Visual working memory comprises object and spatial working memory. Park and Holzman [44] found considerable deficits in visual working memory using spatial delayed-response tasks. In a similar paradigm, the Dot Test [45,46], subjects must indicate, after a delay in which they read words to inhibit verbal mediation, the location of visually presented stimuli. Patients who have schizophrenia are reported to be able to perform this task within normal limits in the no-delay condition, but substantial impairments are typically found in the delay conditions. Impairments are detected in spatial working memory tasks that require even minimal additional processing (simple object alternation) [47], suggesting that these impairments are pervasive. At the same time, a recent study suggested that impairments in object working memory may be an artifact of perceptual deficits, whereas deficits in spatial working memory are consistent with impairments in the working memory system [48]. These impairments may relate to some basic deficits in processing capacity: although patients who have schizophrenia are able to complete working memory tasks at levels consistent with normal performance when the memory load is low, they nevertheless demonstrate aberrant response patterns as measured by functional MRI [49,50]. Studies that compared the relative deficits in storage versus manipulation processes in working memory have demonstrated that the impairment in the manipulation processes of working memory are considerably more severe than those observed in simple storage tasks [51]. Thus, these impairments point to basic deficiencies in processing capacity and short-term storage in patients who have schizophrenia, even with low levels of task demands.

Working memory measures may be associated with both positive and negative symptoms, although some studies have found relatively small correlations [52]. Spatial working memory has been found to be highly associated with psychomotor poverty (ie, negative symptoms) [53] and global negative symptomatology [54]. Keefe and colleagues [55,56] used a source-monitoring paradigm and found more severe delusions and hallucinations were associated with the ability to identify thoughts as self- or other-generated, which could be considered a deficit in working memory. It is likely that this aspect of working memory functions (the inability to hold information on-line for a period of time sufficient to manipulate it, attend to other information, and continuously monitor the content of consciousness) may contribute to schizophrenic symptoms ranging from disorganized behavior to delusional ideation.

In addition to possibly contributing to some of the psychotic symptoms in the illness, deficits in working memory are linked to many functional domains, including impairments in occupational [57] and social behavior [58]. Patients who have working memory deficits are less likely to benefit from psychotherapy designed to teach social skills [59]. Thus, working memory impairments, possibly reflecting reductions in overall information-processing capacity, seem to be among the most important cognitive deficits in the illness.

*Verbal learning and memory*

One of the most consistent findings across studies of neurocognition in schizophrenia is the presence of moderate to severe deficits in verbal learning and memory. A comprehensive assessment of verbal learning and memory requires the subject to learn new information, either by listening to a brief story (paragraph learning) or trying to learn a list of words over a series of trials (multitrial learning). The subject is required to recall the items spontaneously after a delay without prompts or cues (delayed recall) and then to identify the target words with prompts, either from being exposed to a procedure that also contains distractors (delayed recognition) or through some cueing process (cued recall).

Although schizophrenia has been conceptualized as an illness with a global cognitive deficit, substantial variability in ability exists in the verbal learning and memory domain. Overall, deficits tend to be more severe in this domain than in other areas [5,60], especially when rate of learning and delayed recall are considered. Differential impairments exist within this domain, with most patients demonstrating impaired learning rates and delayed recall but relatively intact recognition [61]. Many older schizophrenic patients who have considerable global cognitive impairment demonstrate intact recognition memory [62,63]. Although recognition memory is spared in many schizophrenia patients, some patients evidence lifelong impairments in this area, and declines in this domain in late life are predictive of global worsening in functional status [63].

One of the cognitive processes implicated in the verbal learning and recall deficit observed in schizophrenia is the inefficient use of strategies to learn new episodic information. For example, many list-learning tasks contain semantically related words from superordinate categories such as fruits or clothing. Encoding and then recalling the words according to semantic category, as opposed to the serial order in which the words were presented, is a more efficient strategy. Schizophrenia patients do not use learning strategies as efficiently as healthy subjects [64–67]. Extensive data, however, have suggested that schizophrenia patients benefit from semantic categorization to the same extent as healthy individuals. For instance, if semantic encoding can be induced incidentally, either by requiring some sort of sorting procedure [68] or having the subjects generate a story [69], patients perform consistently with normal control subjects. Thus, it seems that the semantic structure of episodic memory for schizophrenia patients is more intact than the ability to deploy these encoding strategies volitionally. Consistent with the general deficits in recall memory as compared with encoding, volitional deployment of mnemonic strategies seems to be impaired in most patients, whereas more automatically deployed retrieval techniques, such as benefiting from prompts and cues, seem to be intact.

There are some reports that impaired verbal memory is moderately correlated with positive symptoms of schizophrenia [70,71]. Most research, however, has found correlations with negative and general symptoms of psychopathology such as depression, but not with positive symptoms [52,64,72,73].

Impairments in verbal learning and memory are among the most consistent predictors of social, adaptive, and occupational functioning in schizophrenia [74]. The ability to store information adaptively and retrieve it at a later time is crucial for social interactions, occupational performance, and completing everyday activities. Studies have demonstrated a link between impaired verbal learning and memory and skills as specific as shopping [75] and as global as problem solving [76]. In therapy, social skill acquisition is associated with verbal memory [77]. Schizophrenia patients are unlikely to benefit from many aspects of psychosocial therapy if they are unable to retain and recall information that is meant to be learned in therapeutic sessions and then generalized to the external environment. It has been shown that although intact attentional skills are important for initial job success (in the first 3 months), impairments in episodic verbal memory are likely to predict long-term vocational impairment [78].

*Language skills*

The most commonly assessed verbal skills in schizophrenia are phonological and semantic fluency. These measures require the subject to produce words that either start with a specific letter (phonological fluency) or belong to a superordinate category, such as animals or fruits (semantic fluency). Deficits on these tests tend to be mild to moderate in schizophrenia. Schizophrenia patients do not typically reveal impairments on tests of aphasia; in fact, confrontational naming skills are preserved into late life, even in patients who have severe impairments in other domains [79].

Poor storage or loss of access to verbal information may account for verbal fluency impairments in schizophrenia [80]. Even when information is stored, however, schizophrenia patients have difficulty retrieving words with normal efficiency [81]. This inability to access the words efficiently may be caused by a reduced ability to access semantic systems systematically [82,83]. The disorganized semantic system is probably one reason schizophrenia patients do not show the typical pattern of better performance on tests of semantic fluency than of phonemic fluency [84].

Poor performance on tests of verbal fluency is associated with greater negative symptoms but not with positive symptoms [80,85]. More severe negative symptoms are associated with generation of fewer words, although poor verbal fluency is not simply an artifact of depression [86] or thought disorder [87].

The inability to organize semantically related material affects the schizophrenia patient's production of words and results in impairments in communication. Accordingly, impairments in verbal fluency are associated with interpersonal skills [76] and community functions [75] and even with adaptive skills in late life [87].

*Executive functioning*

Executive functioning has been one of the most studied neurocognitive domains in schizophrenia. It is a broad construct encompassing cognitive processes necessary for allocation of attentional resources, goal-directed behavior, and adaptation to environmental changes. Executive functioning tests are sometimes referred to as "frontal lobe" functions. Despite consistent findings of impairment in this domain in patients who have schizophrenia, it has been argued that deficits in these ability areas lack specificity to the frontal lobes [88,89] and lack discriminant validity from other neuropsychologic domains, such as working memory [41]. For example, even one of the most widely used measures of executive functioning in schizophrenia, the Wisconsin Card Sorting Task (WCST), can be adversely affected by impairments in working memory functions, in addition to core problem-solving impairments.

Executive functioning is the ability to solve problems, employ abstract thinking, and coordinate other cognitive skills such as working memory and attentional systems. Although the the WCST is the test most commonly used to assess concept formation and set shifting, and deficits on this test have been well replicated in schizophrenia, executive functioning is actually a multifaceted construct (see ref. [90] for a detailed discussion). When the WCST is used as the reference measure of executive functioning, moderate to severe impairments are detected in several different domains, including the number of conceptual categories attained [91], total efficiency, and perseverative tendencies [92,93].

Other ways to measure executive functioning include tests that require more planning and less interactive reaction to ongoing environmental events. Planning abilities can be measured with tasks that require the subject to reach a goal efficiently, such as the various Tower tasks. These tasks have in common the demand that the subject organize responses efficiently, using as few moves as possible to solve problems of varying complexity. Patients who have schizophrenia perform poorly on these tests [94–96].

Studies of the relationship between neurocognitive domains and functional status consistently identify limitations in executive functioning as one of the important predictors of deficits in basic self-care skills [97], social/interpersonal skills [97], community skills [75,97], and occupational functioning [97–100]. Patients who have executive dysfunction are less likely to use treatment services [101]. Furthermore, even when patients do use treatment services, engagement within therapy sessions [102], therapeutic alliance [103], and compliance with prescribed medication [104,105] are inversely correlated with executive dysfunction. Thus, given the role of executive dysfunction in treatment compliance and participation, it is not surprising that it is related to length of hospitalization [106] and a poorer course of illness. Patients who have executive dysfunction may have less contact with family members and less financial support [107], further increasing their risk for poor outcome.

*Social cognition*

The concept of social cognition as an important and functionally relevant deficit in schizophrenia has gained support recently [108]. This construct is defined broadly as a set of cognitive abilities that allows people to perceive and make sense of their surroundings and the thoughts and actions of themselves and others. In contrast to aspects of cognitive functions that are often referred to as "cold cognition," social cognition refers to the ability to perceive and react to emotional experiences on one's own part and to interpret the emotional displays of other individuals. Social cognition typically is measured with instruments that evaluate the ability to perceive, interpret, and respond in accordance to the emotions and intents of others, while considering one's own emotional reactions as well.

This area of research is less developed than aspects of neurocognition. One of the difficulties in determining the severity of social cognitive deficits in schizophrenia is that the previous studies of social cognition have not adopted a psychometric approach to test development. Many of the tests previously developed lack variance in groups of healthy people. Although on most neurocognitive tests the performance of healthy individuals varies considerably because of attempts to develop tests that elicit normal distributions of test performance, several attempts to measure the social cognitive deficits in individuals who have schizophrenia may have been handicapped by ceiling effects. In fact, some validity studies of social cognitive measures have been published without reference to a healthy control group [109], raising some concern about the ability to these measures to detect discriminating deficits. Some concerns have been raised about whether some widely reported deficits in schizophrenia, such as affect perception, have been unduly influenced by the psychometric properties of the measures [110]. Still, the construct of social cognition has considerable potential importance for functional outcome in schizophrenia, if measurement issues are resolved.

The reason for the potential functional relevance of this cognitive ability is transparent: the inability to perceive, process, and organize social information accurately is likely to affect one's social functioning adversely. Patients who have schizophrenia show deficits in the ability to recognize emotions based on facial expressions or tone of voice; these deficits have been linked to failures in perceptual processing, attention, and verbal memory [111,112] It is becoming increasingly clear that social cognition is a separable factor from schizophrenic symptoms [113]. Social cognition may also serve as a mediating factor in the relationship between neurocognition and social functioning [114]. That is, although neurocognitive functions are necessary for success in many functional domains, these skills may not be of functional use in the absence of other skills, such as the ability to identify social cues. Thus, social cognitive deficits may add incremental predictive power to the understanding of functional impairments in schizophrenia [115].

### Additional considerations

*Substance abuse*

Although substance abuse exacerbates impairment in many neurocognitive domains [116–118], its effects are most pronounced on learning and memory. In both cocaine-abusing [116] and alcohol-abusing [118] patients who have schizophrenia, the rate of acquisition of information across learning trials and the proportion of words recalled after delay are similar to those of schizophrenic patients who do not abuse substances, but the overall number of words learned and recalled is fewer. This phenomenon may reflect a deficit in processing capacity or the amount of information available to be stored, rather than a direct effect on the ability to benefit from learning over trials or to remember information that was stored. It is estimated that as many as 60% of schizophrenics meet diagnostic criteria for a substance-use disorder—excluding nicotine and caffeine—at some point in their lives [119]. Despite the widespread prevalence of substance abuse in schizophrenia, most studies still use substance abuse as an exclusion criterion.

Although it clearly is important to understand the impact of substance use on cognition in schizophrenia and on other aspects of the illness, one of the issues in this area is the tendency for patients who have schizophrenia to abuse more than one substance. Polysubstance abuse makes it difficult to identify specific effects; however, if polysubstance abuse is the norm, then future research would be wise to focus on the multiplicative or additive adverse effects of abuse of these substances. To perform clinically relevant research, researchers should consider controlling for substance abuse at the level of data analysis rather than excluding such patients at the level of recruitment; otherwise, findings will generalize to less than half the population of patients who have schizophrenia.

*Course of cognitive deficits over the lifespan*

Cognitive deficits are detectable before the onset of frank psychosis and when patients first meet criteria for schizophrenia. These deficits are present in multiple areas of cognitive ability, and deficits across these areas typically range from moderate to severe as compared with healthy individuals. With the onset of psychosis, a modest decline in general intellectual functions has been reported [30], and impairment in adulthood is greater than estimates of premorbid cognitive functioning [120]. Although inter- and intraindividual variability exists, cognitive deficits tend to persist from the time of the first episode into middle adulthood without significant change in their topography or severity over short follow-up intervals [3,121,122]. These findings have been interpreted as evidence for a static course throughout the illness [123]. Recent work, however, suggests that the course is more dynamic, at least for a subset of patients. When patients who have schizophrenia are studied into late life, declines in cognitive functions in some patients area as severe as seen in dementia [10–12], although post-mortem analyses of these subjects do not reveal pathology similar to known causes of late-life dementias including Alzheimer's disease [124]. This cognitive decline is not accounted for by medical illness [125]. The course of this decline [10–12] and its cross-sectional profile [122,126] are quite different from that seen in Alzheimer's disease. It is likely that the substantial global cognitive decline observed in the subjects of the Harvey and Friedman studies [10–12,125] are atypical of schizophrenia and apply only to those with a particularly adverse course of illness or a chronic course of treatment-refractory psychosis.

More recent work from multiple laboratories has confirmed a dynamic course of cortical changes beginning even at the time of the first episode [127], with even more drastic changes seen in cases with childhood onset [128] or in middle-aged patients who have refractory psychotic symptoms [129]. These findings suggest that in many patients who have schizophrenia, an active process of cortical change, possibly exacerbated in cases with poorly responsive psychotic symptoms [130], may be present. Thus, cognitive decline may be common in aging schizophrenic patients, with a profile of vulnerability to this decline that is only beginning to be discovered. In older ambulatory patients who have schizophrenia, cognitive declines may be restricted to complex cognitive domains such as executive function [131] and complex information processing [132]. Identification of the specificity and predictors of cognitive decline with aging might lead to reduction in disability as well as understanding of the neuropathologic processes associated with aging in schizophrenia.

*Assessment methods*

With a new priority on measuring cognition in schizophrenia, new concerns have emerged regarding assessment of cognitive functioning. Assessments must be broad enough to capture relevant deficits but retain feasibility. Although some abbreviated instruments, such as the Repeatable Battery for the Assessment of Neuropsychological Status, have adequate psychometric properties, they are not designed specifically to be sensitive to the cognitive impairments of schizophrenia and do not capture important domains such as working memory and executive functioning. Several different abbreviated cognitive assessments have been proposed, including the Brief Assessment of Cognition in Schizophrenia [133] and the Brief Cognitive Assessment [134]. For all abbreviated assessment instruments, more data are required to ensure that these assessments reliably capture the important features of cognitive impairment in schizophrenia.

*The evolving understanding of the relationships between cognitive dysfunction and functional outcome*

Despite adequate control of psychotic symptoms achieved in many patients with the use of antipsychotic medications, less progress has been made in improving functional outcome in schizophrenia since the advent of conventional antipsychotic treatments [135]. An open question in studies of the functional relevance of cognition is whether the relationship is better understood in terms of global cognitive impairment or by examining specific ability areas as predictors of outcome. Not unexpectedly, many neurocognitive variables are highly correlated with each other and share variance in predicting functional domains. Dickinson and colleagues [136] found that among the four Wechsler Adult Intelligence Scale (WAIS) factors, working memory and processing speed accounted for community functioning, but the addition of positive and negative symptoms substantially increased predictive power. Only processing speed survived as a predictor of functional status after controlling for the other WAIS factors. IQ scores, however, are not a comprehensive neuropsychologic assessment; they do not measure executive functions, verbal learning, or episodic memory, all of which are strong predictors of social and adaptive functions in schizophrenia patients.

Evans and colleagues [137] examined seven neurocognitive domains and three symptom domains as correlates of two levels of adaptive functions: basic activities of daily living (eg, eating) and instrumental activities of living (eg, shopping). All seven neurocognitive domains were associated with both aspects of functional skills. Global scores on cognition accounted for most of the variance in both functional skills, even after controlling for negative symptoms. None of the neurocognitive domains were differentially more predictive of functional skills. These data suggest that different cognitive domains have similar relationships to outcome. Prediction of more discrete functional competencies than were used in the study by Evans and colleagues would be necessary to reveal independent neurocognitive predictors [38,74,138].

Although there is general agreement that neurocognition is a strong predictor of social and adaptive functions, there is no consensus on exactly how to measure these functional domains, particularly for treatment studies. Recent developments include performance-based measures of functional skills that can be used in the laboratory setting. The University of California–San Diego Performance-Based Skills Assessment Battery [139] is a laboratory-based measure with adequate psychometric characteristics. Valid assessment of skills in the laboratory may only approximate real world functions, however. Furthermore, the source of information regarding real-world functioning may be critical. Jin and colleagues [140] found an association between self-reported depression and self-reported instrumental functional skills. McKibbin and colleagues [141] found depression, but neither cognition nor or performance-based functional skills, to be associated with self-reported disability in schizophrenia outpatients. Work with other neuropsychiatric groups, such as HIV patients [142], also found a role for depressive symptoms in mediating the relationship between neurocognition and real-world functional skills. Recently, the authors found that the relationship between neurocognition and real-world functional performance was mediated by performance-based assessments of functional skills.

## Treatment of cognitive dysfunction in schizophrenia

Although conventional antipsychotic medications have little effect on neurocognitive functions in schizophrenia, second-generation antipsychotic medications do produce cognitive improvements in some patients [143]. Most changes are modest, particularly given the degree of impairment typically observed in schizophrenia. One of the issues in these studies may be duration of treatment, because most are only 6 to 8 weeks in duration. A recent study found that some patients treated with he atypical antipsychotics olanzapine or ziprasidone benefit to a degree associated with normalization of cognitive performance [144], but these patients were treated for 6 months and enrolled in the study only if they were substantially clinically responsive to short-term treatment. This study highlights the importance of studying the clinical meaningfulness of cognitive change with pharmacotherapy. The cognitive benefits of switching to second-generation antipsychotic medication have not translated into simultaneous functional improvement [145], at least for self-reported measures, although improvements in social cognition and social adjustment may be revealed over time with psychosocial interventions [146]. It will be important to examine whether functional deficits lag behind cognitive improvements that result from antipsychotic medication or whether behavioral or other pharmacotherapy interventions are needed.

The findings of modest cognitive improvements with second-generation antipsychotic medication offer promise but do not resolve cognitive dysfunction in schizophrenia. Behavioral strategies for cognitive improvement are effective in improving neurocognitive deficits, demonstrate durability over time [147,148], and potentially normalize performance [149]. Strategies that help patients who have schizophrenia compensate for their cognitive deficits may lead to functional improvements [150]. Because treatments with second-generation antipsychotic medications may produce modest improvements in neurocognitive functions, they may provide a platform for behavioral interventions that stimulate and extend improvement and facilitate functional recovery.

## Summary

Recent findings support and add to earlier findings of cognitive dysfunction in schizophrenia. Deficits across neurocognitive domains such as attention, working memory, language skills, and executive functioning tend to be moderate, with the most pronounced deficits found in verbal learning and memory. All these neurocognitive domains are related to adaptive and social skills, with executive functions and verbal learning and memory showing more variance across more domains than other neuro-cognitive variables. Negative symptoms and neurocognitive domains, although correlated, are distinct and have differential pathways of change with treatment. General psychopathology symptoms, such as depression and anxiety, may become important treatment targets as strategies are developed for translating cognitive enhancement to real-world functional performance.

## References

[1] Davidson M, Reichenberg A, Rabinowitz J, et al. Behavioral and intellectual markers for schizophrenia in apparently healthy male adolescents. Am J Psychiatry 1999;156(9): 1328–35.

[2] Bilder RM, Goldman RS, Robinson D, et al. Neuropsychology of first-episode schizophrenia: initial characterization and clinical correlates. Am J Psychiatry 2000; 157(4):549–59.

[3] Heaton RK, Gladsjo JA, Palmer BW, et al. Stability and course of neuropsychological deficits in schizophrenia. Arch Gen Psychiatry 2001;58(1):24–32.

[4] Addington J, Addington D, Gasbarre L. Distractibility and symptoms in schizophrenia. J Psychiatry Neurosci 1997;22(3):180–4.

[5] Saykin AJ, Shtasel DL, Gur RE, et al. Neuropsychological deficits in neuroleptic naive patients with first-episode schizophrenia. Arch Gen Psychiatry 1994;51(2):124–31.

[6] Addington J, Addington D. Neurocognitive functioning in schizophrenia: a trial of risperidone versus haloperidol. Can J Psychiatry 1997;42(9):983.

[7] Harvey PD, Siu CO, Romano S. Randomized, controlled, double-blind, multicenter comparison of the cognitive effects of ziprasidone versus olanzapine in acutely ill inpatients with schizophrenia or schizoaffective disorder. Psychopharmacology (Berl) 2004;172(3): 324–32.

[8] Harvey PD, Green MF, McGurk SR, et al. Changes in cognitive functioning with risperidone and olanzapine treatment: a large-scale, double-blind, randomized study. Psychopharmacology (Berl) 2003;169(3–4):404–11.

[9] Keefe RS, Seidman LJ, Christensen BK, et al. Comparative effect of atypical and conventional antipsychotic drugs on neurocognition in first-episode psychosis: a random-ized, double-blind trial of olanzapine versus low doses of haloperidol. Am J Psychiatry 2004;161(6):985–95.

[10] Harvey PD, Parrella M, White L, et al. Convergence of cognitive and adaptive decline in late-life schizophrenia. Schizophr Res 1999;35(1):77–84.

[11] Harvey PD, Silverman JM, Mohs RC, et al. Cognitive decline in late-life schizophrenia: a longitudinal study of geriatric chronically hospitalized patients. Biol Psychiatry 1999; 45(1):32–40.

[12] Friedman JI, Harvey PD, Coleman T, et al. Six-year follow-up study of cognitive and functional status across the lifespan in schizophrenia: a comparison with Alzheimer's disease and normal aging. Am J Psychiatry 2001;158(9):1441–8.

[13] Mishara AL, Goldberg TE. A meta-analysis and critical review of the effects of conventional neuroleptic treatment on cognition in schizophrenia: opening a closed book. Biol Psychiatry 2004;55(10):1013–22.

[14] Spohn HE, Strauss ME. Relation of neuroleptic and anticholinergic medication to cognitive functions in schizophrenia. J Abnorm Psychol 1989;98(4):367–80.

[15] Buchsbaum MS, Nuechterlein KH, Haier RJ, et al. Glucose metabolic rate in normals and schizophrenics during the Continuous Performance Test assessed by positron emission tomography. Br J Psychiatry 1990;156:216–27.

[16] Buchsbaum MS, Haier RJ, Potkin SG, et al. Frontostriatal disorder of cerebral metabolism in never-medicated schizophrenics. Arch Gen Psychiatry 1992;49(12):935–42.

[17] Volz H, Gaser C, Hager F, et al. Decreased frontal activation in schizophrenics during stimulation with the continuous performance test—a functional magnetic resonance imaging study. Eur Psychiatry 1999;14(1):17–24.

[18] Salgado-Pineda P, Baeza I, Perez-Gomez M, et al. Sustained attention impairment correlates to gray matter decreases in first episode neuroleptic-naive schizophrenic patients. Neuroimage 2003;19(2 Pt 1):365–75.

[19] Goldman-Rakic PS. The physiological approach: functional architecture of working memory and disordered cognition in schizophrenia. Biol Psychiatry 1999;46(5):650–61.

[20] Levy R, Goldman-Rakic PS. Segregation of working memory functions within the dorsolateral prefrontal cortex. Exp Brain Res 2000;133(1):23–32.

[21] Callicott JH, Mattay VS, Verchinski BA, et al. Complexity of prefrontal cortical dysfunction in schizophrenia: more than up or down. Am J Psychiatry 2003;160(12): 2209–15.

[22] Bilder RM, Volavka J, Czobor P, et al. Neurocognitive correlates of the COMT Val(158)Met polymorphism in chronic schizophrenia. Biol Psychiatry 2002;52(7):701–7.

[23] Egan MF, Goldberg TE, Kolachana BS, et al. Effect of COMT Val108/158 Met genotype on frontal lobe function and risk for schizophrenia. Proc Natl Acad Sci U S A 2001;98(12): 6917–22.

[24] Goldberg TE, Egan MF, Gscheidle TR, et al. Executive subprocesses in working memory: relationship to catechol-O-methyltransferase Val158Met genotype and schizophrenia. Arch Gen Psychiatry 2003;60(9):889–96.

[25] Blanchard JJ, Neale JM. The neuropsychological signature of schizophrenia: generalized or differential deficit? Am J Psychiatry 1994;151(1):40–8.

[26] Dickinson D, Iannone VN, Wilk CM, et al. General and specific cognitive deficits in schizophrenia. Biol Psychiatry 2004;55(8):826–33.

[27] Kraepelin E. Dementia praecox and paraphrenia. Edinburgh (UK): E. & S. Livingstone; 1919.

[28] Bleuler E. Dementia praecox; or the group of schizophrenias. New York: International Universities Press; 1911.

[29] Cornblatt BA, Erlenmeyer-Kimling L. Global attentional deviance as a marker of risk for schizophrenia: specificity and predictive validity. J Abnorm Psychol 1985;94(4):470–86.

[30] Caspi A, Reichenberg A, Weiser M, et al. Cognitive performance in schizophrenia patients assessed before and following the first psychotic episode. Schizophr Res 2003;65(2–3): 87–94.

[31] Brickman AM, Buchsbaum MS, Bloom R, et al. Neuropsychological functioning in first-break, never-medicated adolescents with psychosis. J Nerv Ment Dis 2004;192(9): 615–22.

[32] Stirling J, White C, Lewis S, et al. Neurocognitive function and outcome in first-episode schizophrenia: a 10-year follow-up of an epidemiological cohort. Schizophr Res 2003; 65(2–3):75–86.

[33] Harvey PD, Docherty NM, Serper MR, et al. Cognitive deficits and thought disorder: II. An 8-month followup study. Schizophr Bull 1990;16(1):147–56.

[34] Green M, Walker E. Attentional performance in positive- and negative-symptom schizophrenia. J Nerv Ment Dis 1986;174(4):208–13.

[35] Walker E, Harvey P. Positive and negative symptoms in schizophrenia: attentional performance correlates. Psychopathology 1986;19(6):294–302.

[36] Goldman RS, Axelrod BN, Tandon R, et al. Neuropsychological prediction of treatment efficacy and one-year outcome in schizophrenia. Psychopathology 1993;26(3–4):122–6.

[37] Green MF, Mintz J, Bowen L, et al. Prediction of response to haloperidol dose reduction by Span of Apprehension measures for treatment-refractory schizophrenic patients. Am J Psychiatry 1993;150(9):1415–6.

[38] Green MF. What are the functional consequences of neurocognitive deficits in schizophrenia? Am J Psychiatry 1996;153:321–30.

[39] Keefe RSE. Working memory dysfunction and its relevance to schizophrenia. In: Sharma T, Harvey PD, editors. Cognition in schizophrenia: impairments, importance and treatment strategies. Oxford (UK): Oxford University Press; 2000. p. 16–50.

[40] Fleming K, Goldberg TE, Gold JM, et al. Verbal working memory dysfunction in schizophrenia: use of a Brown-Peterson paradigm. Psychiatry Res 1995;56(2):155–61.

[41] Gold JM, Carpenter C, Randolph C, et al. Auditory working memory and Wisconsin Card Sorting Test performance in schizophrenia. Arch Gen Psychiatry 1997;54(2):159–65.

[42] McGurk SR, Coleman T, Harvey PD, et al. Working memory performance in poor outcome schizophrenia: relationship to age and executive functioning. J Clin Exp Neuropsychol 2004;26(2):153–60.

[43] Stone M, Gabrieli JD, Stebbins GT, et al. Working and strategic memory deficits in schizophrenia. Neuropsychology 1998;12(2):278–88.

[44] Park S, Holzman PS. Schizophrenics show spatial working memory deficits. Arch Gen Psychiatry 1992;49(12):975–82.

[45] Keefe RS, Roitman SE, Harvey PD, et al. A pen-and-paper human analogue of a monkey prefrontal cortex activation task: spatial working memory in patients with schizophrenia. Schizophr Res 1995;17(1):25–33.

[46] Keefe RS, Lees-Roitman SE, DuPre RL. Performance of patients with schizophrenia on a pen and paper visuospatial working memory task with short delay. Schizophr Res 1997; 26(1):9–14.

[47] Seidman LJ, Yurgelun-Todd D, Kremen WS, et al. Relationship of prefrontal and temporal lobe MRI measures to neuropsychological performance in chronic schizophrenia. Biol Psychiatry 1994;35(4):235–46.

[48] Tek C, Gold J, Blaxton T, et al. Visual perceptual and working memory impairments in schizophrenia. Arch Gen Psychiatry 2002;59(2):146–53.

[49] Kindermann SS, Brown GG, Zorrilla LE, et al. Spatial working memory among middle-aged and older patients with schizophrenia and volunteers using fMRI. Schizophr Res 2004;68(2–3):203–16.

[50] Jansma JM, Ramsey NF, van der Wee NJ, et al. Working memory capacity in schizophrenia: a parametric fMRI study. Schizophr Res 2004;68(2–3):159–71.

[51] Perry W, Heaton RK, Potterat E, et al. Working memory in schizophrenia: transient storage versus executive functioning. Schizophr Bull 2001;27(1):157–76.

[52] Bozikas VP, Kosmidis MH, Kioperlidou K, et al. Relationship between psychopathology and cognitive functioning in schizophrenia. Compr Psychiatry 2004;45(5):392–400.

[53] Pantelis C, Harvey CA, Plant G, et al. Relationship of behavioural and symptomatic syndromes in schizophrenia to spatial working memory and attentional set-shifting ability. Psychol Med 2004;34(4):693–703.

[54] Carter C, Robertson L, Nordahl T, et al. Spatial working memory deficits and their relationship to negative symptoms in unmedicated schizophrenia patients. Biol Psychiatry 1996;40(9):930–2.

[55] Keefe RS, Arnold MC, Bayen UJ, et al. Source-monitoring deficits for self-generated stimuli in schizophrenia: multinomial modeling of data from three sources. Schizophr Res 2002;57(1):51–67.

[56] Keefe RS, Arnold MC, Bayen UJ, et al. Source monitoring deficits in patients with schizophrenia; a multinomial modelling analysis. Psychol Med 1999;29(4):903–14.

[57] McGurk SR, Meltzer HY. The role of cognition in vocational functioning in schizophrenia. Schizophr Res 2000;45(3):175–84.

[58] Smith TE, Hull JW, Goodman M, et al. The relative influences of symptoms, insight, and neurocognition on social adjustment in schizophrenia and schizoaffective disorder. J Nerv Ment Dis 1999;187(2):102–8.

[59] Smith TE, Hull JW, Huppert JD, et al. Recovery from psychosis in schizophrenia and schizoaffective disorder: symptoms and neurocognitive rate-limiters for the development of social behavior skills. Schizophr Res 2002;55(3):229–37.

[60] Saykin AJ, Gur RC, Gur RE, et al. Neuropsychological function in schizophrenia. Selective impairment in memory and learning. Arch Gen Psychiatry 1991;48(7):618–24.

[61] Paulsen JS, Heaton RK, Sadek JR, et al. The nature of learning and memory impairments in schizophrenia. J Int Neuropsychol Soc 1995;1(1):88–99.

[62] Harvey PD, Moriarty PJ, Bowie C, et al. Cortical and subcortical cognitive deficits in schizophrenia: convergence of classifications based on language and memory skill areas. J Clin Exp Neuropsychol 2002;24(1):55–66.

[63] Bowie CR, Reichenberg A, Rieckmann N, et al. Stability and functional correlates of memory-based classification in older schizophrenia patients. Am J Geriatr Psychiatry 2004; 12(4):376–86.

[64] Brebion G, Amador X, Smith MJ, et al. Mechanisms underlying memory impairment in schizophrenia. Psychol Med 1997;27(2):383–93.

[65] Toulopoulou T, Rabe-Hesketh S, King H, et al. Episodic memory in schizophrenic patients and their relatives. Schizophr Res 2003;63(3):261–71.

[66] Iddon JL, McKenna PJ, Sahakian BJ, et al. Impaired generation and use of strategy in schizophrenia: evidence from visuospatial and verbal tasks. Psychol Med 1998;28(5): 1049–62.

[67] Hazlett EA, Buchsbaum MS, Jeu LA, et al. Hypofrontality in unmedicated schizophrenia patients studied with PET during performance of a serial verbal learning task. Schizophr Res 2000;43(1):33–46.

[68] Koh SD. Remembering of verbal materials by schizophrenic adults. In: Schwartz S, editor. Language and cognition in schizophrenia. Hillsdale (NJ): Lawrence Erlbaum Associates; 1978.

[69] Harvey PD. Reality monitoring in mania and schizophrenia. The association of thought disorder and performance. J Nerv Ment Dis 1984;173:67–73.

[70] Norman RM, Malla AK, Morrison-Stewart SL, et al. Neuropsychological correlates of syndromes in schizophrenia. Br J Psychiatry 1997;170:134–9.

[71] Holthausen EA, Wiersma D, Knegtering RH, et al. Psychopathology and cognition in schizophrenia spectrum disorders: the role of depressive symptoms. Schizophr Res 1999; 39(1):65–71.

[72] Stirling JD, Hellewell JS, Hewitt J. Verbal memory impairment in schizophrenia: no sparing of short-term recall. Schizophr Res 1997;25(2):85–95.

[73] Heinrichs RW, Vaz SM. Verbal memory errors and symptoms in schizophrenia. Cogn Behav Neurol 2004;17(2):98–101.

[74] Green MF, Kern RS, Braff DL, et al. Neurocognitive deficits and functional outcome in schizophrenia: are we measuring the "right stuff"? Schizophr Bull 2000;26: 119–36.

[75] Rempfer MV, Hamera EK, Brown CE, et al. The relations between cognition and the independent living skill of shopping in people with schizophrenia. Psychiatry Res 2003; 117(2):103–12.

[76] Addington J, Addington D. Neurocognitive and social functioning in schizophrenia: a 2.5 year follow-up study. Schizophr Res 2000;44(1):47–56.

[77] Smith TE, Hull JW, Romanelli S, et al. Symptoms and neurocognition as rate limiters in skills training for psychotic patients. Am J Psychiatry 1999;156(11):1817–8.

[78] Bryson G, Bell MD. Initial and final work performance in schizophrenia: cognitive and symptom predictors. J Nerv Ment Dis 2003;191(2):87–92.

[79] Bowie CR, Harvey PD, Moriarty PJ, et al. Cognitive assessment of geriatric schizophrenic patients with severe impairment. Arch Clin Neuropsychol 2002;17(7):611–23.

[80] Kerns JG, Berenbaum H, Barch DM, et al. Word production in schizophrenia and its relationship to positive symptoms. Psychiatry Res 1999;87(1):29–37.

[81] Joyce EM, Collinson SL, Crichton P. Verbal fluency in schizophrenia: relationship with executive function, semantic memory and clinical alogia. Psychol Med 1996;26(1):39–49.

[82] Goldberg TE, Aloia MS, Gourovitch ML, et al. Cognitive substrates of thought disorder, I: the semantic system. Am J Psychiatry 1998;155(12):1671–6.

[83] Aloia MS, Gourovitch ML, Weinberger DR, et al. An investigation of semantic space in patients with schizophrenia. J Int Neuropsychol Soc 1996;2(4):267–73.

[84] Gourovitch ML, Goldberg TE, Weinberger DR. Verbal fluency deficits in patients with schizophrenia: semantic fluency is differentially impaired as compared to phonological fluency. Neuropsychology 1996;6:573–7.

[85] Howanitz E, Cicalese C, Harvey PD. Verbal fluency and psychiatric symptoms in geriatric schizophrenia. Schizophr Res 2000;42(3):167–9.

[86] Allen HA, Liddle PF, Frith CD. Negative features, retrieval processes and verbal fluency in schizophrenia. Br J Psychiatry 1993;163:769–75.

[87] Bowie CR, Harvey PD, Moriarty PJ, et al. A comprehensive analysis of verbal fluency deficit in geriatric schizophrenia. Arch Clin Neuropsychol 2004;19(2):289–303.

[88] Anderson SW, Damasio H, Jones RD, et al. Wisconsin Card Sorting Test performance as a measure of frontal lobe damage. J Clin Exp Neuropsychol 1991;13(6):909–22.

[89] Axelrod BN, Goldman RS, Heaton RK, et al. Discriminability of the Wisconsin Card Sorting Test using the standardization sample. J Clin Exp Neuropsychol 1996;18(3): 338–42.

[90] Palmer BW, Heaton RK. Executive dysfunction in schizophrenia. In: Sharma T, Harvey PD, editors. Cognition in schizophrenia: impairments, importance and treatment strategies. Oxford (UK): Oxford University Press; 2000. p. 51–72.

[91] Haut MW, Cahill J, Cutlip WD, et al. On the nature of Wisconsin Card Sorting Test performance in schizophrenia. Psychiatry Res 1996;65(1):15–22.

[92] Koren D, Seidman LJ, Harrison RH, et al. Factor structure of the Wisconsin Card Sorting Test: dimensions of deficit in schizophrenia. Neuropsychology 1998;12(2):289–302.

[93] Pantelis C, Barber FZ, Barnes TR, et al. Comparison of set-shifting ability in patients with chronic schizophrenia and frontal lobe damage. Schizophr Res 1999;37(3):251–70.

[94] Bustini M, Stratta P, Daneluzzo E, et al. Tower of Hanoi and WCST performance in schizophrenia: problem-solving capacity and clinical correlates. J Psychiatr Res 1999;33(3): 285–90.

[95] Goldberg TE, Saint-Cyr JA, Weinberger DR. Assessment of procedural learning and problem solving in schizophrenic patients by Tower of Hanoi type tasks. J Neuropsychiatry Clin Neurosci 1990;2(2):165–73.

[96] Pantelis C, Barnes TR, Nelson HE, et al. Frontal-striatal cognitive deficits in patients with chronic schizophrenia. Brain 1997;120(Pt 10):1823–43.

[97] Velligan DI, Bow-Thomas CC, Mahurin RK, et al. Do specific neurocognitive deficits predict specific domains of community function in schizophrenia? J Nerv Ment Dis 2000; 188(8):518–24.

[98] Lysaker PH, Bell MD, Zito WS, et al. Social skills at work. Deficits and predictors of improvement in schizophrenia. J Nerv Ment Dis 1995;183(11):688–92.

[99] McGurk SR, Mueser KT, Harvey PD, et al. Cognitive and symptom predictors of work outcomes for clients with schizophrenia in supported employment. Psychiatr Serv 2003; 54(8):1129–35.

[100] Evans JD, Bond GR, Meyer PS, et al. Cognitive and clinical predictors of success in vocational rehabilitation in schizophrenia. Schizophr Res 2004;70(2–3):331–42.

[101] McGurk SR, Mueser KT, Walling D, et al. Cognitive functioning predicts outpatient service utilization in schizophrenia. Ment Health Serv Res 2004;6(3):185–8.

[102] McKee M, Hull JW, Smith TE. Cognitive and symptom correlates of participation in social skills training groups. Schizophr Res 1997;23(3):223–9.

[103] Davis LW, Lysaker PH. Neurocognitive correlates of therapeutic alliance in schizophrenia. J Nerv Ment Dis 2004;192(7):508–10.

[104] Robinson DG, Woerner MG, Alvir JM, et al. Predictors of medication discontinuation by patients with first-episode schizophrenia and schizoaffective disorder. Schizophr Res 2002; 57(2–3):209–19.

[105] Jeste SD, Patterson TL, Palmer BW, et al. Cognitive predictors of medication adherence among middle-aged and older outpatients with schizophrenia. Schizophr Res 2003;63(1–2): 49–58.

[106] Jackson CT, Fein D, Essock SM, et al. The effects of cognitive impairment and substance abuse on psychiatric hospitalizations. Community Ment Health J 2001;37(4):303–12.

[107] Fujii DE, Wylie AM, Nathan JH. Neurocognition and long-term prediction of quality of life in outpatients with severe and persistent mental illness. Schizophr Res 2004;69(1):67–73.

[108] Green MF, Nuechterlein KH, Gold JM, et al. Approaching a consensus cognitive battery for clinical trials in schizophrenia: the NIMH-MATRICS conference to select cognitive domains and test criteria. Biol Psychiatry 2004;56(5):301–7.

[109] Corrigan PW, Buican B, Toomey R. Construct validity of two tests of social cognition in schizophrenia. Psychiatry Res 1996;63(1):77–82.

[110] Kerr SL, Neale JM. Emotion perception in schizophrenia: specific deficit or further evidence of generalized poor performance? J Abnorm Psychol 1993;102:312–8.

[111] Kee KS, Kern RS, Green MF. Perception of emotion and neurocognitive functioning in schizophrenia: what's the link? Psychiatry Res 1998;81(1):57–65.

[112] Kohler CG, Bilker W, Hagendoorn M, et al. Emotion recognition deficit in schizophrenia: association with symptomatology and cognition. Biol Psychiatry 2000;48(2):127–36.

[113] Silver H, Shlomo N. Perception of facial emotions in chronic schizophrenia does not correlate with negative symptoms but correlates with cognitive and motor dysfunction. Schizophr Res 2001;52(3):265–73.

[114] Vauth R, Rusch N, Wirtz M, et al. Does social cognition influence the relation between neurocognitive deficits and vocational functioning in schizophrenia? Psychiatry Res 2004; 128(2):155–65.

[115] Penn DL, Spaulding W, Reed D, et al. The relationship of social cognition to ward behavior in chronic schizophrenia. Schizophr Res 1996;20(3):327–35.

[116] Serper MR, Bergman A, Copersino ML, et al. Learning and memory impairment in cocaine-dependent and comorbid schizophrenic patients. Psychiatry Res 2000;93(1):21–32.

[117] Allen DN, Goldstein G, Aldarondo F. Neurocognitive dysfunction in patients diagnosed with schizophrenia and alcoholism. Neuropsychology 1999;13(1):62–8.

[118] Bowie CR, Serper MR, Riggio S, et al. Neurocognition, symptomatology, and functional status of elderly alcohol-abusing schizophrenia patients. Schizophr Bull 2005;31(1):175–82.

[119] Fowler IL, Carr VJ, Carter NT, et al. Patterns of current and lifetime substance use in schizophrenia. Schizophr Bull 1998;24(3):443–55.

[120] Weickert TW, Goldberg TE, Gold JM, et al. Cognitive impairments in patients with schizophrenia displaying preserved and compromised intellect. Arch Gen Psychiatry 2000; 57(9):907–13.

[121] Nopoulos P, Flashman L, Flaum M, et al. Stability of cognitive functioning early in the course of schizophrenia. Schizophr Res 1994;14(1):29–37.

[122] Heaton R, Paulsen JS, McAdams LA, et al. Neuropsychological deficits in schizophrenics. Relationship to age, chronicity, and dementia. Arch Gen Psychiatry 1994;51(6): 469–76.

[123] Rund BR. A review of longitudinal studies of cognitive functions in schizophrenia patients. Schizophr Bull 1998;24(3):425–35.

[124] Purohit DP, Perl DP, Haroutunian V, et al. Alzheimer disease and related neurodegenerative diseases in elderly patients with schizophrenia: a postmortem neuropathologic study of 100 cases. Arch Gen Psychiatry 1998;55(3):205–11.

[125] Friedman JI, Harvey PD, McGurk SR, et al. Correlates of change in functional status of institutionalized geriatric schizophrenic patients: focus on medical comorbidity. Am J Psychiatry 2002;159(8):1388–94.

[126] Davidson M, Harvey P, Welsh KA, et al. Cognitive functioning in late-life schizophrenia: a comparison of elderly schizophrenic patients and patients with Alzheimer's disease. Am J Psychiatry 1996;153(10):1274–9.

[127] DeLisi LE, Sakuma M, Maurizio AM, et al. Cerebral ventricular change over the first 10 years after the onset of schizophrenia. Psychiatry Res 2004;130(1):57–70.

[128] Rapoport JL, Giedd JN, Blumenthal J, et al. Progressive cortical change during adolescence in childhood-onset schizophrenia. A longitudinal magnetic resonance imaging study. Arch Gen Psychiatry 1999;56(7):649–54.

[129] Davis KL, Buchsbaum MS, Shihabuddin L, et al. Ventricular enlargement in poor-outcome schizophrenia. Biol Psychiatry 1998;43(11):783–93.

[130] Lieberman J, Chakos M, Wu H, et al. Longitudinal study of brain morphology in first episode schizophrenia. Biol Psychiatry 2001;49(6):487–99.

[131] Fucetola R, Seidman LJ, Kremen WS, et al. Age and neuropsychologic function in schizophrenia: a decline in executive abilities beyond that observed in healthy volunteers. Biol Psychiatry 2000;48(2):137–46.

[132] Granholm E, Morris S, Asarnow RF, et al. Accelerated age-related decline in processing resources in schizophrenia: evidence from pupillary responses recorded during the span of apprehension task. J Int Neuropsychol Soc 2000;6(1):30–43.

[133] Keefe RS, Goldberg TE, Harvey PD, et al. The brief assessment of cognition in schizophrenia: reliability, sensitivity, and comparison with a standard neurocognitive battery. Schizophr Res 2004;68(2–3):283–97.

[134] Velligan DI, DiCocco M, Bow-Thomas CC, et al. A brief cognitive assessment for use with schizophrenia patients in community clinics. Schizophr Res 2004;71(2–3):273–83.

[135] Hegarty JD, Baldessarini RJ, Tohen M, et al. One hundred years of schizophrenia: a meta-analysis of the outcome literature. Am J Psychiatry 1994;151(10):1409–16.

[136] Dickinson D, Coursey RD. Independence and overlap among neurocognitive correlates of community functioning in schizophrenia. Schizophr Res 2002;56(1–2):161–70.

[137] Evans JD, Heaton RK, Paulsen JS, et al. The relationship of neuropsychological abilities to specific domains of functional capacity in older schizophrenia patients. Biol Psychiatry 2003;53(5):422–30.

[138] Nuechterlein KH, Barch DM, Gold JM, et al. Identification of separable cognitive factors in schizophrenia. Schizophr Res 2004;72(1):29–39.

[139] Patterson TL, Goldman S, McKibbin CL, et al. UCSD Performance-Based Skills Assessment: development of a new measure of everyday functioning for severely mentally ill adults. Schizophr Bull 2001;27(2):235–45.

[140] Jin H, Zisook S, Palmer BW, et al. Association of depressive symptoms with worse functioning in schizophrenia: a study in older outpatients. J Clin Psychiatry 2001;62(10): 797–803.

[141] McKibbin C, Patterson TL, Jeste DV. Assessing disability in older patients with schizophrenia: results from the WHODAS-II. J Nerv Ment Dis 2004;192(6):405–13.

[142] Heaton RK, Marcotte TD, Mindt MR, et al. The impact of HIV-associated neuro-psychological impairment on everyday functioning. J Int Neuropsychol Soc 2004;10(3): 317–31.

[143] Harvey PD, Keefe RS. Studies of cognitive change in patients with schizophrenia following novel antipsychotic treatment. Am J Psychiatry 2001;158(2):176–84.

[144] Harvey PD, Bowie CR, Loebel A. Neuropsychological normalization with long-term atypical antipsychotic treatment: results of a 6-month randomized double-blind comparison of ziprasidone vs. olanzapine. J Neuropsychiatry Clin Neurosci, in press.

[145] Velligan DI, Prihoda TJ, Sui D, et al. The effectiveness of quetiapine versus conventional antipsychotics in improving cognitive and functional outcomes in standard treatment settings. J Clin Psychiatry 2003;64(5):524–31.

[146] Hogarty GE, Flesher S, Ulrich R, et al. Cognitive enhancement therapy for schizophrenia: effects of a 2-year randomized trial on cognition and behavior. Arch Gen Psychiatry 2004; 61(9):866–76.

[147] Wykes T, Reeder C, Williams C, et al. Are the effects of cognitive remediation therapy (CRT) durable? Results from an exploratory trial in schizophrenia. Schizophr Res 2003; 61(2–3):163–74.

[148] Fiszdon JM, Bryson GJ, Wexler BE, et al. Durability of cognitive remediation training in schizophrenia: performance on two memory tasks at 6-month and 12-month follow-up. Psychiatry Res 2004;125(1):1–7.

[149] Wexler BE, Hawkins KA, Rounsaville B, et al. Normal neurocognitive performance after extended practice in patients with schizophrenia. Schizophr Res 1997;26(2–3):173–80.

[150] Velligan DI, Bow-Thomas CC, Huntzinger C, et al. Randomized controlled trial of the use of compensatory strategies to enhance adaptive functioning in outpatients with schizophrenia. Am J Psychiatry 2000;157(8):1317–23.

ELSEVIER
SAUNDERS

Psychiatr Clin N Am 28 (2005) 635–651

PSYCHIATRIC
CLINICS
OF NORTH AMERICA

# Frontal Lobe Seizures

## Barbara C. Jobst, MD, Peter D. Williamson, MD*

*Section of Neurology, Dartmouth Epilepsy Program, Dartmouth-Hitchcock Medical Center,
One Medical Center Drive, Lebanon, NH 03756, USA*

Frontal lobe seizures are relatively common. Approximately 20% of patients admitted to epilepsy surgery programs have frontal lobe seizures [1,2]. They can present with a variety of at least six distinctively different seizure types [3]. Some of these seizure types, such as focal clonic motor seizures, are readily identifiable, others are more difficult to recognize. This article focuses on frontal lobe bizarre hyperactive seizures, supplementary motor area (SMA) seizures, and frontal lobe absence seizures, which in the past, often were confused with nonepileptic events [3–6]. In the case of frontal lobe bizarre hyperactive seizures and SMA seizures, the findings on electroencephalography (EEG) often are normal or nonspecific, both between and during seizures. Clinical presentation and clinical seizure characteristics therefore are used initially to identify these seizure types. In the case of prolonged frontal lobe absence seizures, the routine scalp EEG is crucial for the diagnosis.

The following overview describes the clinical presentation, diagnosis, and treatment of these types of frontal lobe seizures that might be confused with psychogenic disorders. The clinical presentation of psychogenic nonepileptic seizures (NES) also will be examined briefly and compared with frontal lobe seizures.

## Anatomy of the frontal lobes

The frontal lobes are the largest cortical region from which seizures can arise. They comprise approximately 40% of the entire cerebral cortex and reach from the anterior pole of the brain to the sylvian fissure inferiorly and the central sulcus posteriorly. Large orbital and medial cortical surfaces generally are inaccessible to the standard EEG recording. These surfaces are

---

* Corresponding author.
*E-mail address:* peter.d.williamson@hitchcock.org (P.D. Williamson).

doi:10.1016/j.psc.2005.05.012

divided into three anatomical regions [6]: the medial frontal region: consisting of the primary leg motor area, the supplementary motor area: and the remainder of the anterior mesial frontal surface, including the cingulate gyrus (Fig. 1). The remainder of the frontal cortex is divided into the dorsolateral region, the primary motor cortex, with face and hand motor representation, the frontopolar region, and the orbitofrontal region (Fig. 2). Frontal lobe seizures can have different clinical manifestations, depending to some extent, on where in the frontal lobes they arise.

## Clinical characteristics of frontal lobe seizures

### General characteristics of frontal lobe seizures

Frontal lobe seizures can present with a variety of different clinical manifestations, but there are some characteristics that are common to frontal lobe seizures of interest in this discussion. Generally, these frontal lobe seizures are brief, frequent, and occur in clusters [3,5,7]. Seizures often last less than 1 minute. Patients may experience clusters of many seizures in a row, with intermittent relatively seizure-free periods. Studies [3,5,8] have shown that frontal lobe seizures are significantly shorter than temporal lobe seizures are, rarely lasting longer than 1 minute. There often is a definite nocturnal preponderance and an association with sleep. Patients frequently describe seizures recurring throughout the night. Occasionally, seizures are exclusively nocturnal. Laskowitz and colleagues [9] have reported clustering

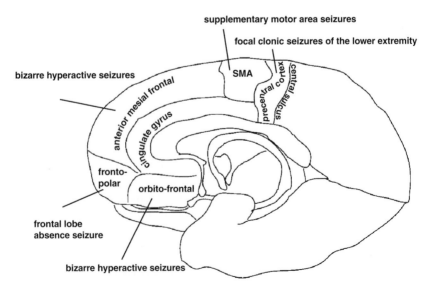

Fig. 1. Medial view of the anatomy of the frontal lobes and related seizures.

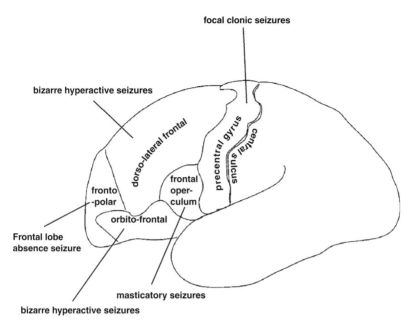

Fig. 2. Lateral view of the anatomy of the frontal lobes and related seizures.

in 50% of patients and a nocturnal preponderance in 38% of patients with frontal lobe seizures, but no daytime seizures were reported.

Frontal lobe seizures of all types tend to be associated with convulsive and nonconvulsive status epilepticus [10,11]. Nonconvulsive status epilepticus with variably altered consciousness lasting for hours or even days, a type of frontal lobe absence, is observed in some patients with frontal lobe seizures [10,12].

In the past, frontal lobe seizures have been described frequently as secondarily generalized [13]. However, recent studies could not confirm this observation. Secondarily generalized seizures are seen with seizure disorders originating in the frontal lobes but do not occur more frequently than seizures originating in other parts of the brain (eg, the temporal lobes) [14,15].

Consciousness often is preserved in certain types of frontal lobe seizures, especially if seizures are brief or do not secondarily generalize or do not spread outside of the frontal lobe [3,5,7]. Often, the patient may be fully conscious but unable to speak. In other patients, vocalization is a prominent part of the seizure. Even when consciousness is impaired, there often is no post-ictal confusion.

There is no specific aura associated with any type of frontal lobe seizure [3,5]. Patients with frontal lobe seizures often describe a nonspecific feeling that is nonlocalized or localized to the head [3]. In a series [3] of 26 patients with frontal lobe seizures, 31% of patients had no aura, whereas the remaining patients reported nonlocalized head feelings, fear, autonomic symptoms, somatosensory symptoms, and sensations localized to the chest. A similar study reported an aura in 56% of patients with frontal lobe seizures [9]. Other authors [16,17] report auras such as visual illusions, dizziness, and epigastric sensations. Quesney and colleagues [17] have associated somatosensory auras with parasagittal seizure onset, but all of the other frontal lobe auras were considered non localizing.

*Bizarre hyperactive seizures (hypermotor or complex partial seizures of frontal lobe origin)*

Bizarre, hyperactive, frontal lobe seizures with complex motor behaviors recently have been better defined, which has helped in identification and diagnosis [3,7]. These seizures also are termed hypermotor seizures or complex partial seizures of frontal lobe origin [18]. Tharp [19] was among the first to recognize these types of seizures in three children who had bizarre motor seizures with presumed seizure onset in the orbitofrontal regions. All three of these children were initially believed to have psychiatric disorders and received prolonged inappropriate treatment before the correct diagnosis was made. Other descriptions of bizarre hyperactive seizures followed shortly thereafter [20,21] and were delineated in detail in the mid 1980s by Williamson and colleagues and Waterman and colleagues [4,5].

The bizarre hyperactive frontal lobe seizures are variably preceded by an unspecific aura. With or without auras, the patients will suddenly and sometimes explosively exhibit behavioral automatisms consisting of very complex behavior. They may jump out of bed, run around, show bicycling movements, pound on objects, rock back and forth, or thrash about the bed. Pelvic thrusting is common (Table 1). Automatisms are repetitive, stereotyped, and frequently have a demonstrative component [7]. During those automatisms, the patient often is awake but unable to control motor behavior [3–5]. The patient may have prominent, sometimes explosive, vocalization, with yelling, screaming, shouted obscenities, growling, barking, and laughing [3,5,9]. Aggressive sexual automatisms can be observed [22], but sexual sensations are never reported. Urinary incontinence may occur. Frontal lobe seizures often end as suddenly as they begin, with little if any post-ictal period [3]. The complex, emotional appearing behaviors could easily suggest the diagnosis of nonepileptic psychogenic events to untrained observers, particularly when there are no surface EEG changes.

Bizarre hyperactive seizures can occur in clusters out of sleep. They can be exclusively nocturnal and disrupt sleep, and they can at times be followed by secondary generalization [3]. Bizarre hyperactive seizures have been associated mostly with seizure onset in the orbitofrontal cortex and the anterior medial frontal regions, including the cingulate gyrus [2,7,23]. However, they also have been described with onset in all other areas of the frontal lobe except the precentral gyrus. Ictal behavior can be the result of

Table 1
Examples of clinical manifestations of bizarre hyperactive seizures in patients who underwent epilepsy surgery

| Age of onset, gender | Clinical manifestations | Average duration of seizures (s) | Other characteristics | Seizure origin | Pathology |
|---|---|---|---|---|---|
| 11 yo F | Fear and "buzzing" feeling localized to head, explosive onset with yelling, squealing, grunting, sexual automatisms, rocking, hand flapping, hopping up and down in bed, need to hug | 17 | Nocturnal, history of nonconvulsive status epilepticus | Orbitofrontal | Ganglioglioma |
| 17 yo M | Claps hands, sitting up, rocking, loud shouting vocalization, thrashing to R, extreme rocking with persistent loud roaring vocalization, staring, speech arrest | 68 | History of nonconvulsive status epilepticus | Orbitofrontal | Cytoarchitectural abnormalities |
| 13 yo F | "Spacey feeling in head" heavy breathing sighs, vocalization, grunting, sighing, mild thrashing, moving on stomach, no impairment of consciousness, occasional urinary incontinence | 27 | Nocturnal | Anterior mesial frontal | Ganglioglioma |
| 12 yo F | Fear and chest pressure, screaming, thrashing, occasional urinary incontinence | 39 | | Frontopolar | Heterotopia |

*Data from* Jobst BC, Siegel AM, Thadani VM, et al. Intractable seizures of frontal lobe origin. Epilepsia 2000;41(9):1139–52.

propagation of the electrical seizure discharge and may not necessarily correlate to the site of seizure origin. Therefore, hyperactive bizarre behavior may be the result of propagation rather than an indication of the site of seizure onset [3].

## Focal clonic seizures and epilepsia partialis continua

Focal clonic seizures consist of clonic movements, commonly of the face but also of unilateral extremities. These are the seizures described originally by Jackson in 1969, who later coined the term "Jacksonian march." The focal clonic activity may spread according to the cortical representation (homunculus of motor function). For example, if seizures start in the hand area of the primary motor cortex, they then may spread caudally to the face area, as well as rostrally to the leg area. Clinically, the seizure may start with clonic movement in the hand and arm that later during the seizure extend to the face, as well as the leg. Those focal clonic seizures tend to persist for longer periods of time. If focal clonic seizures do not subside, the condition is called "epilepsy partialis continua"; this is associated with certain hemispheric syndromes such as Rasmussen's syndrome.

## Tonic (supplementary motor area) seizures

Seizures originating in the SMA have a distinct clinical pattern, with sudden tonic posturing of one or more extremities [24]. Initially, Penfield and Welch [25] described SMA seizures as asymmetrical tonic posturing with the head turning to the side of the extended arm. However, bilateral symmetrical tonic posturing also can be observed (Fig. 3) [3,26]. Head and eye deviation to the side contralateral to the seizure origin is common,

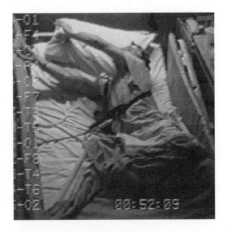

Fig. 3. Bilateral symmetrical upper-extremity tonic posturing in a supplementary motor area seizure that started with tonic activity in the right arm.

therefore the patient's head typically is deviated to the extended arm. Head and eye deviations are not always consistently contralateral and also can occur ipsilateral [27,28]. These seizures usually are brief, lasting 15 to 20 seconds [26,29], and the patient may be fully conscious throughout the seizure. Although speech arrest is the rule, vocalization can occur and, if so, it can be quite loud and explosive. Tonic seizures can be preceded by an aura of unilateral or bilateral sensory symptoms, described as "pulling, pulsing, heaviness, numbness, [and] tingling" [24]. This observation led to the suggestion that these seizures be called "supplementary sensorimotor area seizures" [29]. These brief, frequent seizures often have a nocturnal preponderance and occur in clusters of as many as 100 per night. They often appear to untrained observers as generalized tonic-clonic convulsions. Although tonic-clonic seizures with secondary generalization can occur [3], the brief tonic activity with superimposed clonic movements often does not represent secondary generalization, particularly if the patient remains conscious throughout the entire event.

Although tonic seizures are associated with seizure onset in the supplementary motor area, similar clinical seizure manifestations can be the result of seizure spread to the supplementary motor area from elsewhere [30]. Therefore, not all of these seizures necessarily originate in the supplementary motor area [3,30]. Furthermore, asymmetrical tonic seizures can occur without supplementary motor area involvement [31]. Despite these exceptions, most asymmetrical tonic seizures with nocturnal clustering will originate in the supplementary motor area.

The supplementary motor area is located on the mesial surface of the frontal lobe, and because of this, ictal and inter-ictal EEG findings often do not project to the surface [32]. Even if EEG changes occur during seizures, they often are obscured by muscle and movement artifacts. The absence of EEG findings may erroneously suggest the diagnosis of psychogenic nonepileptic seizures, but the distinct clinical patterns should strongly imply the correct diagnosis, if the investigator is familiar with them [33]. As with bizarre hyperactive frontal lobe seizures, asymmetrical tonic seizures are stereotyped and brief, with a nocturnal preponderance. Therefore, they should be recognizable by history alone. Because asymmetrical tonic seizures usually do not impair consciousness, even when they occur bilaterally, it should not be assumed that bilateral tonic activity without the loss of consciousness is of nonepileptic origin.

## Frontal lobe absence and spike-wave stupor

Frontal lobe seizures can present as simple staring or absence spells. Patients can be completely unresponsive and without motor activity throughout those episodes [7]. Conversely, patients can present with variable responsiveness, appearing to be in a trance-like state with mild confusion, responding to their surroundings, or appearing to move more slowly and to be somewhat disoriented. Frontal lobe absences can be prolonged, lasting minutes, hours, or days. Often, they terminate in a generalized convulsion. These seizures can be confused with encephalopathic states or psychogenic unresponsiveness, but in frontal lobe absence seizures, the EEG always shows a clear, persistent, frontally predominant irregular spike-wave pattern, termed "spike-wave stupor" [4]. Frontal lobe absence seizures are associated with onset in the frontopolar or medial frontal regions. They probably present much more commonly as nonconvulsive status epilepticus than the current literature would suggest.

## Causes and pathophysiology

Frontal lobe seizures can be caused by a variety of intracranial abnormalities involving the frontal lobes (Box 1). Such abnormalities include tumors, vascular malformations, cortical dysplasias or posttraumatic abnormalities (Fig. 4).

Frontal lobe seizures of all types can be observed on MRI of patients who do not have clear abnormalities, which represent a type of cryptogenic epilepsy. It has been speculated that in cryptogenic epilepsy, seizures are caused by subtle abnormalities in neuronal cortical organization that are below the resolution capabilities of conventional MRI.

There is no outstanding risk factor for frontal lobe seizures, nor is there a specific association with febrile seizures or previous cerebral infection [14]. Significant head trauma historically has been considered a significant risk factor for frontal lobe seizures [34], but this was not confirmed by a recent study [3].

A family history of epilepsy is of significance only if the patient suffers from autosomal dominant frontal lobe epilepsy. Frontal lobe seizures can occur in all age groups depending on the underlying cause. Cryptogenic, nonlesional frontal lobe epilepsy and autosomal dominant frontal lobe epilepsy usually manifest during the teenage years, but they can begin during the first decade of life.

### Autosomal dominant nocturnal frontal lobe epilepsy

Autosomal dominant nocturnal frontal lobe epilepsy (ADNFLE) is the only identified genetic syndrome associated with frontal lobe seizures.

---

**Box 1. Causes of frontal lobe seizures**

Autosomal dominant frontal lobe epilepsy (channelopathy)
Cryptogenic (nonlesional)
Rasmussen's encephalitis
Symptomatic (tumor, vascular malformation, posttraumatic)

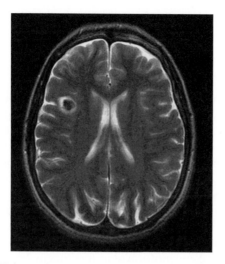

Fig. 4. T2-weighted MR image shows a dysembryoplastic neuroepithelial tumor causing frontal lobe epilepsy.

Clinically, the syndrome presents with typical frontal lobe seizures of the bizarre hyperactive type or with asymmetrical tonic seizures [35]. Seizures are brief, frequent, and nocturnal. Seizures start in the teenage years and usually respond well even to small doses of antiepileptic medications. A dominant family history of frontal lobe seizures is implied with the diagnosis.

Missense mutations of the gene for the neuronal nicotinic acetylcholine receptor $\alpha_4$ subunit (*CHRNA4*) on chromosomes 20q13.2 and 15q24 or the $\beta2$ subunit on chromosome 1 (*CHRNB2*) were found to be responsible for the syndrome [36]. It has been suggested that the ADNFLE mutations reduce $Ca^{2+}$ potentiation of the neuronal nicotinic acetylcholine receptor. Reducing the $Ca^{2+}$ dependence of the acetylcholine response could trigger seizures by increasing $\alpha_4\beta_2$-mediated glutamate release [37]. In this situation, a channelopathy is responsible for localization-related epilepsy.

*Rasmussen's encephalitis*

Rasmussen's encephalitis is an inflammatory disease of the brain that often presents with unilateral focal motor seizures, especially with epilepsia partialis continua. Unilateral clonic motor activity can last from days to weeks. Brain inflammation is unilateral, affecting only one hemisphere, but the disease is progressive, and seizures ultimately become more extensive with more complex motor activity and the loss of consciousness. Cognitive impairment and progressive hemiparesis are later manifestations. Progression ultimately may result in coma and death. The age of onset can vary. On neuroimaging, progressive atrophy of the affected hemisphere can be noted.

The cause of this devastating syndrome is unknown, and an autoimmune cause has been suggested. However treatment trials of steroids and immunoglobulins remain unsuccessful. Only hemipherectomy (removal of one hemisphere) has shown to be effective.

## Diagnostic evaluation

Since frontal lobe seizures of the type discussed here have typical clinical characteristics, they usually can be recognized by the experienced physician by history alone. The importance of a thorough history cannot be overemphasized. A history of stereotyped, brief, nocturnal episodes strongly suggests seizures of frontal lobe origin [3]. Preserved consciousness during bilateral motor activity suggests SMA seizures, although the possibility of NES should also be considered.

EEG can guide in making the diagnosis of frontal lobe seizures, but at times it can be misleading because inter-ictal and ictal EEG changes may be absent or nonspecific. Initial outpatient, standard EEG in any type of focal epilepsy detects only inter-ictal epileptiform abnormalities in 29% to 55% of patients [38–40]. In one study [9], prolonged video-EEG monitoring demonstrated inter-ictal epileptiform abnormalities in 81% of patients in a selected population with frontal lobe seizures. Those abnormalities were restricted to one frontal lobe, although inter-ictal EEG abnormalities can be diffuse and bilateral in frontal lobe seizures. Epileptiform inter-ictal discharges may occur in various multilobar locations [7,9,41] or not be accessible to surface EEG recording, as in seizures originating in the medial frontal cortex [42]. In a series of 11 patients with seizure originating in the supplementary motor area, only one patient had inter-ictal EEG abnormalities [24].

Ictal surface EEG findings can be as variable and misleading as inter-ictal EEG [43] because there are areas of involvement of the frontal lobe that are inaccessible to surface EEG. Also, frontal lobe seizures can be associated with complex prominent motor activity, which is associated with muscle artifact that may obscure EEG findings. Several case series [9,24,43] have reported no ictal EEG change in 33% to 36% of patients. This is more likely to occur if the seizures originate in the medial region or in the bifrontal region and the cingulum [42]. Furthermore, the rapid spread of ictal epileptiform discharges to other areas of the brain can lead to false localization or lateralization of seizure onset. Video-EEG monitoring can be used to better analyze clinical seizure characteristics and the correlation with EEG changes; if there is a lack of EEG correlation, intracranial recording may be indicated, unless neuroimaging or surface EEG recordings provide some localizing information. In summary, it is very important to recognize that a normal or nonspecific EEG, even during obvious clinical seizure activity, can be compatible with the diagnosis of certain types of frontal lobe seizures [26].

Some seizures that originate in the mesial frontal lobe usually have minimal or absent EEG changes. The use of additional montages that record activity over the vertex (transverse montages) may be helpful to localize seizure onset [7]. If seizures originate on the dorsolateral region, ictal EEG is more likely to be abnormal [42]. Various ictal EEG patterns have been described. Voltage attenuation (electrodecremental response) is the most frequent pattern, but other patterns such as rhythmic α or θ activity, diffuse spike, or spike and wave discharges also have been observed. These abnormalities are only infrequently localizing to a specific area within the frontal lobes; more often, they are diffuse and bilateral [5,42–44]. Prolonged frontal lobe absence seizures, however, always have an associated irregular spike-wave pattern [7]. In this situation, ictal EEG will identify these seizures and differentiate them from psychogenic unresponsiveness.

High-resolution MRI, which can identify lesions in the frontal lobe such as tumors or vascular malformations, is imperative for the evaluation of frontal lobe seizures [45]. MRI should include sequences to better identify dysplasias (eg, fluid-attenuated inversion-recovery sequences), vascular malformations, and blood products (eg, proton density imaging). However, the MRI scan often appears normal in patients with frontal lobe seizures compared with patients with temporal lobe seizures [46]. Higher resolution T3-weighted MRI may improve the identification of lesions responsible for frontal lobe seizures [47]. Because frontal lobe seizures often are related to cortical dysplasias, newer multimodal imaging techniques using diffusion tensor imaging [48] and reformatting [49] also can enhance the identification of these lesions.

Other imaging techniques such as fluorode oxyglucose-positron emission tomography (FDG-PET) and ictal single photon emission-computed tomography (SPECT) can be used to help localize frontal lobe seizures. However, those modalities usually are used only if a diagnosis of epilepsy has already been established and the patient is being considered for epilepsy surgery. FDG-PET is much less likely to identify focal abnormalities in patients with frontal lobe seizures compared with patients with temporal lobe seizures [50,51]. Ictal SPECT is logistically difficult to perform, requiring early injection of a radioactive tracer during a seizure. However, if it is properly obtained, SPECT can contribute valuable information to identifying the seizure onset zone, particularly if it is coregistered with MRI [52,53]. MRI is indispensable in any type of neocortical epilepsy.

The gold standard for identifying and characterizing frontal lobe seizures still is video-EEG monitoring. This procedure usually requires admission to a specialized video-EEG monitoring unit [3,5,11]. When seizures are recorded, evaluating clinical manifestations in combination with EEG findings should help to establish the correct diagnosis. Magnetoencephalography is another adjuvant diagnostic test that can identify regions of seizure onset.

## Differential diagnosis and distinction from psychiatric disorders

Frontal lobe seizure can present with bizarre behavioral automatisms or bilateral tonic motor activity with minimal or no EEG findings and no MRI abnormalities. These seizures often can be mistaken for psychogenic non-epileptic events [5,19].

A psychogenic NES is the most important diagnostic consideration in differentiating from frontal lobe seizures. Clinically, NES differ from frontal lobe seizures in that they are less stereotyped and longer in duration and are associated with waxing and waning in-and out-of-phase motor activity with variable responsiveness (Table 2). In psychogenic NES, unresponsiveness often is associated with uncoordinated, violent, and disorganized behavior [54,55]. Conversely, one third of patients can exhibit psychogenic motionless unresponsiveness [56]. Motor activity during NES has been described as being more asynchronous (out of phase) than clonic epileptic activity [55]. Most series report that more women than men have psychogenic NES (4:1 to 3:2 ratio, respectively) [57]. However, two reports describe an equal ratio of men to women [58,59].

Several studies have compared frontal lobe seizures to nonepileptic seizures [60,61]. Saygi and colleagues [61] did not find a statistically

Table 2
Differential diagnosis of bizarre hyperactive seizures and psychogenic non-epileptic seizures

| Characteristics | Bizarre hyperactive frontal lobe seizures | Psychogenic non-epileptic seizures |
| --- | --- | --- |
| Duration | Brief (≤60 s) | Variable |
| Frequency | Frequent, in clusters | Variable, commonly clusters |
| Time of occurrence | Nocturnal preponderance, often out of sleep | Out of wakefulness |
| Motor manifestations | Bizarre but stereotyped | Variable: out-of-phase and in-phase shaking, flailing, jerking common |
| Speech | Explosive vocalization or speech arrest | Slurred speech or other variable vocalization, may be able to talk through event |
| Consciousness | Often preserved | Confusion and altered consciousness, waxing and waning |
| Post-ictal period | Recollection of event if no loss of consciousness; only brief or no post-ictal period | May recall event |
| Associated features | Secondary generalization possible; clonic or tonic features | Pain syndromes, psychiatric disease, especially PTSD |
| Age of onset | Childhood and adolescence | Adulthood ≥ childhood |
| Gender ratio | Male = female | Female ≥ male |
| Psychiatric comorbidity | Depression common | PTSD, conversion, factitious disorder, malingering, depression |
| Spontaneous remission | Uncommon | Possible |
| EEG changes | Common but may lack | Normal |
| MRI | Possibly structural abnormality | Normal |

significant difference in the occurrence of pelvic thrusting, body movements, and side-to-side head movements, but they found that turning to a prone position occurred only with frontal lobe seizures. Nocturnal occurrence, brevity of the seizure, younger age of onset, and stereotypy suggested epileptic events [61]. Because frontal lobe seizures are associated with sleep, it would seem intuitive that events out of sleep would be unlikely to represent psychogenic NES. However, it may be difficult to distinguish whether an event occurs directly out of sleep or after a brief arousal [62]. EEG remains normal throughout NES or often shows muscle artifact. As described previously, EEG and MRI can show normal results in patients with frontal lobe seizures, making the diagnosis at times a challenging one.

There is a high incidence of psychiatric comorbidity in patients with psychogenic NES. Concurrent psychiatric diagnoses are present in 43% to 100% of patients, depending on the study [57]. Psychiatric diagnoses such as posttraumatic stress disorder (PTSD), somatoform disorders, dissociative and personality disorders, and mood disorders have been described in association with NES [54,57]. A history of trauma, especially childhood sexual abuse, has been correlated with NES [63]; however, no well-controlled study has shown a definite relationship.

Whether psychogenic NES are conscious or unconscious phenomena has been debated [63]. However a significant percentage of these patients meets *Diagnostic and Statistical Manual of Mental Disorders, Fourth Edition,* criteria for a conversion disorder. Therefore, the clinician should be strongly cautioned against drawing conclusions, and these patients represent a classic example of a condition in which neurology and psychiatry can work together in providing optimum patient care.

Frontal lobe bizarre hyperactive seizures are stereotypic, brief, and occur in clusters, with a nocturnal preponderance. These features can help to differentiate them from psychogenic NES [33,64]. Tonic seizures originating in the supplementary motor area often are misinterpreted as being psychogenic because they present with brief bilateral tonic activity without the loss of consciousness. The fact that consciousness is preserved during bilateral motor activity is common in these seizures and does not indicate a psychogenic cause. Prolonged frontal lobe absence status can be misinterpreted as a dissociative episode or fugue state. However, it is always associated with clear EEG abnormalities, which can help distinguish it from a psychiatric disease.

Prolactin levels have been used in the past to distinguish psychogenic NES from epilepsy. The prolactin level is elevated up to 10 times the normal level if it is measured 15 to 20 min after a generalized convulsion [65]. It is less frequently abnormal after focal seizures. Frontal lobe seizures may be too brief to result in a change in prolactin levels [66]. Also, there is an increased rate of false-positives in the psychiatric population resulting from the intake of psychotropic medications. Therefore, the clinical value of prolactin levels is limited in this situation. If there is any doubt about the distinction of frontal lobe seizures versus psychogenic NES, video-EEG monitoring should be initiated to assure the correct diagnosis.

Several years ago, paroxysmal nocturnal dystonia was described as a movement disorder that responded well to carbamazepine. However, most of those cases in fact represent a form of frontal lobe epilepsy, possibly a subset of autosomal dominant frontal lobe epilepsy.

Parasomnias, especially night terrors, are an important differential diagnosis in children. Video-EEG monitoring or a sleep study with video monitoring can identify those disorders.

## Treatment

Cryptogenic nonlesional frontal lobe seizures are treated with standard antiepileptic medications. No single antiepileptic medication has been shown to be superior or specific for frontal lobe seizures. Both older antiepileptic medications such as phenytoin, carbamazepine, and valproic acid as well as newer antiepileptic medications like lamotrigine, topiramate, zonisamide, and levetiracetam are effective for frontal lobe seizures, with different side effect profiles. Autosomal dominant frontal lobe epilepsy is treated preferentially with carbamazepine, but other antiepileptic medications are equally effective. Focal motor seizures can be refractory to antiepileptic treatment. Phenobarbital can be very helpful in cases of epilepsia partialis continua.

If frontal lobe epilepsy is refractory to medications, epilepsy surgery should be considered. If the MRI is normal, this condition will require much more extensive diagnostic evaluations with ictal SPECT and intracranial EEG studies. These procedures are performed only at specialized epilepsy centers. If, with the help of intracranial EEG, the seizure onset zone is located and subsequently resected, the success rate for a seizure-free outcome after surgery varies from 50% to 75% [3,32]. If resective surgery cannot be performed, then other adjuvant surgical therapies such as a vagal nerve stimulator implantation or corpus callosotomy can be considered. A vagal nerve stimulator reduces seizure frequency by 50% in 50% of patients. An anterior callosotomy, a procedure in which the anterior two thirds of the corpus callosum is sectioned, can dramatically reduce seizures and the frequency and injuries resulting from falling during seizures.

## Summary

Despite the fact that clinical characteristics of frontal lobe seizures have been recently described better, differentiating seizures of frontal lobe origin from NES on clinical grounds alone is difficult. The difficulty has been compounded by the fact that both inter-ictal and ictal EEG can be normal or nonspecific, and the same is true of imaging studies. A detailed clinical history as well as video monitoring can be helpful diagnostic tools. A multidisciplinary approach is warranted and is at times essential to improve the diagnosis and care of these difficult patients.

## References

[1] Behrens E, Schramm J, Zentner J, et al. Surgical and neurological complications of 708 epilepsy procedures. Neurosurgery 1998;42:675–6.

[2] Manford M, Fish DR, Shorvon SD. An analysis of clinical seizure patterns and their localizing value in frontal and temporal lobe epilepsies. Brain 1996;119:17–40.

[3] Jobst BC, Siegel AM, Thadani VM, et al. Intractable seizures of frontal lobe origin. Epilepsia 2000;41(9):1139–52.

[4] Waterman K, Purves SJ, Kosaka B, et al. An epileptic syndrome caused by mesial frontal lobe foci. Neurology 1987;37:577–82.

[5] Williamson PD, Spencer DD, Spencer SS, et al. Complex partial seizures of frontal lobe origin. Ann Neurol 1985;18:497–504.

[6] Bancaud J, Talairach J. Clinical semiology of frontal lobe seizures. In: Chauvel P, Delgado-Escueta AV, Halgren E, editors. Frontal lobe seizures and epilepsies. New York: Raven Press, Ltd; 1992. p. 3–58.

[7] So NK. Mesial frontal epilepsy. Epilepsia 1998;39(Suppl 4):S49–61.

[8] Niedermeyer E. Frontal lobe epilepsy: the next frontier. Clin Electroencephalogr 1998;29: 163–9.

[9] Laskowitz DT, Sperling MR, French JA, et al. The syndrome of frontal lobe epilepsy: characteristics and surgical management. Neurology 1995;45:780–7.

[10] Williamson PD, Spencer DD, Spencer SS, et al. Complex partial status epilepticus: a depth-electrode study. Ann Neurol 1985;18:647–54.

[11] Williamson PD, Jobst BC. Frontal lobe epilepsy. In: Williamson PD, et al, editor. Advances in neurology. Philadelphia: Lippincott Williams & Wilkins; 2000. p. 215–42.

[12] Kudo T, Sato K, Yagi K, et al. Can absence status epilepticus be of frontal lobe origin? Acta Neurol Scand 1995;92(6):472–7.

[13] Quesney LF, Constain M, Rasmussen T. Seizures from the dorsolateral frontal lobe. In: Chauvel P, et al, editor. Frontal lobe seizures and epilepsies. New York: Raven Press, Ltd; 1992. p. 233–44.

[14] Jobst BC, Neuschwander TB, Thadani VM, et al. Secondarily generalized tonic-clonic seizures: relation to site of seizure origin, pathology and outcome after surgery. Epilepsia 2000;41(Suppl Florence):52.

[15] Herman ST, Walczak TS, Bazil CW. Distribution of partial seizures during the sleep-wake cycle: differences by seizure onset site. Neurology 2001;56:1453–9.

[16] Chauvel P, Delgado-Escueta AV, Halgren E, et al, editors. Frontal lobe seizures and epilepsies: advances in neurology. volume 57. New York: Raven Press, Ltd; 1992.

[17] Quesney LF, Constain M, Fish DR, et al. The clinical differentiation of seizures arising in the parasagittal and anterolaterodorsal frontal convexities. Arch Neurol 1990;47:677–9.

[18] Luders H, Acharya J, Baumgartner C, et al. Semiological seizure classification. Epilepsia 1998;39(9):1006–13.

[19] Tharp BR. Orbital frontal seizures: a unique electroencephalographic and clinical syndrome. Epilepsia 1972;13:627–42.

[20] Geier S, Bancaud J, Talairach J, et al. Automatisms during frontal lobe epileptic seizures. Brain 1976;99:447–58.

[21] Geier S, Bancaud J, Talairach J, et al. The seizures of frontal lobe epilepsy: a study of clinical manifestations. Neurology 1977;27:951–8.

[22] Spencer SS, Spencer DD, Williamson PD, et al. Sexual automatisms in complex partial seizures. Neurology 1983;33(5):527–33.

[23] Ludwig B, Ajmone-Marsan C, Van Buren J. Cerebral seizures of probable orbitofrontal origin. Epilepsia 1972;16:141–58.

[24] Morris HHI, Luders H, Dinner DS, et al. Seizures from the supplementary motor area: clinical and electrographic features. Epilepsia 1987;28:623.

[25] Penfield W, Welch K. The supplementary motor area of the cerebral cortex. AMA Arch Neurol Psychiatry 1951a;66:289–317.

[26] Morris HH, Dinner DS, Lüders H, et al. Supplementary motor seizures: clinical and electroencephalographic findings. Neurology 1988;38:1075–82.

[27] Dinner DS, Lüders H, Morris HH, et al. Human supplementary motor areas (SMA) electrical stimulation study. Epilepsia 1987;28:619.

[28] Wyllie E, Lüders H, Morris HH. The lateralizing significance of versive head and eye movements during epileptic seizures. Neurology 1986;36:606–11.

[29] Bleasel AF, Morris HH. Supplementary sensorimotor area epilepsy in adults. In: Luders HO, editor. Advances in neurology: supplementary sensorimotor area. Philadelphia: Lippincott-Raven; 1996. p. 271–84.

[30] Aghakhani Y, Rosati A, Olivier A, et al. The predictive localizing value of tonic limb posturing in supplementary sensorimotor seizures. Neurology 2004;62(12):2256–61.

[31] Geier S, Bancaud J, Talairach J, et al. Ictal tonic postural changes and automatisms of the upper limb during epileptic parietal lobe discharges. Epilepsia 1977;18:517–24.

[32] Kellinghaus C, Luders HO. Frontal lobe epilepsy. Epileptic Disord 2004;6(4):223–39.

[33] Williamson PD. Psychogenic non-epileptic seizures and frontal seizures: diagnostic considerations. In: Rowan AJ, Gates JR, editors. Non-epileptic seizures. Boston: Butterworth-Heinemann; 1993. p. 55–72.

[34] Pohlmann-Eden B, Bruckmeir J. Predictors and dynamics of posttraumatic epilepsy. Acta Neurol Scandl 1997;95(5):257–62.

[35] Scheffer IE, Bhatia KP, Lopes-Cendes I, et al. Autosomal dominant nocturnal frontal lobe epilepsy: a distinctive clinical disorder. Brain 1995;118(Pt 1):61–73.

[36] Steinlein OK. Nicotinic acetylcholine receptors and epilepsy. Curr Drug Target CNS Neurol Disord 2002;1(4):443–8.

[37] Rodrigues-Pinguet N, Jia L, Li M, et al. Five ADNFLE mutations reduce the Ca2+ dependence of the mammalian alpha4beta2 acetylcholine response. J Physiol 2003;550(Pt 1): 11–26.

[38] Goodin DS, Aminoff MJ, Laxer KD. Detection of epileptiform activity by different noninvasive EEG methods in complex partial epilepsy. Ann Neurol 1990;27(3): 330–4.

[39] Marsan CA, Zivin LS. Factors related to the occurrence of typical paroxysmal abnormalities in the EEG records of epileptic patients. Epilepsia 1970;11(4):361–81.

[40] Salinsky M, Kanter R, Dasheiff RM. Effectiveness of multiple EEGs in supporting the diagnosis of epilepsy: an operational curve. Epilepsia 1987;28(4):331–4.

[41] Westmoreland BF. The EEG findings in extratemporal seizures. Epilepsia 1998;39(Suppl 4): S1–8.

[42] Bautista RE, Spencer DD, Spencer SS. EEG findings in frontal lobe epilepsies. Neurology 1998;50(6):1765–71.

[43] Williamson PD, Spencer SS. Clinical and EEG features of complex partial seizures of extratemporal origin. Epilepsia 1986;27(Suppl 2):S46–63.

[44] Quesney LF, Constain M, Rasmussen T, et al. Presurgical EEG investigation in frontal lobe epilepsy. Epilepsy Res Suppl 1992;5:55–69.

[45] Lorenzo NY, Parisi JE, Cascino GD, et al. Intractable frontal lobe epilepsy: pathological and MRI features. Epilepsy Res 1995;20(2):171–8.

[46] Lawson JA, Cook MJ, Vogrin S, et al. Clinical, EEG, and quantitative MRI differences in pediatric frontal and temporal lobe epilepsy. Neurology 2002;58(5):723–9.

[47] Grant PE. Structural MR imaging. Epilepsia 2004;45(Suppl 4):S4–16.

[48] Dumas de la Roque A, Oppenheim C, Chassoux F, et al. Diffusion tensor imaging of partial intractable epilepsy. Eur Radiol 2005;15(2):279–85.

[49] Bernasconi A. Advanced MRI analysis methods for detection of focal cortical dysplasia. Epileptic Disord 2003;5(Suppl 2):S81–4.

[50] Ryvlin P, Bouvard S, Le Bars D, et al. Clinical utility of flumazenil-PET versus [18F]fluorodeoxyglucose-PET and MRI in refractory partial epilepsy: a prospective study in 100 patients. Brain 1998;12l(Pt 11):2067–81.

[51] Engel JJ, Henry TH, Risinger MW, et al. Presurgical evaluation for partial epilepsy: relative contributions of chronic depth electrode recordings versus FDG-PET and scalp sphenoidal ictal EEG. Neurology 1990;40:1670–7.

[52] Cascino GD, Buchhalter JR, Mullan BP, et al. Ictal SPECT in nonlesional extratemporal epilepsy. Epilepsia 2004;45(Suppl 4):S32–4.

[53] Thadani VM, Siegel A, Lewis P, et al. Validation of ictal single photon emission computed tomography with depth encephalography and epilepsy surgery. Neurosurg Rev 2004;27(1): 27–33.

[54] Meierkord H, Will B, Fish D, et al. The clinical features and prognosis of pseudoseizures diagnosed using video-EEG telemetry. Neurology 1991;41(10):1643–6.

[55] Lesser RP. Psychogenic seizures. Neurology 1996;46(6):1499–507.

[56] Abubakr A, Kablinger A, Caldito G. Psychogenic seizures: clinical features and psychological analysis. Epilepsy Behav 2003;4(3):241–5.

[57] Bowman ES. Psychopathology and outcome in pseudoseizures. In: Ettinger AB, Kanner AM, editors. Psychiatric issues in epilepsy. Philadelphia: Lippincott Williams & Wilkins; 2001. p. 355–78.

[58] Gulick TA, Spinks IP, King DW. Pseudoseizures: ictal phenomena. Neurology 1982;32(1): 24–30.

[59] Leis AA, Ross MA. Psychogenic seizures. Neurology 1992;42(5):1128–9.

[60] Wilkus RJ, Thompson PM, Vossler DG. Bizarre ictal automatisms: frontal lobe epileptic or psychogenic seizures? Journal of Epilepsy 1990;3:207–13.

[61] Saygi S, Katz A, Marks DA, et al. Frontal lobe partial seizures and psychogenic seizures: comparison of clinical and ictal characteristics. Neurology 1992;42:1274–7.

[62] Orbach D, Ritaccio A, Devinsky O. Psychogenic, nonepileptic seizures associated with video-EEG-verified sleep. Epilepsia 2003;44(1):64–8.

[63] Rosenberg HJ, Rosenberg SD, Williamson PD, et al. A comparative study of trauma and posttraumatic stress disorder prevalence in epilepsy patients and psychogenic nonepileptic seizure patients. Epilepsia 2000;41(4):447–52.

[64] Kanner AM, Morris HH, Lüders H, et al. Supplementary motor seizures mimicking pseudoseizures: some clinical differences. Neurology 1990;40:1404–7.

[65] Wyllie E, Luders H, MacMillan JP, et al. Serum prolactin levels after epileptic seizures. Neurology 1984;34(12):1601–4.

[66] Meierkord H, Shorvon S, Lightman S, et al. Comparison of the effects of frontal and temporal lobe partial seizures on prolactin levels. Arch Neurol 1992;49:225–30.

ELSEVIER
SAUNDERS

PSYCHIATRIC
CLINICS
OF NORTH AMERICA

Psychiatr Clin N Am 28 (2005) 653–664

# Nonconvulsive Status Epilepticus: Clinical Features and Diagnostic Challenges

## Silvana Riggio, MD

*Department of Psychiatry, Mount Sinai School of Medicine*
*and Bronx Veterans Medical Center, One Gustave L. Levy Place,*
*Box 1230, New York, NY 10029, USA*

Nonconvulsive status epilepticus (NCSE) is the ultimate condition in which the disciplines of neurology and psychiatry meet and, at times, overlap. The diagnosis may pose a diagnostic challenge, and patient care can greatly benefit from a coordinated approach using the skills brought by multiple specialties. NCSE, once thought to be a relatively rare cause of altered mental status or abnormal behavior, has been described increasingly in the neurology and epilepsy literature, which has heightened awareness of this condition.

Diagnosing NCSE significantly improved in the 1930s when electroencephalography (EEG) became available and allowed a correlation with clinical symptoms. NCSE differs from convulsive status epilepticus in that its presentation is primarily nonmotor, and the outcome is thought to be less grave. The clinical manifestations of NCSE are characterized by a change in behavior that can vary considerably from case to case. These changes range from a mild departure from baseline, to psychotic or affective states, to coma.

Little has been written in the psychiatric literature about NCSE, and only a few texts on neuropsychiatry devote appropriate attention to this entity. NCSE is possibly one of the most frequently missed diagnoses in patients who have a change in mental status. The diagnosis may be missed in part because of the broad range of clinical presentations, in part because of comorbidities, and in part because of limited awareness of this condition. Therefore, a multidisciplinary approach is essential to improve the recognition, diagnosis, and ultimately outcome of NCSE. This article reviews the clinical manifestations of NCSE, its similarities and differences

---

*E-mail address:* silvana.riggio@mssm.edu

0193-953X/05/$ - see front matter © 2005 Elsevier Inc. All rights reserved.
doi:10.1016/j.psc.2005.05.003

with other neurologic and psychiatric conditions, EEG findings, prognosis, and management.

## Definitions

NCSE, like convulsive status epilepticus, is a state of continuous or intermittent seizure activity without a return to baseline lasting more than 30 minutes. In general, NCSE differs from convulsive status epilepticus by the lack of a predominant motor component [1]. The hallmark of NCSE is a change in behavior or mental status that is associated with diagnostic EEG changes.

There are two main types of NCSE: absence status (AS), which is a primary generalized process, and complex partial status (CPS), which is focal in origin. Both AS and CPS are characterized by a change in the level of consciousness and behavior. Onset can be sudden or gradual [2]. The episodes can vary in duration and intensity. In both types of NCSE, abnormal motor activity is either not present or minimal. Unresponsiveness, once thought to be a distinctive feature of CPS [3], has been described in association with AS [4,5], as have cyclic patterns [1]. AS usually is characterized by abrupt clearing of consciousness, although gradual postictal normalization has been reported [2]. CPS is usually followed by a prolonged postictal state with depression.

In early reports, AS was thought to be more common than CPS [6], but this greater prevalence has not been confirmed [1,7]. Rapid generalization of CPS on EEG is the most likely explanation for misdiagnosing cases of CPS as AS, possibly compounded by the relatively limited awareness to this issue [1,8]. AS has been described in children and in adults with differences in both clinical, EEG manifestations and in response to pharmacologic agents. In particular, it has been noted that cases of adult AS have responded to treatment with phenytoin and phenobarbital, which are not known to be efficacious in AS in children. Indeed, anticonvulsants, usually efficacious in the treatment of absence seizures, have not been beneficial in many elderly patients who have AS [9]. There are two possible interpretations for these age-related differences: that the cases diagnosed as AS may actually have been cases of CPS in which the initial focal ictal discharge was not identified because of rapid secondary generalization, or that two distinct entities manifest as AS in the young and the elderly [1].

In summary, considerable overlap is reported in the literature between AS and CPS. The two conditions cannot be differentiated definitively by the timing of the onset or termination of symptoms, cyclic patterns of responsiveness and behavior, intensity of symptoms, the presence or absence of automatisms, or response to specific therapies. Some of the described overlap in clinical presentations may result from misdiagnosis on EEG. Future studies are needed to improve diagnostic accuracy.

## Epidemiology

Generalized convulsive status epilepticus (GCSE) has an incidence of 40 to 80 per 100,000 population. Population-based epidemiologic studies have indicated mortality from GCSE to be almost 22%, and that figure can increase to 30% in the elderly [10]. Although NCSE has been recognized and described for many years, clear data on its true incidence are still lacking. Celesia [6] reported, in a collective review of 2290 patients who had seizures, that 60 patients were in status of which 25% were classified as NCSE. Dunne [11] has reported similar data. Tomson and colleagues [1] found that the yearly incidence of newly diagnosed NCSE in their adult general hospital–based population to be at least 1.5 in 100,000 patients.

Towne and colleagues [8], in a prospective study of 236 patients with coma who had no clinical evidence of seizures, reported that 8% met criteria for NCSE on EEG [8]; DeLorenzo and colleagues [12] found that NCSE was present in 14% of patients after control of GCSE. In a prospective population-based study of status epilepticus, NCSE represented approximately 5% of status epilepticus cases presenting in Richmond, Virginia [13]. In a prospective study of 198 patients who had altered consciousness but no clinical convulsions who were referred for emergency EEG, Privitera and colleagues [14] reported that 37% showed EEG and clinical evidence of NCSE.

NCSE has been reported in all age groups from the very young to the very old and in both sexes without a clear predominance in either sex [8,15–17].

Anywhere from 10% to 100% of patients who present with NCSE do not have a history of seizure disorder [1–3,5,17–19]. It is estimated that 10% of adults with absence seizures will have at least one episode of AS [2,20]. Although AS has been reported most commonly in children, it can present de novo in later life [18,21].

Different precipitating factors have been implicated in NCSE, including metabolic abnormalities, infection, drug toxicity, alcohol intoxication/ withdrawal, pregnancy, central nervous system disturbances, and electro-convulsive treatment [8,21,22]. Different series have indicated that a precipitating factor can be identified in 15% to 70% of cases, emphasizing the importance of assessment in the evaluation of these patients [3,7].

## Clinical characteristics

Clinical manifestations vary considerably, ranging from subtle changes recognizable only to family members, to psychotic or affective states, all the way to delirium or coma [2,3,8,23–26]. The variety of presentations described in the literature include

Mild cognitive disturbances (eg, impaired attention, difficulty in sequential planning of complex motor tasks [27], mild disorientation or confusion [18])

Prolonged confusional states [28]

Mood disturbance [27]

Cortical blindness [29]

Speech disturbance, which can vary from verbal perseveration to reduced verbal fluency, muteness, speech arrest, or aphasia [3,7,27,30]

Echolalia

Confabulation [16]

Bizarre behavior that can be uncharacteristic and deviates from usual (eg, laughing, dancing, and singing inappropriately) [18]

Clear psychotic states [29,31]

Autonomic disturbances such as belching, borborygmus, flatulence

Sensory and psychic phenomena [16]

Symptoms can fluctuate with varying degrees of impairment that at times may obscure the diagnosis.

Motor activity is normal in most cases; however, decreased response time, clumsiness, apraxia, focal jerks, twitching of facial muscles (in particular of the eyelids) and automatisms such as licking, chewing, or picking have been noted [1,31]. When present, automatisms have been thought to be longer in duration and more complex in nature in CPS than in AS [32,33]. Automatisms in the form of gross movements, such as positioning, raising, flexion, or extension of the extremities and head deviation, although not common, have also been noted [1].

The panoply of clinical presentations shows how challenging this diagnosis can be in any circumstance and especially when a patient presents with cognitive impairment at baseline (eg, mental retardation or dementia) or has a history of a psychiatric disorder.

## Diagnostic approach

The differential diagnosis of altered mental status is extensive, and determining the underlying cause on clinical grounds alone is at times almost impossible. Because of the wide range of presentations of NCSE, the diagnosis often is missed, being confused for a psychiatric disorder or a neurologic insult. To put the patient's presentation into the proper context, a detailed history, including change from baseline status, onset and duration of the events, presence or absence of lucid interval, timing in relation to the sleep/wake cycle, and presence or absence of motor activity or automatisms, needs to be obtained. Past medical, neurologic, and psychiatric history, family history, social history, and medication history are additional important components of the diagnostic evaluation.

There are no clear criteria to guide the decision of when an EEG should be requested, but when NCSE is suspected on clinical grounds, an EEG is indicated to confirm the diagnosis and direct management.

In AS, EEG is characterized by continuous or nearly continuous generalized, rhythmic, bilaterally synchronous, spike-and-wave discharges at 3/second intervals with a maximum over the bifrontal region; however, variations in the EEG pattern can occur, including 2 to 3/second spike-wave complexes as well as bursts of rhythmic, slow rhythmic or arrhythmic spike-wave, or polyspike activity [1,17,34,35]. In CPS, various forms of less synchronous seizure activity, rhythmical slowing, rhythmic spikes, and rhythmic sharp and slow waves have been described [1,31,27]. Although several EEG patterns have been described as suggestive of both types of NCSE, a clear pathognomonic pattern has not been defined. When an EEG is performed at the onset of the seizure, a clear focus may be identified that may be critical to differentiating CPS from AS. If secondary generalization is present, either because of rapid spread or because the EEG is performed when a patient has been in CPS for a long period, there is the risk of misclassification [1,19]. Misclassification has significant clinical implications, because long-term pharmacologic management is different for primary and secondary generalized seizure disorders.

## Case presentations

The following cases are selected from the literature to illustrate the diagnostic challenges posed by patients who have NCSE. The cases demonstrate the importance of maintaining a broad-based differential in patients presenting with a change in behavior and emphasize the role of EEG in the evaluation of these patients.

### Case 1

A 64-year-old man had a 2-week history of increasing irritability On the day before admission, his family noticed he was behaving "inappropriately": "the next morning his wife found him sitting in his car, piloting it as if it were an airplane." On arrival at the hospital, he also exhibited delusional ideations, "claiming that he was able to read minds and was in direct communication with God." This patient was diagnosed as having a psychotic disorder and was placed on a psychiatric ward. During admission, the patient continued to exhibit bizarre behavior characterized by intermittent agitation and episodes of motor perseveration such as turning around in circles, tapping his arms, and moving both arms in circular fashion with lucid intervals. He was able to "perform simple tasks even during periods when he was unable to speak." Two days after admission, he suffered from a generalized convulsion. EEG showed generalized 1.5- to 2-Hz bisynchronous multiple spike-and-wave activity with maximal distribution in the frontal region. The patient was given 2 mg diazepam under EEG monitoring with "dramatic clinical improvement and rapid disappearance of epileptiform EEG activity." Two days later, however, the patient experienced a recurrence of clinical symptoms, which were accompanied by EEG changes characterized by intermittent episodes of diffuse, rhythmic, medium-amplitude (1.5–2 Hz) delta activity, which improved after phenytoin and phenobarbital were administered [31].

## Case 2

An 18-year-old woman with a history of seizures presented to the hospital with periods of "fluctuating level of consciousness, ranging from brief periods of responsiveness to deep pain only to a more common trance-like state." Her speech was characterized by stereotyped phrases such as "stop it." She was noticed to have purposeless movements and rare lip smacking. Her extremities could be passively positioned and maintained in an unusual position. She was diagnosed as having catatonic schizophrenia. The EEG showed continuous cyclical pattern of low-voltage rhythmical activity, high-voltage sharp waves, and low-voltage slowing. The patient was treated with antiepileptic drugs with improvement in the EEG pattern and clinical status [29].

## Case 3

A 69-year-old man noted that "for about 10 minutes he was unable to turn off the TV and lights at home." The patient also "felt confused at times and, although he knew what he wanted to do, he was unable to remember how to perform the task." He had several episodes during which he had difficulties deciding what to do with a piece of metal while he was working in his workshop or using a hammer "and was unable to understand what his wife was saying to him." The patient had no history of a seizure disorder but had been treated for lymphocytic lymphoma for 2 years. While in the emergency department, he was noticed to make "random repetitive movements in the air with his hands." The episodes lasted about 2 minutes. An EEG performed 1 day after admission showed continuous generalized 1- to 1.5-Hz multiple spike-and-wave activity, which was maximum bifrontally. While the EEG was being performed, the patient was "mildly confused and unable to carry out manual tasks." An intravenous injection of 2 mg of diazepam was given during EEG monitoring, with resolution of both clinical and EEG changes. During hospitalization, the patient had a recurrence of symptoms; subsequently, he was discharged on phenytoin with no recurrence of his episodes at 4 months follow-up [31].

## Case 4

"The wife of a patient of mine reported that her husband smiled less and lost his sense of humor while the EEG showed florid generalized spike-wave activity" [24].

*Case 5*

A "74-year-old woman who was seen in the [emergency room] ER for cognitive changes characterized by forgetfulness and bizarre behavior: she had gotten on a bus with no money, had left the house without a key, and verbally perseverated on the telephone." While in the emergency department, she was "confused and agitated, repeating her address continually in answer to any question, had catalepsy (waxy limb rigidity) and subtle face and limb myoclonus." EEG showed seizure activity arising from the left frontal region, quickly generalizing and persisting over both frontotemporal regions. The EEG normalized with 3 mg of lorazepam; she remained confused until she fell asleep, but "she woke the next morning alert and oriented" [36].

*Case analysis*

Each of the cases described presented with a constellation of symptoms that should alert the clinician of the potential for NCSE. Case 1 had psychotic features and bizarre behavior. Case 2 had altered mental status and catalepsy with mild automatisms. Case 3 had mild confusion and bizarre behavior characterized by repetitive motor activity. Case 4 had a nonspecific change in behavior recognizable only to family members. Case 5 had a combination of different clinical presentations.

Clearly, NCSE should be suspected in patients who have a change in behavior and who present with even mild automatisms or motor activity. A late onset of psychosis with isolated bizarre delusions in an otherwise well-organized person is suspicious for NCSE rather than an Axis I diagnosis; this suspicion is increased if there is preservation of a warm affect and good interpersonal skills, good work history and social involvement, and no family history of epilepsy or psychiatric illness. At all ages, intermittent episodes of psychosis in the absence of a thought disorder should also raise suspicion of a possible NCSE. Attention should be given to any temporal relation between a psychotic state, an affective state, or altered mental status/behavior and a seizure disorder.

Symptoms temporally related to a convulsive seizure should raise suspicion of the possibility the patient is in NCSE. Postictal or peri-ictal psychosis or mania have been described and should be considered in the differential diagnosis of NCSE [37,38]. When simple or complex motor automatism or repetitive motor activity (eg, kicking or tapping, rocking, pelvic thrusting, genital manipulation, moving the extremities in a circle, running, bicycling, repetitive moaning or vocalizations) is present, the differential diagnosis consists of seizure of frontal or temporal lobe origin versus NCSE versus possible nonepileptic events. Bizarre behavioral or motor manifestations can be characteristic of all three entities. Onset, duration of the event, stereotypicity, lucid intervals, presence of focal findings or automatisms, and sleep-related events help to guide the diagnosis [39–41]. Prolonged episodes that last more than 30 minutes (and which can continue for hours or days) should raise suspicion of NCSE. Lack of stereotypicity and association of several symptoms in addition to bizarre behavior require further investigation, including an EEG. Of note, the scalp EEG can be normal in seizures of frontal lobe origin.

The literature contains many reports similar to the ones given here in which patients initially were labeled as having a psychiatric condition; only later in their evaluations was the correct diagnosis identified, either by EEG or by onset of a convulsive component to the status [2,3,18,31]. It is incumbent for psychiatrists to be aware of this entity so that correct diagnostic and therapeutic measures can be taken.

**Prognosis**

The true incidence of NCSE is not well defined, nor are its morbidity and mortality. Some authors have reported a high morbidity and mortality in NCSE and recommend the use of aggressive therapy [42]. Other series suggest that NCSE is a relatively benign condition [43]. The longest duration of NCSE reported in the literature lasted 9 years; the patient in that case did not exhibit any definite cognitive changes [44].

Research suggests that in convulsive status, even when systemic effects are controlled with paralysis and ventilation, central nervous system damage in the hippocampus occurs relatively quickly [45,46]. The mortality rate ranges from 5% to 50% [47]; aggressive treatment is advocated because the outcome is thought to be related to the duration of the episode as well as to the underlying cause [33]. It has been suggested that neuronal damage may occur in NCSE [47], but controversy still exists regarding the need for aggressive therapy, because there are reports both of complete recovery and of associated transient or permanent cognitive or neurologic deficit [29,48].

Shneker and Fountain [43] found that overall mortality was as high as 27% in patients who had an acute medical problem as the underlying cause of NCSE.

A small prospective series of elderly patients who had NCSE concluded that NCSE had a worse prognosis in elderly patients because of the severity of the underlying cause and because of hospital-acquired infection [49].

The limiting factors in better assessing the true morbidity and mortality of NCSE are the variety of clinical symptoms, potential misinterpretation of EEG patterns, grouping of patients who have different comorbities, and the lack of prior assessment of cognitive or neuropsychologic function for comparison. Because of the lack of well-designed studies, there are no clear guidelines on the treatment of NCSE, and significant controversy still exists regarding the need for aggressive therapy.

In summary, the data suggest that NCSE generally does not result in permanent cognitive or neurologic deficit unless it occurs in the setting of an underlying medical problem. Further controlled, prospective studies and clear guidelines in the management of these difficult patients are needed.

## Treatment

General principles in the management of NCSE include early identification of causative and precipitating factors so they can be corrected as soon as possible. Physiologic stressors including infections, toxins, metabolic abnormalities, structural lesions, drug interactions or withdrawal, and pregnancy should be sought in all patients presenting with either a new seizure or exacerbation of a known disorder.

It is unclear if the morbidity that can occur in NCSE is secondary to NCSE per se or instead is secondary to underlying conditions; thus, there is no consensus to guide timing of interventions. Ultimately, after a careful risk–benefit assessment, treatment is tailored to the individual situation. To assess any correlation between the EEG pattern and clinical symptoms, an intravenous benzodiazepine should be administered during EEG monitoring. Although not always possible, confirmation of NCSE by EEG is recommended before instituting pharmacologic treatment. Some clinicians have opted to give a benzodiazepine without EEG guidance when NCSE is suspected clinically; however, the advantages and disadvantages involved in this practice must be carefully weighed.

Benzodiazepines (eg, diazepam [1,3], lorazepam [36], and clonazepam [1]) have been used as monotherapy or in combination. NCSE has been shown to respond to benzodiazepine, although the response may be delayed or followed by a recurrence within hours or days. Therefore, the use of long-acting antiepileptic drugs may be required to achieve lasting effects [1,29].

Benzodiazepines can be particularly helpful in case of de novo AS when the precipitating factor is secondary to benzodiazepine withdrawal [21] or in cases of Melas syndrome in which valproate and phenytoin are not viable choices because of the underlying impairment of oxidative phosphorylation within the mitochondria and because of carnitine metabolism [50]. The use of benzodiazepines should be considered carefully, because hypotension or respiratory depression may develop, especially in patients who are medically compromised. The response to intravenous benzodiazepines has been reported to be different in AS and CPS; the response is more abrupt in AS and is more variable in CPS [36].

The effect of benzodiazepine often is transient. When long-term treatment is necessary, several options are available. Carbamazepine, phenytoin, phenobarbital, and pirimidone have been used in the treatment of CPS. Valproic acid is the drug of choice in managing patients who have absence seizures [51]. Ethosuximide and clonazepam are alternative choices [52].

Antiepileptic drugs, including viagabatrin and tiagabine, have been reported to play a role in worsening or precipitating NCSE [53].

## Summary

NCSE, once thought to be a rare disorder, should be considered in any patient presenting with an alteration in mental status of indeterminate cause. The psychiatrist needs to be aware of the different clinical characteristics of this disorder as well as similarities and differences from psychiatric disorders. A history of seizure is not necessary for the diagnosis, nor is motor activity necessarily associated with NCSE. An EEG is required to confirm the diagnosis and should be performed when possible, because early recognition and treatment may improve outcome. There is usually a good response to an intravenous benzodiazepine; when response has been delayed, other anticonvulsants have been used as adjuncts. The EEG is necessary to distinguish AS from CPS so that, when indicated, the proper long-term antiepileptic drug therapy can be started. Although NCSE has been described in the literature for many years, there is still a great need for carefully designed prospective studies to help define clear guidelines to assist in clinical and management decision making and, ultimately, to improve outcomes.

## References

[1] Tomson T, Lindbom U, Nilsson B. Nonconvulsive status epilepticus in adults: thirty-two consecutive patients from a general hospital population. Epilepsia 1992;33:829–35.

[2] Andermann F, Robb J. Absence status: a reappraisal following review of thirty-eight patients. Epilepsia 1972;13:177–87.

[3] Guberman A, Cantu-Reyna G, Stuss D, et al. Nonconvulsive generalized status epilepticus: clinical features, neuropsychological testing and long-term follow-up. Neurology 1986;36:1284–91.

[4] Lugaresi E, Pazzaglia P, Tassinari C. Differentiation of absence status and temporal lobe status. Epilepsia 1971;12:77–87.

[5] Tomson T, Svanborg E, Wedlund J. Nonconvulsive status epilepticus: high incidence of complex partial status. Epilepsia 1986;27:276–85.

[6] Celesia G. Modern concepts of status epilepticus. JAMA 1976;235:1571–4.

[7] Ballenger C, King D, Gallagher B. Partial complex status epilepticus. Neurology 1983;33:1545–52.

[8] Towne AR, Waterhouse EJ, Boggs JG, et al. Prevalence of nonconvulsive status epilepticus in comatose patients. Neurology 2000;54:340–9.

[9] Fujiwara T, Watanabe M, Nakamura H, et al. A comparative study of absence status epilepticus between children and adults. Jpn J Psychiatry Neurol 1988;42:497–508.

[10] DeLorenzo RJ, Hauser WA, Towne AR, et al. A prospective, population-based epidemiologic study of status epilepticus in Richmond, Virginia. Neurology 1996;46:1029–35.

[11] Dunne JW, Summers QA, Stewart-Wyne EG. Nonconvulsive status epilepticus: a prospective study in adult general hospital. Q J Med 1987;23:117–26.

[12] DeLorenzo RJ, Waterhouse EJ, Towne AR, et al. Persistent non convulsive status epilepticus after control of convulsive status epilepticus. Epilepsia 1998;38:833–40.

[13] Towne AR, Waterhouse EJ, Morton LD, et al. Unrecognized nonconvulsive status epilepticus in comatose patients. Epilepsia 1998;39(Suppl 6):K07.

[14] Privitera MD, Strawsburg R. Electroencephalographic monitoring in the emergency department. Emerg Med Clin North Am 1994;12(4):1089–100.

[15] Flor HP. Psychosis and temporal lobe epilepsy. A controlled investigation. Epilepsia 1969; 10:363–95.

[16] Husain AM, Horn GC, Jacobson MP. Non-convulsive status epilepticus: usefulness of clinical features in selecting patients for urgent EEG. J Neurol Neurosurg Psychiatry 2003; 74(2):189–91.

[17] Neidermeyer E, Khalifeh R. Petit mal status, an electroclinical appraisal. Epilepsia 1965;6: 250–62.

[18] Lee S. Nonconvulsive status epilepticus: ictal confusion in later life. Arch Neurol 1985;42: 778–81.

[19] Thompson S, Greenhouse A. Petit mal status in adults. Ann Intern Med 1968;68:1271–8.

[20] Hauser W. Status epilepticus: frequency, etiology, and neurological sequelae. In: Delgado-Escueta A, Wasterlain CG, Treiman DM, Porter RJ, editors. Status epilepticus. New York: Raven Press; 1983.

[21] Thomas P, Beaumanoir A, Genton P, et al. 'De novo' absence status of late onset: report of 11 cases. Neurology 1992;42:104–10.

[22] Povlsen UJ, Wildschiodtz G, Hogenhaven H, et al. Nonconvulsive status epilepticus after electroconvulsive therapy. J ECT 2003;19(3):164–9.

[23] Fincham R, Yamada T, Schottelius D, et al. Electroencephalographic absence status with minimal behavior change. Arch Neurol 1979;36:176–8.

[24] Kaplan PW. Assessing the outcomes in patients with nonconvulsive status epilepticus: nonconvulsive status epilepticus is underdiagnosed, potentially overtreated, and confounded by comorbidity. J Clin Neurophysiol 1999;16(4):341–2.

[25] Markand O, Wheeler G, Pollack S. Complex partial status epilepticus. Neurol 1978;28: 189–96.

[26] Audenino D, Cocito L, Primavera A. Non-convulsive status epilepticus. J Neurol Neurosurg Psychiatry 2003;74:1599–600.

[27] Thomas P, Zifkin B, Migneco O. Nonconvulsive status epilepticus of frontal origin. Neurology 1999;52:1174–87.

[28] Fernandez-Torre JL, Gonzales C, Sanchez JM. Nonconvulsive status epilepticus of frontal origin: a case report. Rev Neurol 2000;30(11):1040–3.

[29] Engel J, Ludwig B, Fetell M. Prolonged partial complex status epilepticus: EEG and behavioral observations. Neurology 1978;28:863–9.

[30] Escueta A, Boxley J, Stubbs N, et al. Prolonged twilight state and automatisms: a case report. Neurology 1974;24(4):331–9.

[31] Ellis J, Lee S. Acute prolonged confusion in later life as an ictal state. Epilepsia 1978;19: 119–28.

[32] Belafsky M, Carwille S, Miller P, et al. Prolonged epileptic twilight states: continuous recordings with nasopharyngeal electrodes and videotape analysis. Neurology 1978; 28(3):239–45.

[33] Treiman D, Delgado-Escueta A. Complex partial status epilepticus. In: Delgado-Escueta A, Wasterlain C, Treiman D, et al, editors. Status epilepticus. Advances in neurology vol. 34. New York: Raven Press; 1983. p. 69–81.

[34] Neidermeyer E, Ribeiro M. Consideration of nonconvulsive status epilepticus. Clin Electroencephalogr 2000;31(4):192–5.

[35] Porter R, Penry J. Petit mal status. In: Delgado-Escueta A, Wasterlain C, Treiman D, et al, editors. Status epilepticus. Advances in neurology vol. 34. New York: Raven Press; 1983. p. 61–7.

[36] Kaplan P. Nonconvulsive status epilepticus in the emergency room. Epilepsia 1996;37(7): 643–50.

[37] Savard G, Anderman F, Olivier A, et al. Postictal psychosis after partial complex seizures: a multiple case study. Epilepsia 1991;32(2):225–31.

[38] Ramchandani D, Riggio S. Periictal mania—a case report. Psychosomatics 1992;33: 229–31.

[39] Williamson PD. Frontal lobe epilepsy. Some clinical characteristics. In: Jasper HH, Riggio S, Goldman Rakic PS, editors. Epilepsy and the functional anatomy of the frontal lobe. New York: Raven Press; 1995. p. 127–52.

[40] Williamson PD, Spencer DD, Spencer SS, et al. Complex partial seizures of frontal lobe origin. Ann Neurol 1985;18:497–504.

[41] Riggio S, Harner R. Repetitive motor activity in frontal lobe epilepsy. In: Jasper HH, Riggio S, Goldman Rakic PS, editors. Epilepsy and the functional anatomy of the frontal lobe. New York: Raven Press; 1995. p. 153–66.

[42] Treiman DM, Delgado-Escueta AV, Clark MA. Impairment of memory following complex partial status epilepticus. Neurology 1981;31:109.

[43] Shneker BF, Fountain NB. Assessment of acute morbidity and mortality in nonconvulsive status epileticus. Neurology 2003;61:1066–73.

[44] Gokyigit A, Caliskan A. Diffuse spike-wave status of 9 year duration without behavioral change of intellectual decline. Epilepsia 1995;36:210–3.

[45] Lothman E. The biochemical basis and pathophysiology of status epilepticus. Neurology 1990;40(Suppl 2):13–23.

[46] Simon R, Benowitz N, Culala S. Motor paralysis increases brain uptake of lidocaine during status epilepticus. Neurology 1984;34:384–7.

[47] Treiman DM. Neuron specific enolase and status epilepticus–induced neuronal injury. Epilepsia 1996;37(7):595–7.

[48] Krumholz A, Sung GY, Fisher RS, et al. Complex partial status epilepticus accompanied by serious morbidity and mortality. Neurology 1995;45:1499–504.

[49] Labar D, Barrera J, Soloman G, et al. Nonconvulsive status epilepticus in the elderly: a case series and a review of the literature. J Epilepsy 1998;11:74–8.

[50] Feddersen B, Bender A, Arnold S, et al. Aggressive confusional state as a clinical manifestation of status epilepticus in MELAS. Neurology 2003;61:1149–50.

[51] Porter R. The absence epilepsies. Epilepsia 1993;34(Suppl 3):S42–8.

[52] Berkovic S, Andermann F, Guberman A, et al. Valproate prevents the recurrence of absence status. Neurology 1989;39:1294–7.

[53] Drislane F. Presentation, evaluation, and treatment of nonconvulsive status epilepticus. Epilepsy Behav 2000;1:301–14.

ELSEVIER
SAUNDERS

Psychiatr Clin N Am 28 (2005) 665–683

PSYCHIATRIC
CLINICS
OF NORTH AMERICA

# Delusional Misidentification

Todd E. Feinberg, MD[a,b], David M. Roane, MD[a,b,*]

[a]*Albert Einstein College of Medicine, New York, New York, USA*
[b]*Beth Israel Medical Center, First Avenue at 16th Street, New York, NY 10003, USA*

The delusional misidentification syndrome (DMS) is a condition in which a patient consistently misidentifies persons, places, objects, or events. The most common form of misidentification is the Capgras syndrome. Originally described by Capgras and Reboul-Lachaux [1], this disorder consists of the delusional belief that a person or persons have been replaced by "doubles" or imposters. Another type of misidentification is the Frégoli syndrome [2] in which there is the belief that a person who is well known to the patient is actually pretending to take on the appearance of a relative stranger whom the patient encounters. Vié [3] characterized the Capgras syndrome as the illusion of negative doubles and Frégoli syndrome as the illusion of positive doubles. Christodoulou [4,5] suggested that Capgras syndrome is a "hypo-identification" of a person closely related to the patient, whereas Frégoli syndrome is a "hyperidentification" of a person not well known to the patient. Feinberg and Roane [6–9] concluded that different delusional misidentification syndromes can be separated on the basis of the nature of the changed personal relatedness between the self and other persons, objects, and events. When this approach is used, Capgras syndrome becomes an example of underpersonalized misidentification, and Frégoli syndrome represents overpersonalized misidentification.

Some patients who have DMS reduplicate or double the misidentified entity. For example, a patient with Capgras syndrome may deny the identity of the actual spouse and claim that there are two spouses, the actual and the imposter. Not every patient with DMS reduplicates the misidentified entity, however. For example, in the syndrome of intermetamorphosis, the patient believes that people he or she knows have exchanged identities with each other [10]. Conversely, some patients may claim the existence of a fictitious

---

* Corresponding author. Beth Israel Medical Center, First Avenue at 16th Street, New York, NY 10003.
  *E-mail address:* droane@bethisraelny.org (D.M. Roane).

person or place, often a double of an actual person or place, without any actual misidentification.

The Capgras-type delusion generally has been recognized in the context of psychiatric disorders and often occurs in conjunction with paranoia, derealization, and depersonalization [11–14]. The symptom has been reported in association with a variety of diagnostic entities including schizophrenia, mood disorders, Alzheimer's disease, and other organic conditions.

Capgras syndrome is common. The frequency in schizophrenia has been reported to be as high as 15% [15], with the rate in all psychiatric inpatients ranging from 1.3% to 4.1% [16–17]. Studies in patients who have Alzheimer's disease have demonstrated prevalence between 2% and 30% [18–19].

A broad range of medical and neurologic disorders may manifest with misidentification and reduplication in general. In a review of delusional reduplication in the literature, Signer [20] found various medical comorbidities including drug intoxication and withdrawal, infectious and inflammatory disease, and endocrine conditions. Associated neurologic illnesses included seizures, cerebral infarction, and traumatic brain injury. Forty percent of patients who have identifiable organic conditions had diffuse brain syndromes such as delirium, dementia, and mental retardation. DMS has been seen in association with parkinsonism [21] and, in particular, with dementia with Lewy bodies [22]. Ballard [22] reported that DMS occurred more frequently with Lewy body dementia than with Alzheimer's dementia. Iseki and colleagues [23] found that multiple forms of DMS were common in both dementia with Lewy bodies and levodopa-induced psychosis. DMS may also present as an adverse consequence of electroconvulsive therapy [24] and has been reported in patients receiving diazepam and disulfiram [25].

This article focuses on the relationship between DMS and neurologic illness.

## Delusional misidentification and brain pathology

A review of the range of DMS phenomena that has been reported in the context of localized brain pathology elucidates the neuropsychiatric aspects of this condition.

### Capgras-type misidentifications

Alexander and colleagues [26] reported one of the first cases of Capgras syndrome for persons occurring in the setting of focal brain lesions. They described a 44-year-old man who sustained a traumatic brain injury and right frontotemporal encephalomalacia. This patient claimed that his wife and five children had been replaced by substitutes. Another instance of this disorder involved a 31-year-old man who, years after a traumatic brain injury that resulted in right frontotemporal and parietal damage, claimed that his parents, siblings, and friends were not "real" but were "look-alikes" or "doubles" [27].

Patients have also developed Capgras-type misidentification for their homes. Kapur and colleagues [28] described a patient who claimed his actual home was not his "real" home, although he recognized many ornaments and bedside items as original. Moser and colleagues [29] reported an elderly man with an acute right frontal infarct who called his real home the "twin" of the original.

One further applicable condition is asomatognosia [30,31]. In this syndrome, a patient repeatedly misidentifies a part of the patient's body. Asomatognosia occurs most commonly in a patient with left hemiplegia, caused by a right hemisphere lesion, who denies ownership of the left arm. It typically co-occurs with hemispatial neglect. Early on, Jacques Vié [3,32] recognized that some syndromes, like asomatognosia, although apparently caused by neurologic illness, could not be accounted for simply by confusion. He noted that asomatognosia involved systematic and selective misidentification and resembled delusional syndromes like Capgras syndrome. More recently, Feinberg and Roane [7,9,33] have viewed asomatognosia as a form of Capgras syndrome for the arm in which there is a loss of personal relatedness to the body part. As in Capgras syndrome, in which a person is recognized, but their psychologic identity is not acknowledged, the patient with asomatognosia may be aware that the arm should be his or her arm but denies ownership of the limb.

Asomatognosia generally is seen in association with anosognosia for hemiplegia [34], in that the patient seems unaware of or persistently denies the paralysis of the arm. Both entities appear more frequently after right hemisphere lesions. Anosognosia and asomatognosia are dissociable, however, because not all anosognosic patients deny ownership of the limb, and not all asomatognosic patients deny illness or even hemiplegia.

Patients who have asomatognosia may attribute ownership of the limb to the examining doctor. This simple misattribution often can be reversed when the error is demonstrated to the patient. In other patients, the misidentifications are truly delusional, and patients maintain a fixed belief in the misidentifications when they are confronted with evidence of their errors. Patients may even develop special names for their arms that can be interpreted as personifications [35] or metaphors [36,37]. Descriptions of the arm such as "a piece of rusty machinery" or "my dead husband's hand" communicate an altered relationship between the patient and the arm.

*Frégoli-type misidentification*

The literature includes numerous reports of patients who have brain lesions who develop Frégoli syndrome for persons or places. Ruff and Volpe

[38] described a woman who, after the removal of a right frontal subdural hematoma, claimed that the patient in the bed next to her was her husband. She noted with satisfaction that her husband no longer snored. Feinberg and colleagues [39] described a man who developed numerous Frégoli-type misidentifications at a rehabilitation hospital after suffering a traumatic brain injury with right frontal and left temporoparietal contusions. He insisted that staff members and other patients at the facility were actually his sons, his in-laws, and his coworkers. He identified an ice skater performing on television as himself.

Patients who misidentify their current unfamiliar environment, such as a hospital room or rehabilitation hospital, for a place of close personal significance, such as a home or job site, may be said to have Frégoli syndrome for place. The syndrome was originally described by Pick [40] in 1903 as reduplicative paramnesia, because patients maintained they were in both a correct and an incorrect location, and the disorder was seen with memory impairment. Because many patients have misidentification for place without reduplication, the term Frégoli syndrome for environment is a better descriptor.

## Reduplication without misidentification

Another group of delusional confabulatory patients reduplicate persons or places but do not misidentify the reduplicated entities. Weinstein and colleagues [41] described several patients who had brain lesions and believed that they were the parents of a fictitious child; the investigators termed the condition the "phantom child syndrome." They noted that a recurring aspect of the delusion was that "patients often ascribed to the 'phantom child' the same illness or disability that they themselves had." For example, a woman with a pituitary tumor and blindness claimed she had a child who was "sick and blind," and a young soldier with a head injury and bilateral leg weakness claimed he had a 3-year-old "daughter" who had developed lower limb paralysis from polio. In some cases, the problems of the "phantom child" reflected personal issues of the patient unrelated to the neurologic illness. For instance, a woman who experienced the hospital nurses as abusive believed that she had a baby whom the staff had "harmed and even killed."

An additional case described by Feinberg [6,8] involved a 63-year-old man with a ruptured anterior cerebral artery aneurysm and bilateral frontal infarctions. On neuropsychologic testing, the patient displayed evidence of dysfunction of attention, memory, and executive functioning. He was anosognosic for his impairments, and he denied being a patient in the hospital, declaring that he was "a guest" with the "optimists club." The patient had fathered three children. While in the hospital he developed the delusion that he had an adopted child who was undergoing an evaluation and was being judged unfairly.

## Neuroanatomic pathology

A number of investigators have studied the neuroanatomic correlates of DMS. Joseph [42] reported that 16 of 29 personally examined patients with misidentification for person had abnormal CT scans with bilateral cortical atrophy, including bifrontal atrophy (in 88%), bitemporal atrophy (in 73%), and biparietal atrophy (in 60%). Weinstein and Burnham [43] found that bilateral and diffuse brain involvement, with right hemispheric predominance, were the most typical lesion patterns. Feinberg and Shapiro [44] reviewed the anatomic correlates in a selected series of case reports of patients with misidentification-reduplication. They found that bilateral cortical involvement occurred frequently (in 62% of patients who had Capgras syndrome and in 41% of patients who had reduplication). In considering cases in which cerebral dysfunction was unilateral, they found that right hemispheric predominance in reduplication was highly significant (52% right hemisphere versus 7% left hemisphere), with a statistical trend for more frequent right hemispheric damage in the smaller number of patients who have Capgras syndrome (32% right versus 7% left). Förstl and coworkers [45] reviewed a diverse group of misidentification cases and found right-sided abnormalities in 19 of 20 patients with focal lesions on brain CT scans. Based on three cases of head trauma, Benson and associates [46] proposed a relationship between reduplicative paramnesia and bifrontal impairment in concert with damage to the posterior portion of the right hemisphere. In a prospective study of 50 alcoholic patients, Hakim and coworkers [47] found that three of four reduplicators had acute right hemispheric lesions. They assumed all patients to have chronic bifrontal damage based on chronic alcohol use and neuropsychologic test results. Fleminger and Burns [48] compared right versus left hemispheric asymmetries in CT scans of patients who had misidentification. In one selected group, asymmetry was found, with greater right hemispheric damage in the occipitoparietal area. In the analysis of a second group of patients, greater right hemisphere damage could be detected in frontal, temporal, and parietal lobes.

Forstl and colleagues [49] found that patients who had Alzheimer's disease and misidentification had greater atrophy in the right frontal lobe than did demented controls. Another study involving patients who had Alzheimer's disease demonstrated that those who had DMS had significantly greater hypometabolism in bilateral orbitofrontal and cingulated regions on positron emission tomography than those who did not have DMS [50].

## Case review

To understand further the central aspects of delusional misidentification after focal brain lesions and to clarify the underlying neuropathology of these disorders, the authors recently conducted an analysis of a series of previously published DMS cases plus one unpublished case [51].

Case reports included in this analysis involved patients who demonstrated persistent misidentifications or reduplications of either the Capgras or Frégoli type in the context of focal brain illness. Case descriptions had to provide sufficient clinical and neuroanatomic information to permit analysis. There were 29 applicable reports of DMS involving 27 different individuals (two patients had more than one form of misidentification). In general, all cases were easily divided into Capgras- and Frégoli-type misidentifications, and virtually all delusions involved the patients themselves or highly significant others.

The authors examined the main effects for hemisphere and brain regions. In all 29 cases, the lesion affected the right hemisphere; only 15 (51.7%) involved left hemisphere damage. When cases with bilateral lesions were excluded, there were 14 (48.3%) cases with right hemisphere damage only and no cases with left hemisphere damage only. These data indicate that DMS is strongly associated with right hemisphere damage.

The injury was limited to the frontal lobe in 34.5% of cases. In no case did parietal or temporal damage alone produce DMS. The association between frontal lobe damage and DMS was statistically significant. Consistent with the finding of predominantly right hemisphere pathology, almost all patients who had neuropsychologic testing evidenced a pattern of memory (primarily nonverbal), perceptual, and executive impairments.

## Features of delusional misidentification syndrome

Cases of delusional misidentification associated with brain disease share a number of characteristic features that distinguish these conditions from simple unawareness, confusion, and confabulation in general.

### Alterations in entities of personal significance

Misidentifications and reduplications, almost universally, involve delusions concerning entities of great personal significance such as one's body, family, current location, and job situation.

### Selectivity and consistency

Patients persistently misidentify the same particular aspects of the self and environment. This persistence makes it unlikely that most cases of DMS can be attributed to general impairment in memory or perception.

### Lack of awareness or minimization of illness, functional loss, or personal problem

Many cases of delusional misidentification or reduplication manifest with denial or anosognosia. For patients who have Frégoli-type DMS, the delusions themselves often allow patients to view their situation as being better than it actually is. Thus, patients preferentially locate themselves in pleasant, familiar surroundings such as at home or at work, when actually they are confined in a hospital or rehabilitation setting. If they acknowledge being in a hospital, they tend to believe that the hospital is close to home. Thus, Ruff and Volpe [38] have identified possible wish-fulfilling aspects of the delusions of several patients who have DMS.

### Resistance to correction

Misidentifications are fixed, false beliefs and, therefore, represent true delusions. Even when patients are confronted repeatedly with the illogical nature of the delusion, they maintain their position. Indeed, patients may demonstrate implicit or explicit awareness of their true situation [6,7,9, 38,52,53]. This feature distinguishes DMS from other forms of confabulation (eg, amnestic confabulation) and from unawareness in general. Clearly any causal explanation of DMS must consider the delusional nature of this condition.

### Right hemisphere dysfunction

Right frontal dysfunction predominates in focal and diffuse cases of DMS regardless of the type of delusional misidentification or reduplication.

## Explanations for delusional misidentification syndrome

### Spatial disorientation

Spatial disorientation has been noted to be a causative factor in the production of reduplicative paramnesia [36,38] and is probably associated with virtually any case of delusional misidentification for place. Indeed, visuospatial disorders including hemispatial neglect were noted in nearly all cases in the authors' series, including misidentification for persons. Visuospatial disorientation alone cannot explain the selectivity and delusional quality of DMS, however.

### Anatomic disconnection

Some theories have attributed DMS, especially Capgras syndrome for persons, to anatomic disconnection. Alexander and colleagues [26] argued that a deep right frontal lesion could disconnect temporal and limbic regions functionally from the damaged frontal lobe. This disconnection could result in a disturbance in familiarity of people and places and, in the presence of frontal pathology, could lead to an inability to resolve the cognitive conflict. Staton and colleagues [27] proposed that disconnection of the hippocampus from other parts of the brain important for memory storage could prevent association of new information with previous memories, leading to reduplication.

Some investigators have suggested that Capgras syndrome is caused by visuoanatomic disconnection. Ellis and Young [54], based on the finding that some patients who have prosopognosia have covert (emotional) but not overt recognition of faces [55,56], suggested that patients who had Capgras syndrome have overt recognition of faces without the appropriate emotional reaction. The covert, emotion-laden form of recognition is subserved by a "dorsal route" that runs between the visual cortex and the limbic system through the inferior parietal lobule. A lesion in the dorsal system would allow explicit recognition without the feeling of familiarity and, they suggest, could produce Capgras syndrome. Similarly, Hirstein and Ramachandran [57,58] suggested that a disconnection between the infero-temporal cortex and the amygdala could allow the patient to identify faces correctly but not experience the appropriate emotion connected to familiar faces, leading to delusional misidentification.

In the authors' series of reviewed cases, within the right hemisphere both the temporal and parietal lobes were intact in a majority of the cases of Capgras syndrome for person or place. On the other hand, all eight cases of Capgras syndrome for persons or places had nondominant frontal lesions. Therefore, if anatomic disconnection is important, it seems that a discon-nection of nondominant frontal structures, as suggested by Alexander and colleagues [26], is most likely to play a role in the origin of Capgras syndrome.

Theories such as that of Ellis and Young [54] and Hirstein and Ramachandran [57] emphasizing visuoanatomic disconnection do not account for most cases of Capgras syndrome, because this disorder generally is not limited to the visual modality. In fact, Dietl and colleagues [59] described a case in which a mother developed Capgras syndrome for her daughter during a time that the two had no direct contact. Shah and colleagues [60] have shown through functional imaging that the retrosplenial cortex may be a single anatomic locus for both visual and auditory recognition of familiarity. Still, as Ellis and Lewis [61] note, faulty perceptual experience does not account for the delusional nature of the Capgras syndrome.

When the range of DMS phenomena is considered, explanations that emphasize anatomic disconnection would seem to apply best to the Capgras-type delusions. In these cases, an inability to match current experience with autobiographical memories could result in the under-identification of people and places. Frégoli syndrome, however, is a disorder of overidentification characterized by the confabulation of imaginary resemblances between the misidentified entity and the original. How could a disconnection of current experience from premorbid memory explain over-relatedness to one's environment?

A partial answer to this latter question may come from Rapcsak and colleagues [62] who described a patient without prosopagnosia who displayed false recognition (overidentification) of faces following the surgical removal of a right prefrontal lesion. They attributed the patient's pattern of impairment to an intact reflexive face-recognition system but an impaired reflective or strategic face-processing system, leading this patient to mistake an unknown face for one in memory. This kind of defect might explain some instances of visual overidentification of faces. This account still does not explain selectivity, refractoriness, delusional nature, or multimodality.

### Memory, executive impairment, and confabulation

In addition to the perceptual disturbance seen in the case review, memory and executive impairments were found in nearly all cases in which these functions were assessed. In two other cases of misidentification for the mirrored image reported by Breen and colleagues [63], only one patient had significant face-processing deficits, but both had visual memory and executive dysfunction. Because many of the current cognitive and neuro-psychologic theories of confabulation also involve memory impairment and executive dysfunction [64–67], the possibility of a relationship between DMS and confabulation must be considered. Because patients who have Frégoli-type DMS claim familiarity with unfamiliar persons or places, and patients who confabulate may mistake past for current environmental stimuli [68], it is relevant to consider whether explanations of confabulation account for aspects of DMS.

Confabulation has been defined as the production of erroneous statements made without a conscious effort to deceive [69] or "statements or actions that involve unintentional but obvious distortions" [70]. Korsakoff [71] first discovered that amnesia and confabulation tend to co-occur ("pseudoreminiscences"). Numerous subsequent authors have reported the presence of confabulation in patients who have Korsakoff syndrome [72–77].

Korsakoff [71] observed that, in the course of confabulating, "patients confused old recollections with the present impressions. Thus, they may believe themselves to be in the setting (or circumstances) in which they were 30 years ago, and mistake persons who are around them now for people who were around them at that time" [78]. Kraeplin [79–81] distinguished two subtypes of confabulation. One, which he called simple confabulation, was caused in part by errors in the temporal ordering of real memories. Another form, which he called fantastic confabulation, consisted of bizarre, patently impossible statements unrelated to actual memories. Van Der Horst [74] and Williams and Rupp [75] also noted that many confabulations were based on intact past memories. As an example of this phenomenon, Talland [76] observed that amnestic confabulators tended to misidentify their doctors as old acquaintances.

These observations are consistent with a current theory that confabulation results from temporal context confusion caused by frontal-executive dysfunction. By this explanation, confabulation results from inability to maintain an accurate temporal order of memories [82–86]. Thus, spontaneous confabulation occurs when patients cannot establish the contrast between current experience and memories of past events because of an inability to suppress irrelevant memory traces.

Another theory identifies deficient strategic retrieval as the primary deficit in confabulation [70,87–88]. Strategic retrieval refers to a conscious, effortful, and self-directed mechanism of memory recovery, and it requires frontal functions. According to this theory, confabulation results from a breakdown in strategic retrieval processes involved in memory search, temporal ordering, and output monitoring. Confabulation can occur when a particular cognitive subsystem (eg, memory) is damaged and produces faulty output (eg, failure to remember correctly) in the context of impaired output monitoring (eg, unawareness of response discrepancies).

Cognitively based theories of confabulation could help explain some features of DMS. Temporal context confusion or retrieval defects might allow remote memories to be confused with recent memories, explaining in part why patients who have had DMS believe they are located in previously known locations or are performing well-known social roles. These explanations, however, do not explain why only certain, select entities are misidentified or why persons or places of personal significance are typically the subject of the DMS. General theories of confabulation also fail to explain why most confabulators after anterior communicating artery aneurysms do not display a delusional fabric to their confabulations [67], whereas patients who have DMS are fixed in their delusions. For instance, Paterson and Zangwill [89] noted that their patients who had reduplicative paramnesia, who misidentified their current location as a geographical location closer to their actual homes, were refractory to correction, and their errors could not be explained solely by memory loss. Their patients might accept the correct orientation in an "abstract geographical" sense, such as knowing the correct locale "according to the map," but they still maintained that they "felt" they were located closer to home. Subsequent authors also emphasized the delusional quality of the statements of some patients' misidentifications. Thus, Weinstein [90] referred to instances in which patients adamantly maintained an incorrect orientation in spite of correction as examples of "symbolic or delusional environmental disorientation." These cases suggest that the delusional aspects are an important distinguishing feature between DMS and confabulation in general.

Additional observations support the notion that delusional misidentification is partially dissociated from confabulation in general. Box and coworkers [91] described a woman who developed Frégoli-type misidentifications after a traumatic brain injury. Initially the patient had inconsistent and short-lived confabulations that resolved. Only later did the patient demonstrate more stable Frégoli-type misidentification. Capgras-type DMS can also be dissociated from confabulation. Mattioli and colleagues [92] reported a man with right frontopolar, right temporal, and bilateral frontobasal hypodensities after traumatic brain injury. The patient developed confabulation in both personal recollections and formal long-term verbal memory testing, along with Capgras-like misidentifications for his wife, daughters, and house. One year later, the confabulations were restricted to verbal memory tasks. The delusional misidentification of the wife persisted and remained refractory to correction, however.

Numerous studies have demonstrated that ventromedial frontal damage is critical for the occurrence of spontaneous confabulation [64,67,70,84, 93–98]. There do not seem to be strongly lateralized effects when a broad range of confabulatory patients is considered and when cases with confabulation manifesting as Capgras syndrome, reduplicative paramnesia, and Anton's syndrome are excluded, however [98]. Therefore, the finding of strong right frontal hemisphere predominance in the authors' series indicates that delusional misidentification and reduplication can be distinguished both clinically and neuroanatomically from confabulation.

All these approaches constitute "negative" explanations in a Jacksonian sense [53]. That is, they view neurologic or neuropsychologic deficits as the causal agents for DMS. Many of the negative features discussed are seen commonly in patients who have significant right hemisphere pathology. The question remains why most patients who have right hemisphere lesions, including many with right frontal lesions, do not demonstrate delusional misidentification or reduplication. Following is a discussion of the "positive" mechanisms that may better account for the features of these conditions not explained by the deficits alone. These positive neurologic features result from the functions of the remaining intact brain [53].

In some instances, it is not entirely clear whether a characteristic is a negative or positive feature of a disorder. For example, is the delusional nature of these disorders a positive or negative feature of DMS? Delusions in general have been reported to occur with increased frequency in the presence of right hemisphere pathology [99]. Malloy and Richardson [100], in a review of content-specific delusions that included delusional misidentification, sexual delusions, and somatic delusions, found a high incidence of lesions of the frontal lobes and right hemisphere. Kumral and Özturk [101] found an association between right posterior temporoparietal lesions and delusional ideation, and Sultzer and colleagues [102] found that the severity of delusional thinking in Alzheimer's disease was associated with right prefrontal hypometabolism on positron emission tomographic scans.

Alexander and colleagues [26] attributed the delusional ideation of a patient who had Capgras syndrome to the presence of bilateral frontal deficits leading to a failure to resolve conflicting or competing information. One striking features in the authors' subgroup of Capgras-type misidentification involving persons, however, was that a majority had prior or current paranoia, suspiciousness, or depression. Indeed, in the case reported by Alexander and coworkers [26], the patient suffered from "grandiose and paranoid delusions, and had auditory hallucinations" before the brain injury that led to his Capgras-type delusions. This observation raises the possibility that premorbid psychopathology subserved by brain areas left undamaged by cortical lesions, including paranoia, may play a positive role in the production of DMS. Several of the cases with Frégoli-type delusions for persons in the authors' review had paranoia, but this association was not as strong as with Capgras-type delusions for persons.

An entirely different picture emerges in the cases with Frégoli-type delusions for place. In this group, no patients were reported to be paranoid or to demonstrate other evidence of psychopathology. In every instance, however, the patients' conviction that they were close to or actually in their homes could not be corrected. Patterson and Zangwill [89] hypothesized that the failure of patients to accept evidence that conflicted with their delusional disorientation was related to the patients' desire to return home. They argued that "a strong desire was actively inhibiting the cognitive mechanisms which normally subserve orientation," and that these patients were oblivious to the conflict presented by their dual orientation and would confabulate explanations when confronted with the disparity. The authors attributed the delusional disorientation to the negative features of anterograde and retrograde amnesia, restriction of perception, and defective judgment in which there is a failure to correct incompatible interpretations, as well as to the positive features of motivation.

Ruff and Volpe [38] also suggested that motivation might play a role in the maintenance of delusional disorientation. These authors described four patients who misidentified the location of their hospital rooms and claimed the hospital was located within their homes or that the hospital had been moved into their house. These authors suggested that a multiplicity of neurologic and psychologic factors created the delusional beliefs; these factors included "right parietal or frontal cerebral lesion, impaired spatial perception and visual memory, confusion or apathy early in the hospital course, and a strong desire to be at home." Therefore, within the Frégoli group, there is evidence that motivation or wish fulfillment is important in the creation and maintenance of the delusion.

Turk and colleagues [103] proposed that the functioning left hemisphere's attempt to make sense of or to interpret faulty information might account for DMS. That is, when the injured right hemisphere cannot produce the appropriate emotional response to a patient's spouse, the left hemisphere concludes the spouse has been replaced by an imposter.

Finally, a disturbance in ego functions may be involved in the creation of delusional misidentification. For instance, in the delusional asomatognosia cases, the arm is not simply misidentified, it is projected onto another person close to the patient. Further, in the cases with delusional reduplication without misidentification, the patients' own disabilities often are projected onto external fictitious or reduplicated persons. Thus, these cases demonstrate the potential role of psychologic projection in DMS, often in association with anosognosia.

## Delusional misidentification and the self

To account for the various features of delusional misidentification, the authors propose the following hypothesis. In addition to perceptual, memory, and executive impairments, patients who have delusional mis-identification and reduplication suffer from a disturbance of self and self-related functions. That is, the right hemisphere may be dominant for the self, and right hemisphere damage may result in a disorder of ego boundaries and ego functions. This disorder could explain why delusional misidentifications are almost universally and selectively about aspects of the self or others of personal significance.

This hypothesis is consistent with the idea that delusional misidentification syndromes should be viewed as disorders of personal relatedness and the self [6–8,33,104]. This explanation also may account for disorders involving either under-relatedness or over-relatedness. Consistent with the finding of the frequent presence of right frontal damage in DMS, a growing body of research indicates that the right hemisphere is integral to the function of self-representation [105,106]. In a study of self-face presentation using functional MRI, Kircher and coworkers [107] found that self-faces activated almost twice as much area in the right hemisphere compared with unfamiliar faces and 1.3 times greater activation when compared with familiar faces. Another study [108] employed patients who had epilepsy anesthetized during a presurgical Wada test. These subjects were presented with a morphed face generated from a composite formed from their own face and that of a famous person. Under the condition of left hemisphere inactivation, with the right hemisphere functioning, subjects tended to identify the morphed face as their own. In contrast, with right hemisphere inactivation, they identified the face as a famous person. Right hemisphere dominance also has been demonstrated for self-face recognition [106,109] and for other functions related to the self such as autobiographical memories [110–114].

In the authors' view, right frontal hemisphere damage creates a deficit in the ego functions that mediate the relationship between the self and the world for personally significant incoming afferent information and for self-generated affects and drives. Thus, there is a two-way relationship between the self and the environment with regard to personal relatedness that, when disturbed, can result in disorders of both under- and over-relatedness to the environment. Without the intact functioning of right frontal regions that subserve certain self-related functions, personally significant incoming information may be disconnected from a feeling of familiarity [26] or personal relatedness [6,8]. Conversely, when internal motives, such as the desire to be home, are not monitored appropriately by the ego functions of the right frontal regions, the patient may view the wish as an externalized reality. Similarly, in delusional asomatognosia, when the right frontal regions fail to establish appropriate ego boundaries, the feelings of alienation from the limb can result in an actual denial of ownership of the limb. Finally, in the case of delusional reduplication without misidentification, as occurs in the "phantom child syndrome," personal affects are projected onto fictitious others in the environment.

Spatial cognition may play a special role in linking right hemisphere pathology to disturbed ego boundaries. An accurate representation of the self–nonself boundary requires intact spatial cognition, because this boundary depends fundamentally on a concrete spatial distinction. Right hemisphere damage that impairs spatial cognition may therefore lead to disturbances of ego boundaries. These disturbances consist of deficits of veridical self–nonself space representation and in the release of more primitive (affectively driven) representations of ego boundaries whereby the self represents space according to wishes rather than to unwelcome current reality [115].

## Treatment considerations

The treatment of the specific form of delusion discussed in this article has not been studied systematically. For patients manifesting any psychotic disorder in the context of a neurologic illness, atypical antipsychotics are generally recommended because of the decreased risk of adverse neurologic effects. With patients who have progressive dementia, such as dementia with Lewy bodies, in which DMS is common, cholinesterase inhibitors have demonstrated some ability to reduce psychiatric symptoms [116]. Wells and Whitehouse [117] have emphasized the importance of distinguishing true delusions such as DMS from confabulations, arguing that the latter do not respond to pharmacotherapy. Pihan and coworkers [118], however, described patient with an anterior communicating artery aneurysm patient who had both DMS and spontaneous confabulation whose delusions and confabulations both improved with risperidone treatment.

## Summary

The Capgras syndrome and other forms of delusional misidentification may be encountered frequently in neuropsychiatric settings. DMS can occur in the presence of idiopathic psychiatric illness, in diffuse brain illness such as dementia, and in focal neurologic disease. In patients who have focal lesions, there is evidence that right hemisphere damage is necessary for the production of DMS. Although DMS is associated with a pattern of neuropsychologic impairments in the domains of memory, perception, and executive function, these impairments alone do not account for the selectivity and delusional nature of DMS. Therefore, other factors such as premorbid psychopathology, motivation, and loss of ego functions may be important in determining which vulnerable patients develop DMS and which do not.

## References

[1] Capgras J, Reboul-Lachaux J. L'illusion des "sosies"dans un delire systematize. Bull Soc Clin Med Ment 1923;11:6–16.
[2] Courbon P, Fail G. Syndrome "d'illusion de Fregoli" et schizophrenie. Ann Med Psychol (Paris) 1927;85:289–90.
[3] Vié J. Un trouble de l'identification des personnes: L'illusion des sosies. Ann Med Psychol (Paris) 1930;88:214–37.
[4] Christodoulou GN. Delusional hyper-identifications of the Fregoli type. Acta Psychiatr Scand 1976;54:305–14.
[5] Christodoulou GN. The syndrome of Capgras. Br J Psychiatry 1977;130:556–64.
[6] Feinberg TE. Some interesting perturbations of the self in neurology. Semin Neurol 1997; 17:129–35.
[7] Feinberg TE, Roane DM. Anosognosia, completion and confabulation: the neutral-personal dichotomy. Neurocase 1997;3:73–85.
[8] Feinberg TE. Altered egos: how the brain creates the self. New York: Oxford University Press; 2001.
[9] Feinberg TE, Roane D. Misidentification syndromes. In: Feinberg TE, Farah MJ, editors. Behavioral neurology and neuropsychology. New York: McGraw-Hill; 2003. p. 373–81.
[10] Courbon P, Tusques J. L'illusion d'intermetamorphose et de charme. Ann Med Psychol 1932;90:401–6.
[11] Kimura S. Review of 106 cases with the syndrome of Capgras. Bibl Psychiatr 1986;164: 121–30.
[12] Todd J, Dewhurst K, Wallis G. The syndrome of Capgras. Br J Psychiatry 1981;139: 319–27.
[13] Christodoulou GN. Role of depersonalization-derealization phenomena in the delusional misidentification syndromes. In: Christodoulou GN, editor. The delusional misidentification zyndromes. Basel: Karger; 1986.
[14] Spier SA. Capgras' syndrome and the delusions of misidentification. Psychiatr Ann 1992; 22:279–85.
[15] Dohn H, Crews E. Capgras syndrome: a literature review and case series. Hillside J Clin Psychiatry 1986;8:56–74.
[16] Tamam L, Karatas G, Zeren T, et al. The prevalence of Capgras syndrome in a university hospital setting. Acta Neuropsychiatrica 2003;15:290–5.
[17] Kirov G, Jones P, Lewis SW. Prevalence of delusional misidentification syndromes. Psychopathology 1994;27:148–9.
[18] Harwood DG, Barker WW, Ownby RL, et al. Prevalence and correlates of Capgras syndrome in Alzheimer's disease. Int J Geriat Psychiatry 1999;14:415–20.
[19] Silva JA, Leong GB, Weinstock R, et al. Delusion misidentification and aggression in Alzheimer's disease. J Forensic Sci 2001;46:581–5.
[20] Signer SF. Psychosis in neurologic disease: Capgras symptom and delusions of reduplication in neurologic disorders. Neuropsychiatr Neuropsychol Behav Neurol 1992; 5:138–43.
[21] Roane DM, Rogers JD, Robinson JH, et al. Delusional misidentification in association with parkinsonism. J Neuropsychiatry Clin Neurosci 1998;10:194–8.
[22] Ballard C. Psychiatric morbidity in dementia with Lewy bodies: a prospective clinical and neuropathological comparative study with Alzheimer's disease. Am J Psychiatry 1999;156: 1039–45.

[23] Iseki E, Marui W, Nihashi N, et al. Psychiatric symptoms typical of patients with dementia with Lewy bodies—similarity to those of levodopa induced psychosis. Acta Neuropsychiatrica 2002;14:237–41.

[24] Hay GG. Electroconvulsive therapy as a contributor to the production of delusional misidentification. Br J Psychiatry 1986;148:667–9.

[25] Stewart JT. Capgras syndrome related to diazepam treatment. South Med J 2004;97:65–6.

[26] Alexander MP, Stuss DT, Benson DF. Capgras syndrome: a reduplicative phenomenon. Neurology 1979;29:334–9.

[27] Staton RD, Brumback RA, Wilson H. Reduplicative paramnesia: a disconnection syndrome of memory. Cortex 1982;18:23–36.

[28] Kapur N, Turner A, King C. Reduplicative paramnesia: possible anatomical and neuropsychological mechanisms. Neurol Neurosur Psychiatry 1988;51:579–81.

[29] Moser DJ, Cohen RA, Malloy PF, et al. Reduplicative paramnesia: longitudinal neurobehavioral and neuroimaging analysis. J Geriatr Psychiatry Neurol 1998;11:174–81.

[30] Feinberg TE, Haber LD, Leeds NE. Verbal asomatognosia. Neurology 1990;40:1391–4.

[31] Meador KJ, Loring DW, Feinberg TE, et al. Anosognosia and asomatognosia during intracarotid amobarbital inactivation. Neurology 2000;55:816–20.

[32] Vié J. Les meconnaissances systematiques. Ann Med Psychol (Paris) 1944;102:410–55.

[33] Feinberg TE, Roane D. Misidentification syndromes. In: Feinberg TE, Farah M, editors. Behavioral neurology and neuropsychology. New York: McGraw-Hill; 1997. p. 391–7.

[34] Weinstein EA, Kahn RL. Denial of illness. Springfield (IL): Charles C. Thomas; 1955.

[35] Critchley M. Personification of paralyzed limbs in hemiplegics. BMJ 1955;30:284–7.

[36] Weinstein EA, Friedland RP. Behavioral disorders associated with hemi-inattention. In: Weinstein EA, Friedland RP, editors. Advances in neurology. New York: Raven Press; 1977. p. 51–62.

[37] Weinstein EA. Anosognosia and denial of illness. In: Prigatano GP, Schacter DP, editors. Awareness of deficit after brain injury: clinical and theoretical issues. New York: Oxford University Press; 1991. p. 240–57.

[38] Ruff RL, Volpe BT. Environmental reduplication associated with right frontal and parietal lobe injury. Neurol Neurosurg Psychiatry 1981;44:382–6.

[39] Feinberg TE, Eaton LA, Roane DM, et al. Multiple Fregoli delusions after traumatic brain injury. Cortex 1999;35:373–87.

[40] Pick A. On reduplication paramnesia. Brain 1903;26:260–7.

[41] Weinstein EA, Kahn RL, Morris GO. Delusions about children following brain injury. J Hillside Hospital 1956;5:290–8.

[42] Joseph AB. Focal central nervous system abnormalities in patients with misidentification syndromes. In: Christodoulou GN, editor. The delusional misidentification syndromes. Basel: Karger; 1986. p. 68.

[43] Weinstein EA, Burnham DL. Reduplication and the syndrome of Capgras. Psychiatry 1991;54:78–88.

[44] Feinberg TE, Shapiro RM. Misidentification-reduplication and the right hemisphere. Neuropsychiatr Neuropsychol Behav Neurol 1989;2:39–48.

[45] Förstl H, Almeida OP, Owen A, et al. Psychiatric, neurological and medical aspects of misidentification syndromes: a review of 260 cases. Psychol Med 1991;21:905–50.

[46] Benson DF, Gardner H, Meadows JC. Reduplicative paramnesia. Neurology 1976;26:147–51.

[47] Hakim H, Verma NP, Greiffenstein MF. Pathogenesis of reduplicative paramnesia. Neurol Neurosurg Psychiatry 1988;51:839–41.

[48] Fleminger S, Burns A. The delusional misidentification syndromes in patients with and without evidence of organic cerebral disorder: a structured review of case reports. Biol Psychiatry 1993;33:22–32.

[49] Forstl H, Burns A, Jacoby R, et al. Neuroanatomical correlates of clinical misidentification and misperception in senile dementia of the Alzheimer type. J Clin Psychiatry 1991;52:268.

[50] Mentis MJ, Weinstein EA, Horwitz B. Abnormal brain glucose metabolism in the delusional misidentification syndrome: A positron emission tomography study in Alzheimer disease. Biol Psychiatry 1995;38:438–49.

[51] Feinberg TE, DeLuca J, Giacino JT, et al. Right hemisphere pathology and the self. In: Feinberg TE, Keenan JP, editors. The lost self: pathologies of the brain and identity. New York: Oxford University Press; in press.

[52] Weinstein EA, Friedland RP, Wagner EE. Denial/unawareness of impairment and symbolic behavior in Alzheimer's disease. Neuropsychiatr Neuropsychol Behav Neurol 1994;7:176–84.

[53] Taylor J, editor. Selected writings of John Hughlings Jackson. New York: Basic Books; 1958.

[54] Ellis HD, Young AW. Accounting for delusional misidentification. Br J Psychiatry 1990;57: 239–48.

[55] Bauer RM. Autonomic recognition of names and faces: a neuropsychological application of the Guilty Knowledge Test. Neuropsychologia 1984;22:457–69.

[56] Bauer RM. The cognitive psychophysiology of prosopagnosia. In: Ellis H, Jeeves M, Newcombe F, et al, editors. Aspects of face processing. Dordrecht (The Netherlands): Martinus Nijhoff; 1986. p. 253–67.

[57] Hirstein W, Ramachandran VS. Capgras syndrome: a novel probe for understanding the neural representation of the identity and familiarity of persons. Proc R Soc Lond B Biol Sci 1997;264:437–44.

[58] Ramachandran VS. Consciousness and body image: lessons from phantom limbs, Capgras syndrome and pain asymbolia. Philos Trans R Soc Lond B Biol Sci 1998;353: 1851–9.

[59] Dietl T, Herr A, Brunner H, et al. Capgras syndrome—out of sight, out of mind. Acta Psychiatr Scand 2003;108:460–3.

[60] Shah NJ, Marshall JC, Zafiris O, et al. The neural correlates of person familiarity: a functional magnetic resonance imaging study with clinical implications. Brain 2001;124: 804–15.

[61] Ellis HD, Lewis MB. Capgras delusion: a window on face recognition. Trends Cogn Sci 2001;5:149–56.

[62] Rapcsak SZ, Polster MR, Glisky ML, et al. False recognition of unfamiliar faces following right hemisphere damage: neuropsychological and anatomical observations. Cortex 1996; 32:593–611.

[63] Breen N, Caine D, Coltheart M. Mirrored-self misidentification: two cases of focal onset dementia. Neurocase 2001;7:239–54.

[64] Stuss DT, Alexander MP, Lieberman A, et al. An extraordinary form of confabulation. Neurology 1978;28:116–72.

[65] Kopelman MD. Two types of confabulation. Neurol Neurosurg Psychiatry 1980;43:461–3.

[66] Deluca J. Predicting neurobehavioral patterns following anterior communicating artery aneurysm. Cortex 1993;29:639–47.

[67] DeLuca JA. Cognitive neuroscience perspective on confabulation. Neuro-Psychoanalysis 2000;2:119–32.

[68] Levin M. Delirious disorientation: the law of the unfamiliar mistaken for the familiar. J Mentl Sci 1945;91:447–53.

[69] Berlyne N. Confabulation. Br J Psychiatry 1972;120:31–9.

[70] Moscovitch M, Melo B. Strategic retrieval and the frontal lobes: evidence from confabulation and amnesia. Neuropsychologia 1997;35:1017–34.

[71] Victor M, Yakovlev PI. SS Korsakoff's psychic disorder in conjunction with peripheral neuritis: a translation of Korsakoff's original article with brief comments on the author and his contribution to clinical medicine. Neurology 1955;5:394–406.

[72] Bonhoeffer K. Die akuten Geisteskrankheiten der Gewohnheitstrinker. Jena (Germany): Gustav Fischer; 1901.

[73] Bonhoeffer K. Der Korsakowsche Symptomenkomplex in seinen Beziehungen zu den verschiedenen Krankheitsformen. Allg Z Psychiatr 1904;61:744–52.
[74] Van Der Horst L. Uber die Psychologie des Korsakowsyndroms. Monatsschr Psychiatry Neurol 1932;83:65–84.
[75] Williams HW, Rupp C. Observations on confabulation. Am J Psychiatry 1938;95:395–405.
[76] Talland GA. Confabulation in the Wernicke-Korsakoff syndrome. J Nerv Ment Dis 1961; 131:361–81.
[77] Talland GA. Deranged memory. New York: Academic Press; 1965.
[78] Victor M, Adams RD, Collins GH. The Wernicke-Korsakoff syndrome and related neurological disorders due to alcoholism and malnutrition. 2nd edition. Philadelphia: Davis; 1989.
[79] Kraepelin E. Lectures on clinical psychiatry. London: Bailliere, Tindall, & Cox; 1904. [Johnstone T, Trans.]
[80] Kraepelin E. Clinical psychiatry: a textbook for students and physicians. New York: MacMillan; 1907. [Diefendorf AR, Trans.]
[81] Kraepelin E. Dementia praecox and paraphrenia. Edinburgh (UK): E. & S. Livingstone; 1919. [Barclay RM, Trans.]
[82] Schnider A, von Daniken C, Gutbrod K. Disorientation in amnesia. A confusion of memory traces. Brain 1996;119:1627–32.
[83] Schnider A, Gutbrod K, Hess CW, et al. Memory without context: amnesia with confabulations after infarction of the right capsular genu. J Neurol Neurosurg Psychiatry 1996;61:186–93.
[84] Schnider A, Ptak R. Spontaneous confabulators fail to suppress currently irrelevant memory traces. Nat Neurosci 1999;2:677–81.
[85] Schnider A, Ptak R, von Daniken C, et al. Recovery from spontaneous confabulations parallels recovery of temporal confusion in memory. Neurology 2000;55:74–83.
[86] Schnider A. Spontaneous confabulation and the adaptation of thought to ongoing reality. Nat Rev Neurosci 2003;4:662–71.
[87] Moscovitch M. Confabulation and the frontal systems: strategic vs. associative retrieval in neuropsychological theories of memory. In: Roediger HL, Craik FM, editors. Varieties of memory and consciousness: essays in honour of Endel Tulving. Hillsdale (NJ): Lawrence Erlbaum; 1989. p. 133–60.
[88] Moscovitch M. Confabulation. In: Schacter DL, editor. Memory distortion: how minds, brains and societies reconstruct the past. Cambridge (MA): Harvard University Press; 1995. p. 226–51.
[89] Patterson A, Zangwill OL. Recovery of spatial orientation in the post-traumatic confusional state. Brain 1944;67:54–68.
[90] Weinstein EA. Symbolic aspects of confabulation following brain injury: influence of premorbid personality. Bull Menninger Clin 1996;60:331–50.
[91] Box O, Laing H, Kopelman M. The evolution of spontaneous confabulation, delusional misidentification and a related delusion in a case of severe head injury. Neurocase 1999;5: 251–62.
[92] Mattioli F, Miozzo A, Vignolo LA. Confabulation and delusional misidentification: a four year follow-up study. Cortex 1999;35:413–22.
[93] Alexander MR, Freedman M. Amnesia after anterior communication artery aneurysm rupture. Neurology 1984;34:752–7.
[94] Vilkki J. Amnesic syndromes after surgery of anterior communicating artery aneurysms. Cortex 1985;21:431–44.
[95] Fischer RS, Alexander MP, D'Esposito M, et al. Neuropsychological and neuroanatomical correlates of confabulation. J Clin Exp Neuropsychol 1995;17:20–8.
[96] Ptak R, Schnider A. Spontaneous confabulations after orbitofrontal damage: the role of temporal context confusion and self-monitoring. Neurocase 1999;5:243–50.

[97] Feinberg TE, Giacino JT. Confabulation. In: Feinberg TE, Farah MJ, editors. Behavioral neurology and neuropsychology. New York: McGraw-Hill; 2003. p. 363–72.

[98] Johnson MK, Hayes SM, D'Esposito M, Raye CL. Confabulation. In: Grafman J, Boller F, editors. Handbook of neuropsychology. 2nd edition. Amsterdam: Elsevier Science; 2002. p. 383–407.

[99] Levine DN, Grek A. The anatomic basis for delusions after right cerebral infarction. Neurology 1984;34:577–82.

[100] Malloy PF, Richardson ED. The frontal lobes and content-specific delusions. J Neuropsychiatry Clin Neurosci 1994;6:455–66.

[101] Kumral E, Özturk Ö. Delusional state following acute stroke. Neurology 2004;62:110–3.

[102] Sultzer DL, Brown CV, Mandelkern MA, et al. Delusional thoughts and regional frontal temporal cortex metabolism in Alzheimer's disease. Am J Psychiatry 2003;160:341–9.

[103] Turk DJ, Heatherton DF, Macrae CN, et al. Out of contact, out of mind: the distributed nature of the self. Ann N Y Acad Sci 2003;1001:65–78.

[104] Feinberg TE. Anosognosia and confabulation. In: Feinberg TE, Farah MJ, editors. Behavioral neurology and neuropsychology. New York: McGraw-Hill; 1997.

[105] Keenan JP, Wheeler MA, Gallup GG, et al. Self-recognition and the right prefrontal cortex. Trends Cogn Sci 2000;4:338–44.

[106] Keenan JP, Gallup GG, Falk D. The face in the mirror: the search for the origins of consciousness. New York: Harper Collins/Ecco; 2003.

[107] Kircher TT, Senior C, Phillips ML, et al. Recognizing one's own face. Cognition 2001;78: B1–15.

[108] Keenan JP, Nelson A, O'Connor M, et al. Self- recognition and the right hemisphere. Nature 2001;409(6818):305.

[109] Sugiura M, Kawashima R, Nakamura K, et al. Passive and active recognition of one's own face. Neuroimage 2000;11:36–48.

[110] Calabrese P, Markowitsch HJ, Durwen HF, et al. Right temporofrontal cortex as critical locus for the ecphory of old episodic memories. J Neurol Neurosurg Psychiatry 1996;61: 304–10.

[111] Fink GR, Markowitsch HJ, Reinkemeier M, et al. Cerebral representation of one's own past: neural networks involved in autobiographical memory. J Neurosci 1996;16:4275–82.

[112] Markowitsch HJ, Thiel A, Reinkemeier M, et al. Right amygdalar and temporofrontal activation during autobiographic, but not during fictitious memory retrieval. Behav Neurol 2000;12:181–90.

[113] Nakamura K, Kawashima R, Sugiura M, et al. Neural substrates for recognition of familiar voices: a PET study. Neuropsychologia 2001;39:1047–54.

[114] Decety J, Sommerville JA. Shared representations between self and other: a social cognitive neuroscience view. Trends Cogn Sci 2003;12:527–33.

[115] Kaplan-Solms K, Solms M. Clinical studies in neuro-psychoanalysis. London: Karnac Books; 2000.

[116] McKeith I, Del Ser T, Spano P, et al. Efficacy of rivastigmine in dementia with Lewy bodies: a randomized, double-blind, placebo-controlled international study. Lancet 2000;356: 2031–6.

[117] Wells CE, Whitehouse PJ. Cortical dementia. In: Fogel BS, Schiffer RB, editors. Neuropsychiatry. Baltimore (MD): Williams & Wilkins; 1996. p. 871–94.

[118] Pihan H, Gutbrod K, Baas U, et al. Dopamine inhibition and the adaptation of behavior to ongoing reality. Neuroreport 2004;15:709–12.

ELSEVIER
SAUNDERS

PSYCHIATRIC
CLINICS
OF NORTH AMERICA

Psychiatr Clin N Am 28 (2005) 685–700

# Neurobehavioral Aspects of Cerebral White Matter Disorders

## Christopher M. Filley, MD[a,b,*]

[a]Departments of Neurology and Psychiatry, University of Colorado School of Medicine,
Denver, CO, USA
[b]Denver Veterans Affairs Medical Center, Denver, Colorado, USA

White matter, the densely packed collection of myelinated axons coursing between widely dispersed gray matter areas, occupies nearly one half the human brain and plays a vital role in the distributed neural networks subserving higher function [1,2]. The white matter is also vulnerable to a wide range of neuropathologic insults from disease or injury, and the clinical syndromes resulting from these lesions may require the expertise of both neurologists and psychiatrists. In both the healthy and the disordered brain, therefore, the white matter is an essential neural constituent that contributes to all realms of human behavior. In recent years, a growing recognition of the importance of white matter has emerged in the clinical and basic neurosciences, and information on this often-neglected area is rapidly accumulating. This article summarizes the understanding of white matter and its disorders from the perspective of behavioral neurology [1,2].

## Background

White matter was first distinguished from gray matter by the Renaissance anatomist Andreas Vesalius in 1543 [2]. As the neurosciences developed, the role of white matter in providing structural and functional connections between gray matter areas within the brain became apparent [2]. In the nineteenth century, Jean Martin Charcot greatly advanced the understanding of white matter with his detailed studies of multiple sclerosis, the most important demyelinative disease of the central nervous system. In 1965,

---

* Correspondence. Behavioral Neurology Section, Department of Neurology, UCHSC
B-183, 4200 East Ninth Avenue, Denver, Colorado 80262.
 E-mail address: Christopher.Filley@uchsc.edu

Norman Geschwind [3] proposed the notion of cerebral disconnection as a mechanism of neurobehavioral dysfunction, thus strongly suggesting the importance of white matter lesions in brain–behavior relationships. At the turn of the twenty-first century, the notion of distributed neural networks as championed by M-Marsel Mesulam [4] has become widely accepted, further suggesting that the white matter occupies a central place in the elaboration of human behavior [5]. In parallel with this development has been the impressive growth of modern neuroimaging that enables the viewing of white matter and its functional specializations in increasingly elegant detail. Today, there is an explosion of information on the white matter, its role in normal brain function, and its relevance to human illness.

## Anatomy and physiology

At the microscopic level, cerebral white matter consists of collections of closely apposed axons that are wrapped concentrically in myelin, the insulation of nerve cells made up of roughly 70% lipid and 30% protein. Oligodendrocytes, the glial cells that myelinate the axons, are numerous, as are astrocytes, ependymal cells, and blood vessels. Macroscopically, the white matter can be seen to form fiber collections known as tracts, fasciculi, bundles, peduncles, and lemnisci. The three major fiber systems are the projection fibers, the association fibers, and the commissural fibers. For this discussion, the most critical tracts are the association fibers that travel within the hemispheres and the commissural fibers that course between them (Fig. 1). Many other smaller tracts, such as the fornix and the median forebrain bundle, also merit attention. In general, however, with the exception of the corpus callosum and some of the association systems, little is known of the neurobehavioral affiliations of these tracts [2].

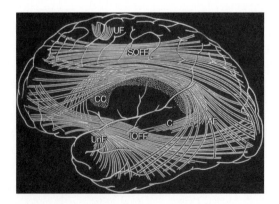

Fig. 1. Major white matter tracts in the human brain. AF, arcuate fasciculus; C, cingulum; CC, corpus callosum; IOFF, inferior occipitofrontal fasciculus; SOFF, superior occipitofrontal fasciculus; UF, U fiber; UnF, uncinate fasciculus.

Understanding the function of white matter begins with a consideration of its cellular physiology. Myelin forms a sheath that encircles the axon in such as a way that small regions, known as nodes of Ranvier, are left unwrapped; these regions permit the phenomenon of saltatory conduction, whereby the propagation of the action potential along the axon is dramatically enhanced. This feature contributes to the vastly increased conduction velocity of myelinated axons in comparison with those that are unmyelinated. Thus, the normal white matter ensures that rapid and efficient neuronal conduction occurs and contributes to the speed of information processing that typifies normal cognition [2]. At the macroscopic level, a striking feature is the abundance of white matter in the frontal regions of the brain. The frontal lobes have the highest degree of connectivity of any lobe of the brain and are positioned uniquely to exert an integrative influence by means of white matter tracts on mental operations performed by other cerebral regions [5].

## Development and aging

The white matter manifests a unique pattern of development through the life span. In early life, brain myelination is not complete for many years, perhaps past the second decade, in contrast to the full complement of brain neurons, which are present at birth [2]. Conversely, in the later decades of life, there is slow but steady loss of white matter that may in fact be more crucial than the loss of neurons, which now is thought to be not as pronounced as once believed [2].

Important clinical implications of this developmental trajectory may soon emerge. In children and adolescents, for example, the maturation of white matter, particularly in the frontal lobes, has been proposed to correlate with the acquisition of mature aspects of personality such as motivation, comportment, and executive function [1,2]. These attributes, well known to reflect the function of the frontal lobes, may signify the myelination of white matter tracts connecting the frontal lobes to other brain regions and thus contributing to the mature behavioral repertoire of adults [1,2]. In addition, a variety of psychiatric disorders in childhood may be influenced by abnormal white matter maturation [6].

In contrast, the aging process may involve a progressive diminution of white matter. In an autopsy study of normal brains from age 20 to 90 years, white matter volume loss was 28%, whereas neocortical volume loss was just 12% [7]. This selective tissue loss may account for normal cognitive changes in aging such as slowed speed of information processing, diminished attentional capacity, and forgetfulness [8]. Normal age-related changes in white matter loss may also contribute to the development of mild cognitive impairment [9], a controversial concept recently proposed to represent a transitional stage between normal aging and dementia. Although mild cognitive impairment most often is considered a precursor of Alzheimer's disease [9], the neuropathologic basis of mild cognitive impairment is unclear and may be explained by white matter changes in some individuals [10]. Even if mild cognitive impairment becomes established as a harbinger of Alzheimer's disease, age-related changes in white matter cannot be ignored as having a potential impact on cognitive function in older persons. Normal aging changes in myelin must also be considered when the impact of superimposed disease or injury, such as infarction or traumatic brain injury, further damages the white matter.

## Neuroimaging

Although the appearance of CT in the 1970s vastly improved the clinical visualization of the brain, it was the advent of MRI in the 1980s that first permitted the detailed interpretation of the structure of white matter. MRI quickly became the method of choice for providing detailed images of the white matter and its disorders, and the diagnosis of multiple sclerosis and many other problems was revolutionized. Older disorders were better understood, and many new ones were recognized with MRI, leading to a proliferation of clinical research. One of the major benefits of this research was the opportunity to seek correlations of clinical features with white matter pathology on MRI, particularly with regard to higher functions [2].

More recently, additional MRI techniques have been developed that further refine the depiction of white matter. Diffusion tensor imaging measures the diffusion of water in white matter tracts, which normally occurs anisotropically in the direction of tracts. In contrast, isotropic diffusion is less directional and is typical of damaged white matter. Diffusion tensor imaging thus offers the prospect of tractography, which can help characterize the connectivity of both abnormal and normal white matter regions [11,12]. MR spectroscopy is a technique that allows determination of the chemical composition of white matter regions [13]. Often referred to as a noninvasive biopsy, MR spectroscopy can be used to measure certain metabolites in selected regions and provide data regarding myelin and axonal integrity. Studies are increasingly showing, for example, that white matter alterations can be found by MR spectroscopy even in areas that appear normal on conventional MRI. Finally, magnetization transfer imaging is based on the interactions of protons and macromolecules and generates data on the fine structure of white matter [14]. The most commonly used magnetization transfer imaging parameter, the magnetization transfer ratio, is used as a marker of myelin integrity, so that a low magnetization transfer ratio suggests myelin injury. As with MR spectroscopy, magnetization transfer imaging can detect changes in white matter that appears normal on standard MRI.

In parallel with these advances in structural neuroimaging, studies examining brain function have been equally impressive. The cerebral cortex has been the focus of these methods because of its high degree of metabolic activity. The first method used in this regard was positron emission tomography (PET), in which a radiolabeled isotope is injected into the bloodstream, and brain metabolic activity is then measured [15]. A less expensive but also less elegant technique of this type is single-photon emission computed tomography (SPECT) [16]. Most recently, functional MRI has been added to the armamentarium of functional imaging methods. This method exploits the degree of blood oxygenation in relation to cognitive activity and has more favorable spatial resolution than PET and SPECT. Whereas some technical issues remain problematic, functional MRI does offer the prospect of more refined analyses of brain–behavior correlations [17].

The advantages of structural and functional neuroimaging are proving complementary in the pursuit of understanding the architecture of higher function. Whereas PET and functional MRI can identify cortical regions involved in cognitive processing, the various MRI methods available can establish the connectivity between these areas. If distributed neural networks consist of both gray and white matter structures linked into coherent arrays, it should be possible to combine the techniques that can characterize both of these components to formulate a unifying picture [18]. The goal of mapping neural networks is currently motivating a major effort in cognitive neuroscience and related disciplines.

## Disorders of white matter

The cerebral white matter is vulnerable to a wide range of neuropathology (Table 1). These diseases and injuries of white matter vary greatly in terms of cause, pathogenesis, extent and location of pathology, natural history, prognosis, and treatment [2]. Details of the neurology of these disorders can be found in standard neurologic textbooks, and some familiarity with them assists in appreciating their neurobehavioral

Table 1
White matter disorders

| Category | Example |
| --- | --- |
| Genetic | Metachromatic leukodystrophy |
| Demyelinative | Multiple sclerosis |
| Infectious | AIDS dementia complex |
| Inflammatory | Systemic lupus erythematosus |
| Toxic | Toluene leukoencephalopathy |
| Metabolic | Cobalamin deficiency |
| Vascular | Binswanger's disease |
| Traumatic | Traumatic brain injury |
| Neoplastic | Gliomatosis cerebri |
| Hydrocephalic | Normal pressure hydrocephalus |

consequences. The objective here is to develop common themes that occur in these disorders, because from this synthetic approach much can be learned about higher brain function.

Some neuropathologic overlap exists between the white matter disorders and those primarily involving gray matter. In multiple sclerosis, for example, demyelination can be seen in cortical gray matter areas to a variable extent [19]; conversely, in Alzheimer's disease there is damage to white matter tracts, most likely secondary to Wallerian degeneration that accompanies neuronal loss in the cerebral cortex [20]. Although this complexity may suggest that study of white matter disorders as a group is unproductive, much overlap of this kind exists in neurology, psychiatry, and indeed all branches of medicine. There is as much utility in examining details of various white matter disorders as there is in pursuing fine distinctions between degenerative diseases of the cortex such as Alzheimer's disease and frontotemporal dementia, or the subtleties of bipolar disorder in contrast to schizophrenia. The focus on white matter serves to introduce a host of testable hypotheses and also to inform the investigation of distributed neural networks that necessarily involve integrated systems of gray and white matter structures working in concert.

The cerebral white matter disorders can be classified as genetic, demyelinative, infectious, inflammatory, toxic, metabolic, vascular, traumatic, neoplastic, and hydrocephalic (Table 1) [2]. Each category involves a fundamentally distinct pathophysiologic basis, and even the entities within these categories can vary in many clinical and neuropathologic respects. Nevertheless, a consideration of the white matter disorders as a whole points out commonalities in their effects on neurobehavioral function. Remarkably, after careful review of available clinical literature, all of these disorders—of which there are more than 100—can be seen to be associated with some form of cognitive or emotional dysfunction [2]. This observation alone validates the emphasis on white matter; in addition, similarities in neurobehavioral dysfunction cut across all etiologic categories, further justifying an emphasis on the white matter as a substrate of higher function in humans.

A brief survey of selected white matter disorders can highlight the diversity of clinical phenomena. In infants and children, genetic diseases such as metachromatic leukodystrophy illustrate the failure of brain myelin to develop normally, and the subsequent dysmyelination leads to early disability and death, or, in occasional older individuals, a common sequence of psychosis followed by dementia [21,22]. In contrast, young adults are at high risk for the demyelinative diseases such as multiple sclerosis, in which inflammatory destruction of myelin leads to neurologic and neurobehavioral disability [23]. A number of infectious diseases that produce cognitive decline may affect the white matter, including the AIDS dementia complex [24] and progressive multifocal leukoencephalopathy [25]. Similarly, noninfectious inflammatory diseases such as systemic lupus erythematosus can affect the white matter by immune-related processes, and the multiple manifestations of neuropsychiatric lupus are being recognized increasingly [26]. In the category of toxic disorders, a large and growing number of white matter toxins have been identified, among them the common industrial and household solvent toluene. Detailed studies of toluene leukoencephalopathy in solvent abusers has disclosed dramatic white matter disease on MRI that correlates with the severity of dementia produced [27–29]. Metabolic disorders of white matter have been noted, among them the dementia of vitamin $B_{12}$ (cobalamin) deficiency [30]. One of the most common white matter disorders is the variant of vascular dementia referred to as Binswanger's disease or subcortical ischemic vascular dementia [31,32]. Closely related to Binswanger's disease is the genetic disease, cerebral autosomal dominant arteriopathy with subcortical infarcts and leukoencephalopathy (CADASIL) [33,34]. Traumatic brain injury qualifies as a white matter disorder because of the common white matter lesion known as diffuse axonal injury in patients who have traumatic brain injury [35]. A variety of brain neoplasms also primarily affect white matter, and the entity gliomatosis cerebri serves especially well to illustrate the adverse consequences of neoplastic white matter infiltration on neurobehavioral status [36]. Finally, hydrocephalus from any cause exerts its major effect on the periventricular white matter, and examples in children (early hydrocephalus) and adults (normal-pressure hydrocephalus) indicate that white matter damage of this sort can result in major neurobehavioral sequelae [37,38].

## Prognosis and treatment

Because of the great variety of white matter disorders, summary statements about prognosis and treatment can be given only in general terms. Textbooks of neurology and medicine can provide details of individual disorders; the aim here is to suggest principles pertaining to all of them in an effort to understand the neurobiology of white matter as a whole.

The prognosis of white matter disorders depends on many factors, including the nature of the neuropathologic insult, the extent and location of white matter damage, the chronicity of the disorder, the age of the patient, and the coexistence of other neurologic and medical disorders. Despite this complex clinical picture, one consistent theme on outcome is that there seems to be a spectrum of severity in white matter disorders, from mild and reversible white matter changes to severe and irreversible necrosis, that generally correlates with prognosis [2,28]. This phenomenon has been most evident in the toxic leukoencephalopathies [28] but probably applies to other white matter insults as well. For example, there is considerable evidence that when the neuropathology is severe enough to cause axonal loss, a less favorable outcome can be expected in many white matter disorders, including leukodystrophies, multiple sclerosis, central pontine myelinolysis and other metabolic encephalopathies, the AIDS dementia complex, Binswanger's disease, and CADASIL [39].

The observation that white matter pathology can be mild and reversible suggests that, in general, the prognosis of white matter disorders is more optimistic than that of gray matter disorders, most notably Alzheimer's disease, in which cell bodies, synapses, and receptors are destroyed by the primary disease process. In many cases, such as subtle toxic leukoencephalopathies characterized by myelin edema alone, full recovery can be expected after withdrawal of the offending agent because the myelin and axons have not been permanently damaged [28]. Even when there is significant myelin damage, substantial recovery often can be predicted if axons are spared [28].

For clinicians, these observations suggest that prevention and early treatment after diagnosis have the best potential for improving clinical care and outcome. Preventive efforts are of course to be encouraged for many disorders, including infectious, metabolic, toxic, vascular, and traumatic causes of white matter damage [2]. Early treatment of individuals who develop many of the white matter disorders can retard, arrest, or reverse the neuropathologic process before axonal loss occurs [2]. As medical and surgical treatments for the various white matter disorders continue to improve, opportunities for effective early intervention should expand [2]. It has been encouraging, for example, that treatment of multiple sclerosis with immunomodulatory agents such as interferon-beta-1a seems to have a beneficial effect on cognition [40]. Exciting possibilities using gene therapy [41] and stem cells [42] now are being considered for many white matter disorders. Additional options may include neuropharmacologic approaches for these patients, such as stimulants for cognitive slowing [43] and cholinesterase inhibitors for attention and memory loss [44].

## White matter dementia

Among the wide array of cerebral white matter disorders, cognitive dysfunction is the most common neurobehavioral syndrome that can be related to white matter pathologic burden. In many cases, this disturbance is sufficiently severe to merit the term dementia. The prevalence of cognitive dysfunction and dementia resulting from white matter disorders as a group is unknown because epidemiologic data of this nature are unavailable, but much clinical experience favors this view [1,2]. Moreover, the typically diffuse distribution of white matter neuropathology suggests that syndromes reflecting widespread white matter dysfunction are far more common than syndromes reflecting isolated regions of white matter involvement [1,2]. Evidence that focal neurobehavioral syndromes are considerably less common is available from studies of multiple sclerosis, in which cognitive dysfunction or dementia may afflict as many as 65% of patients [45], whereas aphasia occurs in less than 1% [46]. Similarly, although neuropsychiatric syndromes such as depression are common in patients who have white matter disorders, the prevalence of these syndromes remains debatable; in any case, because they may result from many causes, there is a less secure association with white matter pathology. Thus, cognitive impairment may be a major source of clinical distress and functional disability that relates directly to damage in the cerebral white matter.

White matter dementia is a term introduced to call attention to the morbidity caused by disabling cognitive loss in patients who have white matter disorders [47]. Although, in early stages, milder cognitive dysfunction is more common than dementia and may be the presenting feature of the disease [48], a level of severity sufficient to merit the diagnosis of dementia often follows. In multiple sclerosis, for example, estimates hold that 10% to 20% of patients develop dementia in the course of the disease [49]. Because the understanding of the origin and prevention of dementia are such high priorities, the term white matter dementia is intended to alert clinicians and researchers to these issues in the context of white matter and its many disorders.

In clinical practice, the recognition of early cognitive dysfunction in the white matter disorders may be far from straightforward. Many patients who have these disorders present with subtle cognitive symptoms and signs, frequently commingled with other neurologic or medical features of their disease, that challenge the clinician to interpret the relationship of white matter pathologic burden to cognitive status. The range of clinical features heralding the onset of cerebral white matter involvement is impressively broad and may include inattention, executive dysfunction, confusion, memory loss, personality change, depression, somnolence, lassitude, and fatigue. The nonspecific clinical profile of many affected patients often suggests a primary psychiatric disorder, and indeed, in retrospect, many patients who have white matter dementia have had early psychiatric dysfunction that antedated measurable cognitive impairment [2]. This interdigitation of cognitive and emotional features in many patients renders the category of white matter disorders particularly relevant to the growing field of neuropsychiatry. There is, however, no adequate nosology to describe the complex presentation of white matter disorders, and a new term may be needed to describe this still rather obscure area of clinical dysfunction. One suggestion is to consider the descriptor "dysmentia," a term introduced in 1978 and meaning "disordered" (Greek *dys*) "mind" (Latin *mens*) [50]. Properly defined and standardized, dysmentia could become a useful term to describe the early cognitive impairment in white matter disorders, much as mild cognitive impairment [9] is becoming accepted for the description of early cognitive loss that may precede the development of the gray matter disorder Alzheimer's disease.

Because the problem of cognitive dysfunction and dementia is important and underappreciated, a deeper understanding of its clinical manifestations is imperative. Thus, considerable effort has been devoted to developing an understanding of the profile of deficits and strengths (Box 1) that can be used in diagnosis, counseling, rehabilitation, and research on new

---

**Box 1. Characteristics of white matter dementia**

Sustained attention deficit
Executive dysfunction
Memory retrieval deficit
Visuospatial impairment
Psychiatric dysfunction
Normal language
Normal extrapyramidal function
Normal procedural memory

---

therapeutic strategies [1,2]. Although more work needs to be done, preliminary data suggest that this specific combination differs from that seen with cortical dementia such as Alzheimer's disease [1,2,51] and from subcortical gray matter dementias such as Huntington's disease [1,2,52]. Thus, the cerebral white matter may have a unique role in the organization of cognition and emotion.

Sustained attention deficits, executive dysfunction, and memory retrieval deficits may be particularly salient. These problems are typical of patients who have white matter disorders and relate to a general slowing of cognition, often called impaired speed of information processing [2]. Neuroanatomically, sustained attention (concentration, vigilance), executive function, and memory retrieval are all closely associated with frontal lobe function, and most white matter disorders show a predilection for the frontal white matter [2]. Even when white matter lesions are situated in more posterior cerebral locations, frontal lobe functions are still affected [53], probably because of the dense connectivity between frontal and other regions. Visuospatial skills also are affected in white matter disorders [2], and a wide variety of psychiatric concerns can be implicated as well, as discussed later. In contrast, language typically is normal or mildly affected because of the sparing of language-related cortex [2], a fact that may lead the clinician to overlook cognitive dysfunction that involves nonlinguistic function. Extrapyramidal function also tends to be intact in white matter disorders, in keeping with the relative sparing of deep gray matter structures [2]. For the same reason, procedural (skill) memory is spared, and although this domain cannot be routinely tested in clinical settings, the theoretical implications of intact procedural memory can be useful in guiding research on brain function [52,54].

### Focal neurobehavioral syndromes

The syndrome of white matter dementia vividly illustrates the impact of white matter disorders on cognition, but other neurobehavioral syndromes also can be ascribed to white matter lesions of the brain. In addition to cognitive loss and dementia, a wide range of focal neurobehavioral syndromes has been described (Box 2) [2]. These disturbances are classic syndromes in behavioral neurology such as aphasia and amnesia, and although such syndromes correctly are considered to be more common with cortical lesions, recent findings have confirmed that they may also follow white matter damage. Focal syndromes are associated with discrete, isolated white matter lesions, in contrast with white matter dementia that results from the more typical widespread pathology of white matter disorders. As examples of this principle, reports have documented isolated amnesia associated with bilateral mamillothalamic tract infarction [55] and conduction aphasia related to an acute multiple sclerosis plaque in the left arcuate fasciculus [56]. Although uncommon in comparison with the syndromes caused by diffuse white matter damage, the focal neurobehavioral syndromes illustrate the importance of white matter tracts in all domains of higher function. Further observations of these syndromes and their neuroanatomic correlates can be expected, steadily contributing to the understanding of the many neural networks that subserve the higher functions.

---

**Box 2. Focal neurobehavioral syndromes**

Amnesia
Aphasia
   Broca's
   Transcortical motor
   Conduction
   Wernicke's
   Global
   Mixed transcortical
Apraxia
Alexia
   Pure alexia
   Alexia with agraphia
Developmental dyslexia
Gerstmann's syndrome
Agnosia
   Visual
   Auditory
Visuospatial dysfunction
Akinetic mutism
Executive dysfunction
Callosal disconnection

**Neuropsychiatric syndromes**

Abnormalities of cerebral white matter also have been associated with a wide spectrum of emotional disturbances, comprising a group referred to as the neuropsychiatric syndromes. This category, however, is less securely defined than the neurobehavioral syndromes discussed previously, because the correlation of white matter pathology with psychiatric syndromes is far less clear. Some suggestion exists that the burden of white matter pathology contributes to emotional dysfunction, but other factors also play a role, and the origin of psychiatric impairment must be considered multifactorial. Nevertheless, much information on the role of white matter in emotional function has been adduced recently, and new insights are illuminating the white matter disorders themselves and many psychiatric diseases as well.

It is useful to consider these neuropsychiatric syndromes in two general groups: the psychiatric features described in patients who have known white matter disorders, and the psychiatric diseases in which white matter abnormalities have been implicated (Table 2). In patients who have known white matter disorders, numerous reports have documented the presence of depression, mania, psychosis, pathologic affect, euphoria, and fatigue [2]. The correlations between these syndromes and measures of white matter dysfunction are uncertain, however, leaving open the possibilities that psychiatric syndromes may be related only indirectly or not at all to the specific white matter disorder. A complex interplay of many factors, including white matter injury, may contribute to emotional distress, and further investigation clearly is needed in this area [2].

In considering primary psychiatric diseases that typically are considered idiopathic and unrelated to structural brain damage, a number of intriguing reports have recently appeared that exploit MRI techniques to examine the structure of white matter. In schizophrenia, for example, conventional MRI, diffusion tensor imaging, and magnetization transfer imaging all detect microstuctural white matter abnormalities; widespread myelin and oligo-dendrocyte dysfunction leading to altered cerebral connectivity has been implicated [57]. Much evidence also supports an association between white matter changes in geriatric depression [58], although a firm correlation has

Table 2
Neuropsychiatric syndromes

| Psychiatric syndromes in white matter disorders | Psychiatric disorders with white matter abnormalities |
| --- | --- |
| Depression | Schizophrenia |
| Mania | Depression |
| Psychosis | Bipolar disorder |
| Pathologic affect | Attention deficit hyperactivity disorder |
| Euphoria | Autism |
| Fatigue | Aggression |

yet to be established [2]. MRI white matter hyperintensities are more common in patients who have bipolar disorder than in the general population [59]. A diminished volume of right frontal white matter has been found to correlate with impaired sustained attention in children who have attention deficit hyperactivity disorder [60]. In contrast, an increased volume of hemispheric white matter in all lobes has been observed in autism [61]. Finally, diffusion tensor imaging studies of schizophrenic men have found a correlation of inferior frontal lobe white matter abnormalities with impulsive aggression [62]. These studies indicate that detailed examination of the white matter may offer important new insights into psychiatric disease by concentrating on disruption of the neural networks devoted to emotional function [2,63].

## The behavioral neurology of white matter

The white matter is a major constituent of the brain (Fig. 1), and the syndromes discussed here illustrate the profound effect that white matter disorders may exert on cognition and emotion. White matter dementia seems to be the most important of these syndromes because of its frequency and major clinical impact. Regardless of the specific neurobehavioral syndrome produced, however, the white matter disorders bear directly on the notion of distributed neural networks. These networks, consisting of widespread ensembles of neurons dedicated to discrete neurobehavioral functions, have recently come to dominate thinking about the higher functions in general. White matter, providing the connectivity in all these networks, plays a pivotal role in the organization of human mental life. In a general sense, although the gray matter of the brain subserves information processing, the white matter provides for information transfer; both are critical for the efficient operations of the neural network responsible for a specific mental domain. In the presence of damaged white matter, information processing occurs only in a slowed and inefficient manner; if the white matter is severely impaired, there may be no processing at all. Such considerations suggest an evolving behavioral neurology of white matter, an organizing framework that can stimulate further study and insight.

## Summary

The study of higher function in humans requires a consideration of all the neural tissues in the brain. Long neglected as a contributor to the organization of cognitive and emotional operations, the cerebral white matter is now the subject of substantial effort to improve understanding. Among the many approaches that can address this area usefully, the study of individuals with white matter disorders offers a wealth of clinical insights that exploits the time-tested lesion method of behavioral neurology. This process is complemented by sophisticated neuroimaging techniques that increasingly enable detailed visualization of white matter tracts as they participate in the cognitive and emotional operations of distributed neural networks. In practical terms, an appreciation of the neurobehavioral importance of white matter disorders can be of great benefit for patients seen by neurologists and psychiatrists alike, especially because early recognition and treatment often can have an important influence on outcome. In theoretical terms, a focus on the white matter and its disorders promises to expand knowledge of the brain as an extraordinarily complex organ in which the connectivity provided by white matter is central to cognition, emotion, and consciousness itself [64]. As the details of white matter structure and function become clarified, a more complete portrait of the organ of the mind can be anticipated.

## References

[1] Filley CM. The behavioral neurology of cerebral white matter. Neurology 1998;50:1535–40.
[2] Filley CM. The behavioral neurology of white matter. New York: Oxford University Press; 2001.
[3] Geschwind N. Disconnexion syndromes in animals and man. Brain 1965;88:237–94, 585–644.
[4] Mesulam M-M. Large-scale neurocognitive networks and distributed processing for attention, language, and memory. Ann Neurol 1990;28:597–613.
[5] Mesulam M-M. Behavioral neuroanatomy: large-scale neural networks, association cortex, frontal syndromes, the limbic system, and hemispheric specializations. In: Mesulam M-M. Principles of behavioral and cognitive neurology. 2nd edition. New York: Oxford University Press; 2000. p. 1–120.
[6] Durston S, Hulshoff Pol HE, Casey BJ, et al. Anatomical MRI of the developing human brain: what have we learned? J Am Acad Child Adolesc Psychiatry 2001;40:1012–20.
[7] Pakkenberg B, Gundersen HJG. Neocortical neuron number in humans: effect of sex and age. J Comp Neurol 1997;384:312–20.
[8] Filley CM, Cullum CM. Attention and vigilance functions in normal aging. Appl Neuropsychol 1994;1:29–32.
[9] Petersen RC, Smith GE, Waring SC, et al. Mild cognitive impairment: clinical characterization and outcome. Arch Neurol 1999;56:303–8.
[10] Maruyama M, Matsui T, Tanji H, et al. Cerebrospinal fluid tau protein and periventricular white matter lesions in patients with mild cognitive impairment. Implications for 2 major pathways. Arch Neurol 2004;61:716–20.
[11] Wakana S, Jiang H, Nagae-Poetscher LM, et al. Fiber tract-based atlas of human white matter anatomy. Radiology 2004;230:77–87.
[12] Moseley M, Bammer R, Illes J. Diffusion-tensor imaging of cognitive performance. Brain Cogn 2002;50:396–413.
[13] Ross B, Michaelis T. Clinical applications of magnetic resonance spectroscopy. Magn Reson Q 1994;10:191–247.
[14] van Buchem MA. Magnetization transfer: applications in neuroradiology. J Comp Assist Tomogr 1999;23(Suppl 1):S1–18.
[15] Cabeza R, Nyberg L. Imaging cognition: an empirical review of PET studies with normal subjects. J Cogn Neurosci 1997;9:1–26.
[16] Alavi A, Hirsch LJ. Studies of central nervous system disorders with single photon emission computed tomography and positron emission tomography. Semin Nucl Med 1991;21:58–81.

[17] Prichard JW, Cummings JL. The insistent call from functional MRI. Neurology 1997;48: 797–800.

[18] Werring DJ, Clark CA, Parker GJ, et al. A direct demonstration of both structure and function in the visual system: combining diffusion tensor imaging with functional magnetic resonance imaging. Neuroimage 1999;9:352–61.

[19] Amato MP, Bartolozzi ML, Zipoli V, et al. Neocortical volume decrease in relapsing-remitting patients with mild cognitive impairment. Neurology 2004;63:89–93.

[20] Bozalli M, Falini A, Francheschi M, et al. White matter damage in Alzheimer's disease assessed in vivo using diffusion tensor imaging magnetic resonance imaging. J Neurol Neurosurg Psychiatry 2002;72:742–6.

[21] Filley CM, Gross KF. Psychosis with cerebral white matter disease. Neuropsychiatry Neuropsychol Behav Neurol 1992;5:119–25.

[22] Hyde TM, Zeigler JC, Weinberger DR. Psychiatric disturbances in metachromatic leukodystrophy. Insights into the neurobiology of psychosis. Arch Neurol 1992;49:401–6.

[23] Feinstein A. The clinical neuropsychiatry of multiple sclerosis. Cambridge (UK): Cambridge University Press; 1999.

[24] Bencherrif B, Rottenberg DA. Neuroimaging of the AIDS dementia complex. AIDS 1998; 12:233–44.

[25] Berger JR, Concha M. Progressive multifocal leukoencephalopathy: the evolution of a disease once considered rare. J Neurovirol 1995;1:5–18.

[26] West S. Neuropsychiatric lupus. Rheum Dis Clin North Am 1994;20:129–58.

[27] Filley CM, Heaton RK, Rosenberg NL. White matter dementia in chronic toluene abuse. Neurology 1990;40:532–4.

[28] Filley CM, Kleinschmidt-DeMasters BK. Toxic leukoencephalopathy. N Engl J Med 2001; 345:425–32.

[29] Filley CM, Halliday W, Kleinschmidt-DeMasters BK. The effects of toluene on the central nervous system. J Neuropathol Exp Neurol 2004;63:1–12.

[30] Kealey SM, Provenzale JM. Tensor diffusion imaging in $B_{12}$ leukoencephalopathy. J Comp Assist Tomogr 2002;26:952–5.

[31] Caplan LR. Binswanger's disease—revisited. Neurology 1995;45:626–33.

[32] Kramer JH, Reed BR, Mungas D, et al. Executive dysfunction in subcortical ischemic vascular disease. J Neurol Neurosurg Psychiatry 2002;72:217–20.

[33] Filley CM, Thompson LL, Sze C-I, et al. White matter dementia in CADASIL. J Neurol Sci 1999;163:163–7.

[34] Harris JG, Filley CM. CADASIL: neuropsychological findings in three generations of an affected family. J Int Neuropsychol Soc 2001;7:768–74.

[35] Hurley RA, McGowan JC, Arfanakis K, et al. Traumatic axonal injury: novel insights into evolution and identification. J Neuropsychiatry Clin Neurosci 2004;16:1–7.

[36] Filley CM, Kleinschmidt-DeMasters BK, Lillehei KO, et al. Gliomatosis cerebri: neuro-behavioral and neuropathological observations. Cogn Behav Neurol 2003;16:149–59.

[37] Fletcher JM, Bohan TP, Brandt ME, et al. Cerebral white matter and cognition in hydrocephalic children. Arch Neurol 1992;49:818–24.

[38] Del Bigio MR. Neuropathological changes caused by hydrocephalus. Acta Neuropathol 1993;85:573–85.

[39] Medana IM, Esiri MM. Axonal damage: a key predictor of outcome in human CNS diseases. Brain 2003;126:515–30.

[40] Fischer JS, Priore RL, Jacobs LD, et al, and the Multiple Sclerosis Collaborative Group. Neuropsychological effects of interferon beta-1a in relapsing multiple sclerosis. Ann Neurol 2000;48:885–92.

[41] Hsich G, Sena-Esteves M, Breakefield XO. Critical issues in gene therapy for neurologic disease. Hum Gene Ther 2002;13:579–604.

[42] Rice CM, Halfpenny CA, Scolding NJ. Stem cells for the treatment of neurological disease. Transfus Med 2003;13:351–61.

[43] Weitzner MA, Meyers CA, Valentine AD. Methylphenidate in the treatment of neuro-behavioral slowing associated with cancer and cancer treatment. J Neuropsychiatry Clin Neurosci 1995;7:347–50.

[44] Arciniegas DB, Adler LE, Topkoff J, et al. Attention and memory function after traumatic brain injury: cholinergic mechanisms, sensory gating, and a hypothesis for further investigation. Brain Inj 1999;13:1–13.

[45] Rao SM. Cognitive function in patients with multiple sclerosis: impairment and treatment. Int J MS Care 2004;1:9–22.

[46] Lacour A, De Seze J, Revenco E, et al. Acute aphasia in multiple sclerosis: a multicenter study of 22 patients. Neurology 2004;62:974–7.

[47] Filley CM, Franklin GM, Heaton RK, et al. White matter dementia: clinical disorders and implications. Neuropsychiatry Neuropsychol Behav Neurol 1988;1:239–54.

[48] Franklin GM, Nelson LM, Filley CM, et al. Cognitive loss in multiple sclerosis: case reports and review of the literature. Arch Neurol 1989;46:162–7.

[49] Rao SM. White matter disease and dementia. Brain Cogn 1996;31:250–68.

[50] Hachinski V. Cerebral blood flow: differentiation of Alzheimer's disease from multi-infarct dementia. In: Katzman R, Terry RD, Bick KL, editors. Alzheimer's disease: senile dementia and related disorders. New York: Raven Press; 1978. p. 97–103.

[51] Filley CM, Heaton RK, Nelson LM, et al. A comparison of dementia in Alzheimer's disease and multiple sclerosis. Arch Neurol 1989;46:157–61.

[52] Lafosse JM, Corboy JR, Leehey MA, et al. Neuropsychological support for the concept of white matter dementia. Neurology 2002;58(Suppl 3):A355–6.

[53] Tullberg M, Fletcher E, DeCarli C, et al. White matter lesions impair frontal lobe function regardless of their location. Neurology 2004;63:246–53.

[54] Gabrieli JD, Stebbins GT, Singh J, et al. Intact mirror-tracing and impaired rotary-pursuit skill learning in patients with Huntington's disease: evidence for dissociable memory systems in skill learning. Neuropsychology 1997;11:272–81.

[55] Yoneoka Y, Takeda N, Inoue A, et al. Acute Korsakoff syndrome following mammillo-thalamic tract infarction. AJNR Am J Neuroradiol 2004;25:964–8.

[56] Arnett PA, Rao SM, Hussain M, et al. Conduction aphasia in multiple sclerosis: a case report with MRI findings. Neurology 1996;47:576–8.

[57] Davis KL, Stewart DG, Friedman JI, et al. White matter changes in schizophrenia. Evidence for myelin-related dysfunction. Arch Gen Psychiatry 2003;60:443–56.

[58] Alexopoulos GS, Kiosses DN, Choi SJ, et al. Frontal white matter microstructure and treatment response of late-life depression: a preliminary study. Am J Psychiatry 2002;159:1929–32.

[59] Lenox RH, Gould TD, Manji HK. Endophenotypes in bipolar disorder. Am J Med Genet 2002;114:392–406.

[60] Semrud-Clikeman M, Steingard RJ, Filipek P, et al. Using MRI to examine brain-behavior relationships in males with attention deficit disorder with hyperactivity. J Am Acad Child Adolesc Psychiatry 2000;39:477–84.

[61] Herbert MR, Zeigler DA, Makris N, et al. Localization of white matter volume increase in autism and developmental language disorder. Ann Neurol 2004;55:530–40.

[62] Hoptman MJ, Volavka J, Johnson G, et al. Frontal white matter microstructure, aggression, and impulsivity in men with schizophrenia: a preliminary study. Biol Psychiatry 2002;52:9–14.

[63] Filley CM. Neurobehavioral anatomy. 2nd edition. Boulder (CO): University Press of Colorado; 2001.

[64] Mesulam M-M. Brain, mind, and the evolution of connectivity. Brain Cogn 2000;42:4–6.

PSYCHIATRIC
CLINICS
OF NORTH AMERICA

Psychiatr Clin N Am 28 (2005) 701–711

ELSEVIER
SAUNDERS

# Management of the Acutely Violent Patient

## Jorge R. Petit, MD[a,b]

[a]*Bureau of Program Services, The New York City Department of Health and Mental Hygiene,
93 Worth Street, Room 200A, New York, NY 10013, USA*
[b]*Department of Psychiatry, Mount Sinai School of Medicine, New York, NY 10029, USA*

Violence, constantly highlighted and sensationalized in the news media, television, music, video games, and movies, has, lamentably, not spared the workplace. Although the US Justice Department data [1] have shown that the nation's murder rate in 2001 and 2002 was 5.6 per 100,000 population, similar to the rates seen in the late 1960s, violence seems to have become a daily occurrence and will be encountered in some fashion by a health professional working in an acute care setting.

Recently published studies show that thousands of assaults occur in American hospitals each year; the mental health sector and emergency departments are becoming serious occupational hazard sites [2,3]. It is well documented that mental health workers are at an increased risk of experiencing work-related violence, and studies conducted on board-certified psychiatrists have shown that there is a 5% to 48% chance of being physically assaulted by a patient during their careers [4]. Surveys conducted on psychiatry residents have found that assaults are twice as high among psychiatry residents as among medical residents. Studies have shown that 40% to 50% of psychiatry residents will be attacked physically during their 4-year training program [5]. In a survey of psychiatry residents, two thirds of the residents felt either untrained or undertrained in dealing with violent patients [6]. Even in the prehosptial sector, emergency medical service providers are at an increased risk for encountering violence; factors highly associated with episodes of violence were male gender, age, and hour of the day [7]. As the front-line staff in patient care, nurses also are at an increased risk of experiencing emotional, verbal and even physical abuse by not only the patients but family members and visitors as well [8,9].

*E-mail address:* jpetit@health.nyc.gov

Acute care settings such as emergency departments, psychiatric emergency rooms, and inpatient or outpatient psychiatric settings should be considered high-risk work sites, given the degree of acuity and potential for seeming chaos. These settings are prime examples of workplaces that can create or exacerbate volatile situations, potentially ending in violent acts. Because these are volatile work places, potentially fraught with danger and at times violence, it is imperative that safety is a top priority and that education and continuous inservice training of all staff is an ongoing part of an acute care setting. Studies have shown that educational programs can help to reduce the number of violent events, especially when the events are focused at staff who are less experienced or have less formal training. Violence prevention management, inservice training on the use of restraints, careful screening of violence-prone individuals, and security personnel training and response are methods that have been recognized to be effective in improving safety and increasing awareness among staff [10]. Many studies have shown that some form of pre- and post-critical incident stress management can significantly reduce staff assaults [11].

Additionally, psychiatrists are frequently required to assess violent patients, especially in acute care settings. Because all of these settings are different in terms of size, staff composition, room and patient allocation, and security presence and especially in training institutions (with the presence of new and untrained staff), the following principles are discussed as general recommendations in the assessment and management of the violent patient. First, basic safety considerations are crucial, and it is imperative to have a clear management approach when dealing with these situations and patients. There are some basic tenets of safety that must be adhered to at all times when in an acute care setting (Table 1) [12,13]. The key is to make sure at all times that patients', staff members', and personal safety are maintained and that patients are always monitored for possible violence. It is the adequate and prompt assessment of the situation and the implementation of well-coordinated management responses to a potentially violent patient that maximize the outcome for the patient and safety for the staff.

Agitation, aggression, impulsivity, and violence are behaviors that may arise from innate drives or as a response to frustration, and they can be manifested by destructive and attacking behaviors or covert attitudes of hostility and obstruction. These behaviors sometimes can manifest as a verbal assault or physical action directed toward others, such as hospital staff or other patients. They can be triggered by a trivial event or may be unprovoked and find an external expression; they also can fluctuate and overlap with many other conditions. These behaviors additionally cut across both medical and psychiatric conditions.

Violence, more specifically, is defined as the behaviors used by individuals that intentionally threaten or attempt to or actually inflict harm on others. Over the years there has been a reported increase in the number of aggressive and violent patients who present to emergency departments [14].

Table 1
Ten safety do's and don'ts

| Do... | Do not... |
|---|---|
| Search all patients for contraband and remove dangerous objects. | Allow patients to keep objects that are potentially dangerous. |
| Keep the door open when interviewing patients. | Allow patients to have hot beverages, glass, or sharp objects. |
| Make sure your environment is uncluttered and "safe." | Allow yourself to become trapped or cornered in a room by a patient. |
| Make sure personal belongings are tucked away or are in sight. | Feel embarrassed or intimidated to ask for help. |
| Position yourself with a rapid means of egress. | Feel you cannot have assistance or help when conducting a patient interview. |
| Know how to get help. | Allow splitting or inconsistencies. |
| Know where your panic buttons or alarms are located. | Conduct an interview if you feel menaced or frightened. |
| Trust your "gut" feeling about patients and potentially dangerous situations. | Lay hands on or attempt to restrain the patient if you are alone or the patient is too agitated. |
| Ask patients about suicidal plans and or homicidal thoughts. | Use the most restrictive measures before trying less invasive techniques. |
| Ask patients about access to a weapon and remove weapons immediately. | Allow a patient to be alone or unattended if the patient is agitated. |

Patients may voice threats of violence, from unspecified, vague threats (eg, "I just feel like I want to hurt or kill someone") to targeted homicidal threats toward an individual (eg, "I am going to kill my wife"). Patients who are violent are not a homogenous group, although there are some common characteristics and risk factors. Table 2 lists factors associated with violence, and Table 3 cites common correlates and predictors of violence. The most important predictor is a history of violence, regardless of diagnosis, which indicates an increased risk of subsequent violent behavior [13].

Violence and homicidal threats are not unique symptoms seen only by a psychiatrist; they can be symptoms or findings in many other disorders. Table 4 shows primary psychiatric and nonpsychiatric disorders associated with violence [13]. Antisocial personality disorders, alcohol or drug intoxication, borderline personality disorder, intermittent explosive disorder, patients with mental retardation, conduct disorder, personality changes due to a general medical condition (aggressive type) are just a few possible psychiatric disorders that are associated with violence.

Patients who exhibit agitation, aggressive behavior, impulsivity, and especially violence are at risk to hurt themselves and others and require quick assessment and treatment. Safety is the number-one priority, and all efforts should be made to assess the immediate situation and try to prevent further escalation. An important task, once safety has been achieved, is the medical work-up of violent patients. This is fundamental to establishing a diagnosis and future treatment recommendations. Observations of disorientation, abnormal vital signs, head trauma, alteration in levels of consciousness, and

Table 2
Factors associated with aggression and violence

| Factors | Examples |
| --- | --- |
| Genetic | Possible sex chromosome abnormalities, such as XXX, XXY, or XYY. Genetic metabolic disorders such as Sanfilipo's or Vogt syndrome or phenylketonuria have been associated with aggressive personalities. |
| Hormonal | Certain hormonal changes have been associated with onset of violent acts, such as thyroid storm or Cushing's disease. Androgens, estrogens, and progestins and their regulation also have been implicated. |
| Environmental | Unpleasant surroundings, air pollution, loud and irritating noises, and overcrowded situations can enhance the likelihood of violence. |
| Historical | History of early violence, battered or abused as children, poor parental models, limited availability of significant others, poor schooling, and previous violent episodes are linked to violence. |
| Interpersonal | Low frustration tolerance, direct provocation, exposure to violence |
| Biochemical | γ-Aminobutyric acid and serotonin have been linked with impulsivity and aggression. |
| Neurologic | Brain lesions such as tumors, trauma, or seizures, eg, complex partial seizures and post-ictal states, and temporal, frontal, or limbic lesions |

no psychiatric history should lead to the consideration of "organic" causes. Even patients with a psychiatric history should undergo a complete medical work-up to rule out medical conditions. First and foremost, a serum glucose level should be determined immediately for all patients. Second, consider the following tests: complete blood count, automated serum chemistry analysis (eg, SMA-7), calcium level, creatine phosphokinase level, alcohol and drug screen, and CT or MRI as needed. Chest radiography, arterial blood gas, lipoprotein, liver and thyroid function tests should be ordered as indicated clinically.

The signs and symptoms encountered in a patient who is agitated and potentially violent are enumerated below, listed on a spectrum of severity from least agitated to outright violence. It is crucial to assess the patient in the earlier stages of agitation to institute some measure of containment and hopefully de-escalate the possibility of violence. The sooner escalating violence is responded to and resolved, the safer it will be for the patient and the staff. When a patient crosses the limit into violence and poses a threat to others, it is time to act decisively. Changes or shifts in behavior observed in the patient should be cues that escalation to full-blown violence may occur. The rule should be "ACT FAST" [12,13,15–17].

Pacing
Psychomotor agitation
Threatening remarks
Combative posture and stance
Acting-out behavior
*Violent Outcome*

Guardedness
Suspiciousness
Paranoid ideation
Paranoid delusions
Carrying or access to weapons
*Violent Outcome*
Poor impulse control or low frustration tolerance
Emotional lability
Irritability and/or impulsivity
*Violent Outcome*

Violent outcomes can be considered screaming, cursing, yelling, spitting, biting, throwing objects, hitting or punching at self or others, or attacking or assault behavior [13].

There are no diagnostic measures to determine violence, but because a history of violence is the best predictor of future violence, promptly recognizing patients with histories of violence (if the patient is known to the hospital) at triage or registration is important [18]. Many hospitals have

Table 3
Common correlates and predictors of violence

| Correlates | Examples |
| --- | --- |
| History | Childhood abuse or neglect; history of suicide attempts or self-mutilation; previous violence and/or family violence |
| Age and gender | Young (13 to 25 years old) |
| | Male |
| Psychiatric factors | Active symptoms of psychiatric disorders (eg, command auditory hallucinations, paranoid delusions, psychotic disorganization of thought, excitability) |
| | Combination of serious mental illness and substance abuse |
| | Personality disorders |
| | Substance-related disorders such as intoxication and/or withdrawal (IMPORTANT: Chronic alcoholism is more predictive of violence than immediate alcohol use, and the higher the number of comorbid psychiatric disorders the greater the rate of violence.) |
| Emotional factors | "Acting out" behavior |
| | Angry or rageful affects |
| | Emotional lability |
| | Irritability and/or impulsivity |
| | Poor frustration tolerance |
| Social factors | Limited or poor social supports |
| | Low socioeconomic status |
| | Medication noncompliance |
| Neurobiologic factors | Delirium (eg, HIV/acquired immuno deficiency syndrome) |
| | Mental retardation |
| | Neurologic diseases |
| | Seizures; structural brain abnormalities |
| | Traumatic brain injury |

Table 4
Disorders associated with violence

| Disorders | Other causes |
| --- | --- |
| Primary psychiatric disorders (Diagnostic and Statistical Manual of Mental Disorders, Fourth Edition) | Antisocial personality disorders |
| | Borderline personality disorders |
| | Conduct disorder |
| | Delirium |
| | Dementia |
| | Dissociative disorders |
| | Intermittent explosive disorders |
| | Mental retardation |
| | Oppositional defiant disorder |
| | Personality change caused by a general medical condition, aggressive type |
| | Post-traumatic stress disorders |
| | Premenstrual dysphoric disorder |
| | Schizophrenia, paranoid type |
| | Sexual sadism |
| | Substance abuse disorders (alcohol-related disorders, amphetamine, inhalant, and phencyclidine intoxication) |
| Other causes | Intracranial pathology (eg, trauma, infection, neoplasm, anatomic defect, vascular malformation, cerebrovascular accident, degenerative disease) causing dementia, delirium, affective, and psychotic syndromes or personality changes |
| | Medications |
| | Seizure or seizure-like syndromes, including behaviors occurring during ictal, post-ictal and inter-ictal periods |
| | Systemic disorders causing dementia, delirium, affective, and psychotic syndromes or personality changes (eg, metabolic, endocrine, infectious, and environmental) |

some system to identify patients at high risk and thus take the necessary safety measures from the start, whether that means enhanced observation status, a thorough search, or a security observation. The recognition of these patients from the outset can raise a clinician's level of awareness and minimize the possibilities of acting out and thus catching people off guard. The removal of all weapons by security, whether through a manual search or with a metal detector, will vary according to each institution's policies but must be performed.

It is imperative to directly question the patient about their intent to harm themselves or harm others, possession of a weapon, formulation of a definitive plan, recent violence, current alcohol or drug use, adherence with aftercare and medication management, and associated psychiatric or medical conditions By asking these questions, preliminary information can be gathered and a relationship with the patient can be established. Remember that the higher the awareness and level of suspicion for acting out, agitated, or violent behavior there is, the less likely an explosive situation will occur—do not be caught off guard or by surprise.

The management of violent patients can be divided into four progressive unified approaches that are neither mutually exclusive nor absolute in their order of implementation: environmental manipulation, de-escalation techniques, physical restraint or seclusion, and pharmacological interventions. A stepwise approach should be used to manage the violent patient with the least restrictive yet effective means of control being selected. This is known as the least restrictive alternative doctrine.

## Environmental manipulation

When agitation is present, it is essential that precautions be taken to ensure the immediate safety of other patients and staff. There are several environmental variables that can be controlled or modified to decrease the potential for escalation of violence. These include: patient comfort, relative isolation, decreased time of waiting, staff attitude, and decreased stimuli. The patient should be made as comfortable and safe as possible. A quiet room or an individual examination room can decrease external stimuli, which in turn can assist in the de-escalation of a patient. Offering the patient a chair on which to sit or a stretcher on which to lie down or something to drink, such as a cup of water or juice, conveys caring and respect and can improve a potentially volatile situation.

Physicians should never place themselves or any other staff member in an unsafe situation (eg, in a closed room or where access to doors is blocked or other compromising locations). All items or objects that can be potentially dangerous should be removed or at least accounted for by the staff to prepare and minimize the danger of injury. There are certain staff approaches that should be monitored carefully especially when dealing with a violent patient. It is important both to maintain a safe distance from an agitated patient and to respect the patient's personal space. Prolonged or intense direct eye contact can be perceived as menacing by the patient. Body language and positions such as crossed arms or hands behind the back or hidden also can be considered confrontational and threatening. The most important approach is always to maintain a stance that is calm and in control. Staff should closely monitor the patient's behavior for any changes in mood, speech, and psychomotor activity (any of the above can signal an impending loss of control).

## De-escalation

Techniques of verbal de-escalation ("defusing" or "talking down") should be used as the first approach with any agitated patient, including all of the verbal and nonverbal responses used to defuse or reduce a potentially violent situation. The overriding interventional principles are that the staff conveys their professional concern for the well being of the patient, their assurance that no harm will come to the patient, and that they are in control of the situation.

The staff must appear calm and in control, speaking to the patient in a nonprovocative, nonconfrontational manner, and using a calm and soothing voice. Staff must remain at a safe distance from the patient, be prepared for potential violence, and be familiar with emergency or "panic" alarms or buttons, if the institution has them. Overt anger or hostility should never be expressed toward an agitated patient. Use empathic statements such as, "I understand you're not feeling well and that you're having a hard time," or "it sounds like you're in pain and confused." These statements can place an agitated patient at ease, especially when the statements are made in the context of genuine concern by using phrases such as, "you're here to get help, and we're going to try to figure out what's going on," or "let us help you, don't be afraid." Staff should reinforce the feeling that the patient is in a safe environment and that everyone is there to assist in the patient's evaluation and treatment. At the same time, the limits on patient behavior and consequences of present and future actions need to be verbalized. The patient should be told decisively and emphatically that the staff will ensure and maintain control and that he or she will not be allowed to harm him- or herself or others. The clinician should provide reasonable positive reinforcements and propose alternatives to aggressive behavior, such as talking with staff or making a phone call. Staff should be consistent in their approach: manipulative patients may attempt to split staff who do not have a unified strategy.

**Restraints and seclusion**

Restraints and seclusion are used as a final response to emergent and imminently dangerous behavior. Seclusion and restraints are never to be used as a means of punishment or retribution for an agitated, demanding, or disruptive patient, for the convenience of staff, or as a substitute for a treatment program. It is crucial to preserve the patient's rights and dignity at all times. This can be achieved by ensuring the patient's privacy as much as possible, allowing for participation in care decisions by the patient or significant others, and by providing ongoing assessment and monitoring and the provision of physical care and comfort during the time the patient is in restraints and seclusion.

Once the decision has been made to proceed with restraints or seclusion, a team leader must be identified who has experience in the implementation of restraints or seclusion. There must be sufficient and trained personnel so that the procedure can be performed safely and effectively, especially if physical force becomes warranted. At all times, the staff must convey confidence and calmness and proceed with implementation as if it were a standard and familiar procedure [19–21].

## Pharmacologic interventions

Pharmacologic management of the violent or agitated patient may serve as a primary therapy or as an adjunct to other efforts at de-escalation. If the behavior is extreme or continues to deteriorate despite other management efforts, medications must be offered. Whenever possible, the patient should be given the option or choice of medication type or route, which often can assist in their ability to regain some measure of control, thus potentially defusing further escalation. The choices of possible agents and routes first must be discussed by the staff, and a unified approach must be taken when discussing these options with an agitated patient. Ideally, the patient will agree to take the medication voluntarily. Oral administration can potentially address control issues and permit the patient to retain control and dignity; if not, parenteral routes should be used. In the event that the involuntary administration of intramuscular (IM) medication is required, security and other staff must be present, and all efforts should be taken to ensure a safe and rapid intervention. The choice of IM location can be left up to the patient, (eg, deltoids, buttocks, or other sites). A thorough note should be written that describes the preceding events, the least restrictive measures attempted, the actual intervention, and patient outcome or effect.

Rapid tranquilization has become a standard of care that has been shown to be safe and effective. The goal of rapid tranquilization is simply to regain behavioral control without oversedation [22]. Traditional approaches use a typical antipsychotic such as haloperidol, with or without the use of benzodiazepines such as lorazepam. Rapid tranquilization that combines a benzodiazepine and an antipsychotic drug offers the theoretical advantage of minimizing the amount of any single drug and combining the sedation of the benzodiazepine with the behavioral modification of the antipsychotic [23,24]. Haloperidol has become the standard for rapid tranquilization because of its strength and desirable side-effect profile; it is a powerful antipsychotic with minimal sedating and cardiovascular effects. It has been shown repeatedly to be safe and effective for the control of agitated behavior in the acute setting [25]. The newer atypical agents, used widely in practice, have slower titration schedules or dose-limiting adverse effects that prevent them from becoming first-line options. Newer preparations, such as oral liquid forms, rapidly dissolving tablets (risperidone and olanzapine), and parenteral (IM) forms of ziprasidone, risperidone, and olanzapine, are becoming important and useful alternatives for the management of violence in the acute setting. Preliminary data suggest that these agents are better tolerated, have fewer side effects, are effective in reducing agitation and psychosis, and make the transition from intramuscular to oral route easier and better tolerated [26–29]. Recent studies also have shown that valproate can be effective in the management of violence, with significant decreases in the violent behaviors, especially in patients with "organic" causes, dementias, mental retardation, or bipolar disorder and manic type [30].

The use of benzodiazepines as an adjunct or alone in the management of agitated behavior has been shown to be effective, especially lorazepam, which has the advantage of safety, rapid IM absorption and reliability [31,32].

Ultimately, the decision about the medications to be used, alone or in combination, is a clinical one and is best discussed and reviewed among the team members when they are confronted with a potentially explosive situation. Each physician, as well as the patient, will need to be comfortable with their choice, and the implementation of chemical restraints needs to be carefully thought out, ordered, and documented. Least restrictive alternatives must be considered and documented before acute psychopharmacologic interventions are used. Remember, always use sound clinical judgment when making these decisions.

## Summary

Violence in the work place is a new but growing problem for our profession. It is likely that at some point a psychiatrist will be confronted with a potentially violent patient or need to assess a violent patient. Understanding predictors and associated factors in violence as well as having a clear and well-defined strategy in approaching and dealing with the violent patient, thus, are crucial. Ensuring patient, staff, and personal safety is the most important aspect in the management of a violent patient. All of the staff must be familiar with management strategies and clear guidelines that are implemented and followed when confronted with a violent patient. The more structured the approach to the violent patient, the less likely a bad outcome will occur. Manipulating one's work environment to maximize safety and understanding how to de-escalate potentially mounting violence are two steps in the approach to the violent patient. Restraint, seclusion, and psychopharmacologic interventions also are important and often are necessary components to the management of the violent patient.

## References

[1] Homicide trends in the United States: 2002 Update, November 2004 NCJ 204885. US Department of Justice Web site. Available at: www.ojp.usdoj.gov/bjs/homicide/homtrnd. htm.

[2] Flannery RB, et al. Characteristics of staff victims of patient assault: ten year analysis of the Assaulted Staff Action Program (ASAP). Psychiatr Q 2001;72(3):237–48.

[3] Snyder W. Hospital downsizing and increased frequency of assaults on staff. Psychiatr Serv (Hospital & Community Psychiatry) 1994;45:378–80.

[4] Erdos BZ, Hughews DH. A review of assaults by patients against staff at psychiatric emergency centers. Psychiatr Serv 2001;52:1175–7.

[5] Black KJ, et al. Assaults by patients on psychiatric residents at three training sites. Psychiatr Serv (Hospital & Community Psychiatry) 1994;45:706–10.

[6] Schwartz TL, Park TL. Assaults by patients on psychiatric residents: a survey and training recommendations. Psychiatr Serv 1999;50:381–3.

[7] Grange JT, Corbett SW. Violence against emergency medical services personnel. Prehosp Emerg Care 2002;6(2):186–90.

[8] May DD, Grubbs LM. The extent, nature and precipitating factors of nurse assault among three groups of registered nurses in a regional medical center. J Emerg Nurs 2002;28(1):11–7.

[9] Presley D, Robinson G. Violence in the emergency department: nurses contend with prevention in the healthcare arena. Nurs Clin North Am 2002;37(1):161–9 [abstract p. viii–ix].

[10] Fernandes CM, et al. The effect of an educational program on violence in the emergency department. Ann Emerg Med 2002;39(1):47–55.

[11] Flannery RB. The assaulted staff action program (ASAP): ten year empirical support for critical incident stress management (CISM). Int J Emerg Ment Health 2001;3(1):5–10.

[12] Hill S, Petit J. The violent patient. Emerg Med Clin North Am 2000;18:301–15.

[13] Petit J. Handbook of emergency psychiatry. Philadelphia (PA): Lippincott Williams & Wilkins; 2004.

[14] Citrome L, Volvaka J. Violent patients in the emergency setting. Psychiatr Clin North Am 1999;23:789–801.

[15] Hughes DH. Assessment of the potential for violence. Psych Ann 1994;24:579–83.

[16] Kao LW, Moore GP. The violent patient: clinical management, use of physical and chemical restraints, and medicolegal concerns. Emergency Medicine Practice 1999;1:1–23.

[17] Tardiff K. Management of the violent patient in an emergency situation. Psychiatr Clin North Am 1988;11:539–49.

[18] Tardiff K. Prediction of violence. Jrnl Prac Psych and Behav Hlth 1998:12–9.

[19] Currier GW, Allen MH. Physical and chemical restraints in the psychiatric emergency service. Psychiatr Serv 2000;51:717–9.

[20] American Psychiatric Association. Seclusion and restraint (Task Force report no. 22). Washington (DC): APA; 1984.

[21] Bell CC, Palmer JM. Survey of the demographic characteristics of patients requiring restraints in the psychiatric emergency service. J Natl Med Assoc 1983;75:981.

[22] Dubin WR, Feld JA. Rapid tranquilization of the violent patient. Am J Emerg Med 1989;7: 313.

[23] Hillard JR. Choosing antipsychotics for rapid tranquilization in the ER. Curr Psychiatry Rep 2002;1:22–9.

[24] Currier GW, Trenton A. Pharmacological treatment of psychotic agitation. CNS Drugs 2002;16(4):219–28.

[25] Donlon PT, Hopkin J, Tupin JP. Overview: safety and efficacy of rapid neuroleptization method with injectable haloperidol. Am J Psychiatry 1979;136:273.

[26] Currier GW. Atypical antipsychotic medications in the pscyhiatric emergency service. J Clin Psychiatry 2000;61(Suppl 14):S21–6.

[27] Daniel DG, Potkin SG, Reeves KR, et al. Intramuscular (IM) ziprasidone 20 mg is effective in reducing acute agitation associated with psychosis: a double-blind, randomized trial. Psychopharmacology (Berl) 2001;155:128–34.

[28] Kinon BJ, Roychowdhury SM, Milton DR, et al. Effective resolution with olanzapine of acute presentation of behavioral agitation and positive psychotic symptoms in schizophrenia. J Clin Psychiatry 2001;62(Suppl 2):S17–21.

[29] Lesem MD, Zajecka JM, Swift RH, et al. Intramuscular ziprasidone, 2 mg versus 10 mg, in the short-term management of agitated psychotic patients. J Clin Psychiatry 2001;62:12–8.

[30] Lindenmayer JP, Kotsaftis A. Use of sodium valproate in violent and aggressive behaviors: a critical review. J Clin Psychiatry 2000;61:123–8.

[31] Bodkin JA. Emerging uses for high potency benzodiazapines in psychotic disorders. J Clin Psychiatry 1990;51(Suppl):S41.

[32] Salzman C, Green A, Rodriguez-Villa F, et al. Benzodiazepines combined with neuroleptics for management of severe disruptive behavior. Psychosomatics 1986;27(Suppl 1):S17–22.

ELSEVIER
SAUNDERS

PSYCHIATRIC
CLINICS
OF NORTH AMERICA

Psychiatr Clin N Am 28 (2005) 713–735

# Chronic Pain: Physiological, Diagnostic, and Management Considerations

## Brian Hainline, MD[a,b,*]

[a]*Department of Neurology, New York University School of Medicine, NY, USA*
[b]*Neurology and Integrative Pain Medicine, ProHEALTH Care Associates,*
*2 ProHEALTH Plaza, Lake Success, NY 11042, USA*

The following descriptions of pain by patients who suffer with chronic pain syndromes suggest the complexity of the conscious experience of chronic pain:

> "I feel as if someone has pulled the skin off of my left leg, and is then constantly rubbing salt into my leg."
> "I feel as if my leg is on fire. My skin feels burnt, and it is as if someone is taking claws and tearing into my skin twenty-four hours a day."
> "I feel as if someone has taken a hot poker knife and is jabbing it deep in my right eye. If I could pull my eye out, only to remove this sensation, I would gladly do so."

The suffering experienced by patients who have chronic pain is immense. Something distinguishes their perception of pain from the simpler sensory experience of acute pain: chronic pain is processed within the nervous system in a more complex manner than acute pain.

Acute pain is a universal experience and is biologically protective. Acute pain is generally short lived, although, when there is an ongoing component of tissue injury, the pain may persist for days or weeks as the body attempts to heal from the initial insult. Acute pain is an appropriate response to an inciting event associated with actual or potential tissue damage.

Chronic pain is pain that persists more than 1 month longer than might be reasonably expected following an inciting event and is sustained by aberrant somatosensory nervous system processing. Chronic pain can last for months, years, and even decades. Chronic pain may be considered a pain sensation that arises from within the nervous system rather than from an

---

* ProHEALTH Care Associates, 2 ProHEALTH Plaza, Lake Success, NY 11042.
  *E-mail address:* bhainline@prohealthcare.com

external source [1]. This salient feature of chronic pain becomes the basis for differentiating it from acute pain and for understanding that patients who suffer from chronic pain are suffering from dysfunction of the nervous system.

## Pain processing and perception

The International Association for the Study of Pain has defined pain as "an unpleasant sensory and emotional experience which we primarily associate with tissue damage or describe in terms of such damage, or both" [2]. An analysis of this definition makes it clear that the experience of pain is multimodal, including physical, sensory, emotional, and cognitive experiences, as well as a perception that may or may not be related to actual tissue insult [3–5]. The quotations given above give evidence of this experience.

Acute pain essentially arises from activation of peripheral pain receptors called nociceptors. Activation of nociceptors alone is not sufficient for the experience of pain, because there are central nervous system modifiers for the processing of nociceptive pain [6]. Illustrative of this concept are the familiar wartime stories of soldiers who are severely injured, but who are also in imminent danger, and who experience no pain until they reach safety. Thus, pain is a subjective experience that depends on the state of the nervous system.

The normal processing of acute, nociceptive pain begins in the peripheral nervous system in primary afferent neurons. These neurons, known as nociceptors, distinguish noxious from innocuous events. The transmitting nerves may be lightly myelinated or unmyelinated and are specialized to respond to mechanical, heat, thermal, and chemical stimuli. Threshold activation of nociceptive afferent neurons leads to afferent transmission of signals into the spinal cord. Most afferent input occurs by way of the dorsal root (Fig. 1), although some fibers traverse the ventral route. Nociceptive input can be modified within the spinal cord. Both nociceptive-specific neurons and more nonspecific, wide-dynamic-range cells can be activated from these afferent sensory pathways [7]. In the most simplistic view of pain processing, nociceptive-specific cells in the spinal cord ascend to the contralateral thalamus by way of the neocorticospinal thalamic tract. From the thalamus, afferent pathways then activate both primary and secondary somatosensory cortices (Fig. 1).

Pain-processing pathways, however, are more complex than previously realized. Wide-dynamic-range cells, which are activated by innocuous and noxious stimuli, can amplify afferent stimuli. In addition, more widespread ascending pathways from the spinal cord to the brain activate multiple brainstem and subcortical regions, limbic pathways, and both ipsilateral and contralateral cortical brain regions (Fig. 1) [6]. These pathways intermingle with regions of the brain that mediate emotions, autonomic activity, attention and localization, motor planning, and cognition [8].

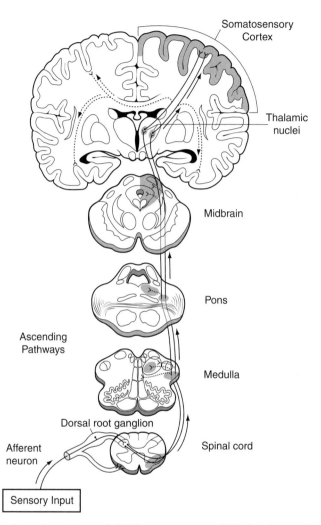

Fig. 1. Ascending pain pathways. Solid lines represent established pathways. Broken lines represent putative pathways.

Several descending pain pathways influence the perception of pain (Fig. 2). The best-studied descending pathway originates from the midbrain periaqueductal gray matter [6]. This brain region subserves the endogenous opiate system. The endogenous opioids comprise endorphins and enkephalins, which regulate the pain response, homeostasis, immune function, and the normal stress response. Activation of the periaqueductal gray matter leads to inhibition of dorsal horn neurons and subsequent analgesia, primarily through an excitatory connection with the dorsal raphe nucleus. The dorsal raphe nucleus (serotonergic) and locus ceruleus (noradrenergic) are two other brainstem centers that relay key descending pain-inhibitory

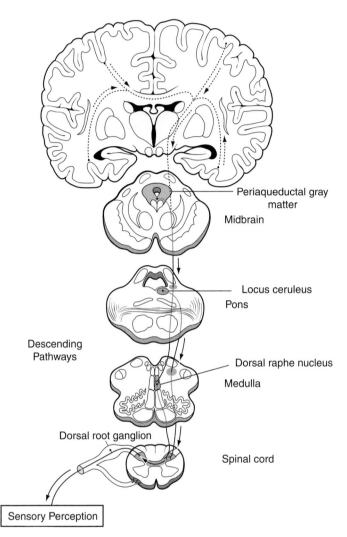

Fig. 2. Descending pain pathways. Solid lines represent established pathways. Broken lines represent putative pathways.

pathways (Fig. 2). These brainstem centers are modified by cortical, subcortical, and limbic pathways.

Additional brain regions are intimately involved in pain modulation through the activation of endogenous neurotransmitters, including acetylcholine, γ-aminobutyric acid (GABA), vasoactive intestinal peptide, oxytocin, somatostatin, cholecystokinin, vasopressin, histamine, prolactin, and cannabinoids [9–11]. Indeed, a host of endogenous neurotransmitters either inhibits or augments pain perception, but the manner in which these pathways become activated is poorly understood. These pain-modulating pathways and their neurochemical substrate become one basis for the pharmacologic management of chronic pain.

Functional brain imaging studies have furthered the understanding of pain processing. In control situations, noxious stimuli lead to somatotopic activation of the contralateral primary and secondary somatosensory cortex. Additional activation occurs in the contralateral insular cortex, anterior cingular and prefrontal cortices, and ipsilateral secondary somatosensory and parietal cortices [12]. These diverse but interlinked pathways demonstrate that simple physical pain processing is an outdated concept; pain perception is mediated by attentional, cognitive, emotional, and motor planning brain responses [8,12].

Neuropathic pain responses demonstrate recruitment of brain areas other than the control network. Whether or not an individual with neuropathic pain presents with a well-defined lesion, functional brain imaging studies consistently reveal abnormalities in the ipsilateral hemisphere, including the somatosensory cortex, the insular, motor, and premotor cortices, and the anterior cingulate cortex [12]. Activation of the contralateral posterior parietal cortex develops in patients who have mechanical allodynia [13], and left temporal and anterior cingulate cortex dysfunction is described in patients who experience chronic pain after thoracotomy when compared with surgical controls who heal uneventfully (H. Nemoto MD, personal communication, December 2004).

Such complex pain processing demonstrates that the central nervous system may reorganize after injury or perception of injury. Thus plasticity, which is the ability of the central nervous system to adapt to or to reorganize in response to new internal or external environmental requirements, may underlie the basis of neuropathic pain [14]. The cause of such reorganization is unclear, and the search for explanations must move beyond a simplistic lesion-oriented and single–pain pathway model to an appreciation of the conscious and nonconscious processing of pain.

There may be genetic predispositions to developing chronic pain involving the $N$-methyl-D-aspartic acid (NMDA) receptors within the spinal cord and brain [15], but such evidence is tentative. Psychologic maladaptations may be a significant factor for some individuals who develop chronic pain. Studies have demonstrated that patients who suffer with neuropathic pain have a statistically significantly increased incidence of childhood abuse [16–19]. Such statistics, however, do not lay a foundation for a causal relationship between childhood abuse and neuropathic pain and should not lead to an assumption that patients who have chronic pain have an underlying psychologic or psychosomatic illness. Ultimately, the dysfunction and misprocessing that occur in individuals who suffer from neuropathic pain need to be understood in terms of biologic predisposition and central processing of internal and external perception [8].

An understanding of the complexity of the central processing of pain, coupled with the clinical observation that patients who have chronic pain are not experiencing pain as a result of simplistic processing of nociceptive input, leads to the acceptance of the definition of neuropathic pain. Understanding neuropathic pain is the cornerstone of effective diagnosis and management. Investigators have argued about the definitions of chronic pain versus central pain versus neuropathic pain [20]. In this article, chronic pain, central pain, and neuropathic pain are considered interchangeable terms.

The International Association for the Study of Pain defines neuropathic pain as "initiated or caused by a primary lesion or dysfunction in the nervous system" [2]. Although some argue that the term "dysfunction" makes this definition too vague, others believe that this term allows a better understanding that neuropathic pain is not simply the result of a localizable anatomic lesion [21,22]. For example, complex region pain syndrome is a well-defined clinical entity in which patients present with severe, unrelenting pain and autonomic dysfunction but with no lesion that accounts for the pain. Essentially, neuropathic pain represents a dysfunction in pain processing and perception and involves multiple nervous system sites.

## Comorbidities

Neuropathic pain affects every aspect of a patient's being. In many ways, the patient defines his or her life by pain rather than by a more soulful sense of being. In other words, the patient identifies himself primarily as one who has pain; virtually every aspect of life becomes associated with a maladaptive response. Whereas the purported initial injury or insult that leads to chronic pain may seem simplistic, the ultimate course, outcome, and cost of chronic pain are affected by a multitude of factors, including emotional, social, economic, and environmental factors [23].

Depression is the most common comorbidity between chronic pain and Axis I disorders in the *Diagnostic and Statistical Manual IV*. Indeed, some studies find a prevalence rate approaching 100% [24]. The relationship between depression and pain is complex. Although depression is not an independent risk factor for developing neuropathic pain, patients who have depression report higher levels of pain than do patients who do not have depression [25,26]. Depression augments the impairment associated with chronic pain, and there is a very low likelihood of successfully treating neuropathic pain if depression is not treated as well [23].

Anxiety similarly has a high comorbid association with chronic pain, and some postulate that chronic neuropathic pain may be an expression of chronic posttraumatic stress disorder [27–30]. Functional and metabolic similarities exist between neuropathic pain and posttraumatic stress disorder [31,32]. Some patients adapt to prior traumatic stress with chronic behavioral strategies and then develop complex regional pain syndrome after a seemingly innocuous inciting event years later. Thus, investigation must focus both on the injury or inciting event per se that leads to chronic pain and on the meaning or perception of that event within the context of the individual's life experience [8].

Sleep deprivation is common among chronic pain patients, and sleep deprivation alone causes a hyperexcitability state that amplifies the pain response [23]. Social support systems for patients who have chronic pain may be dysfunctional both at home and at work, and self-esteem can be diminished considerably. Some patients believe that they deserve to suffer with pain and place such reasoning within a religious or metaphysical context. Patients who have chronic pain often develop several maladaptive physical responses that then predispose to perpetuating the cycle of chronic pain.

### Examples of neuropathic pain syndromes

An exhaustive discussion of various chronic pain syndromes is beyond the scope of this article. Following is a brief discussion of some common chronic pain syndromes.

*Low back pain*

Although chronic low back pain is ubiquitous, there is no single satisfactory treatment regimen for this problem. Too often, back pain is viewed as a biomechanical problem that can be fixed by either local injections or surgical therapy. It is more useful, however, to view chronic low back pain as neuropathic pain. Chronic low back pain may comprise elements of acute biomechanical pain and active nerve root entrapment.

Patients who have chronic low back pain without active biomechanical symptomatology complain of essentially constant pain that is independent of position. Pain may be across the lower back and may radiate into one or both legs. The pain can have a burning quality but may also be described as stabbing or cramplike, as a deep pressure, or, less often, with other pain characteristics described later. Some patients describe position-dependent pain superimposed on chronic pain. For example, patients who have segmental lumbar instability complain of acute, severe pain occurring with sudden positional changes. Patients with lumbar stenosis develop progressively severe low back pain, with or without leg pain, upon walking greater than one block. Patients with active facet syndrome complain of sudden pain with back extension. It is important to distinguish these variations when obtaining a history. Treatment may combine interventions targeted at the acute, biomechanical pain while addressing the overall chronic pain syndrome.

The multitude of failed back surgeries is a testament that low back surgery, including laminectomy/discectomy, spinal fusion, and disc replacement, is not the answer for patients who suffer with chronic low back pain [33]. Similarly, to label all chronic low back pain as myofasciitis does not advance the scientific and clinical understanding of chronic low back pain [34]. As with all neuropathic pain syndromes, chronic low back pain represents a transformation from acute pain into a chronic somatosensory processing disorder. The clinician's management should shift so that the chronic nature of the pain becomes the guiding principle for multidisciplinary management.

## Postherpetic neuralgia

Postherpetic neuralgia is one of the better-studied chronic pain syndromes and is a clear example of how a peripheral nerve insult can lead to dysfunction of the central nervous system. Postherpetic neuralgia is caused by reactivation of the varicella zoster virus along a single dermatome related to either a spinal dorsal root ganglion or a brainstem cranial nerve ganglion. Pain develops along the same dermatome as the rash. The initial pain of postherpetic neuralgia is an appropriate, nociceptive response to irritation of the peripheral nerve. In a substantial number of individuals, however, postherpetic neuralgia becomes transformed into chronic pain. Such chronic pain, like other neuropathic pain syndromes, affects multiple aspects of life including affect, physical activities, social interactions, self-esteem, and sleep.

The transition from nociceptive pain to chronic neuropathic pain may result from deafferentation of the second-order neurons of the spinothalamic tract because of primary sensory neuronal death. This possibility has not been conclusively demonstrated, however, and pain transformation may involve other aspects of sensory processing, including an alteration in descending inhibitory signals. The key point in all neuropathic pain syndromes is that the transition from acute pain to chronic pain is probably multifactorial and differs from individual to individual. In terms of the final syndrome, it is irrelevant whether the transforming event is a lesion with subsequent deafferentation, in the classic lesion-oriented model of allopathic medicine, or the transforming event is one of processing, thus raising the possibility that the transformation is physiologically based. Ultimately, the central nervous system expression of chronic pain involves similar pathways, and the overlap between physiologic dysfunction and physical dysfunction becomes blurred, both causally and from a management viewpoint.

Patients who suffer with postherpetic neuralgia typically describe a burning, stabbing, or lancinating pain along the affected dermatome. Pain is unremitting and hypersensitive to touch, leading to considerable behavioral changes to protect this region of the body. As with all neuropathic pain states, treatment directed to the peripheral nerve alone is unrewarding; successful management involves a multidisciplinary approach.

## Diabetic peripheral neuropathy

Approximately one quarter of the 17 million diabetic Americans develop a peripheral neuropathy. A substantial number of such patients experience neuropathic pain, but there is no clear peripheral nerve feature distinguishing patients who have diabetic neuropathic pain from those who have nonpainful peripheral neuropathy [35]. Diabetic peripheral neuropathy is another example of a peripheral nerve lesion transforming into a chronic, sustaining pain mediated by dysfunction of the nervous system.

Patients with painful diabetic neuropathy and other painful peripheral neuropathies typically complain of pain in a stocking distribution. The pain is often burning and may be sharp or lancinating. Often, the pain is worse in a recumbent position and is somewhat better with weight bearing. There may be associated allodynia, thus leading to avoidance-type behavior. Patients often have severe interruption of sleep, because the pain typically is worse at nighttime. As with all neuropathic pain syndromes, other aspects of the patient's life can be affected in a cascade in the breakdown of affect, social support, and self-esteem. Treatment directed simply at the peripheral nerves is not successful.

*Complex regional pain syndrome*

Complex regional pain syndrome, formerly known as reflex sympathetic dystrophy, is a poorly understood chronic condition. Unlike low back pain, postherpetic neuralgia, and diabetic neuropathy, the initial inciting event of complex regional pain syndrome may not be evident. Often, the inciting event is a seemingly innocuous injury to the soft tissue, but the injury then becomes transformed into an unrelenting, debilitating pain syndrome. The term reflex sympathetic dystrophy, although still commonly in use, was changed to complex regional pain syndrome because it is not clear that the pain of complex regional pain syndrome is simply related to dysfunction of the sympathetic nervous system. Also, dystrophic changes are not universal, and the transformation from an inciting event into chronic pain is not reflexive. Complex regional pain syndrome is divided into type I (no evidence of peripheral nerve injury) and type II (documented peripheral nerve injury).

Complex regional pain syndrome illustrates the enormous complexity of neuropathic pain. Often, the inciting event is a seemingly trivial trauma. Indeed, the inciting event can be so trivial that patients often are led to believe they are fabricating the pain. Additionally, because there is no clear cut, satisfactory pathophysiologic explanation for the severe transformed pain, some authors have even doubted the neuropathic nature of this syndrome and have concluded that complex regional pain syndrome is a somatoform disorder [36]. Complex regional pain syndrome has been described as a peripheral nerve insult that results in one of the following: local peripheral nerve trauma with secondary ephaptic conduction and ectopic pacemaker activity; cross talk between unmyelinated C-fibers and interlinked sympathetic fibers; or wide-dynamic-range neuron hypersensitivity in the spinal cord from prolonged, intense nociceptive input [37].

Complex regional pain syndrome is diagnosed using the following four criteria [38]:

1. There has been an initiating noxious event for a cause of immobilization.
2. There is continuing pain, allodynia, or hyperalgesia that is disproportionate to any inciting event.
3. There is evidence at some time of edema, changes in skin blood flow, or abnormal sudomotor activity in the region of the pain.
4. The condition is excluded by the existence of a condition that otherwise would account for the degree of pain and dysfunction.

Thus, the diagnosis is made purely on clinical grounds, taking into account objective, autonomic nervous system pathophysiology. The changes in the autonomic nervous system led to sympathetic blockade becoming one of the hallmarks of treatment. Although pain relief from sympathetic blockade helps support the diagnosis of complex regional pain syndrome, sympathetically independent pain may develop early in the course of this condition and is unresponsive to peripheral sympathetic blockade [39,40].

Although there is unusual autonomic activity early in the course of complex regional pain syndrome, and this activity may be caused by dysregulation of the sympathetic nervous system, the condition quickly becomes transformed into neuropathic pain. In other words, the pain becomes sustained by dysfunction in somatosensory processing and is not simply secondary to sympathetic nervous system dysfunction. There is some controversy concerning this latter point: some authors have argued that complex regional pain syndrome has nothing to do with the sympathetic nervous system, confusing the difference between transient sympathetic nervous system dysfunction and long-lasting neuropathic pain [41,42].

The sometimes seemingly trivial inciting event of complex regional pain syndrome has led some to speculate that this condition is emotionally based. Whereas there may be truth in this supposition, it is likewise true that all neuropathic pain syndromes have a component of emotional dysfunction. On the one hand, depression and anxiety coexist almost universally with neuropathic pain syndromes. On the other hand, there may be a fundamentally important emotional processing component in the transformation from simple pain to more complex, chronic pain. It would be more useful to break down the arbitrary barriers between psychiatry and neurology, mind and body, and emotionality and physicality and to consider neuropathic pain as a neuropsychiatric disorder, instead of dividing chronic pain syndromes into emotionally based or physically based problems.

## Pain secondary to central nervous system injury

A variety of chronic pain states have been described following well-documented central nervous system injury, including trauma, multiple sclerosis, cerebrovascular accidents, infections, spinal cord syrinx, neo-plasms, and others [43–47]. All have in common a well-documented lesion of the central nervous system. It is not clear, however, how some patients who have such lesions develop a transformed pain syndrome, whereas others with the same lesion develop a neurologic deficit without such pain. The only thing that is known with certainty is that the clinical manifestation of pain can become the overwhelming chronic presentation in such patients, and they develop the same comorbidities as individuals with other neuropathic pain syndromes. Pain usually develops weeks to months after the insult to the central nervous system, indicating that central nervous system reorganization may develop over time [45].

## Diagnosis

### History

Clinicians can make a diagnosis of neuropathic pain with confidence by taking a careful history, performing a focused physical examination, and judiciously using ancillary diagnostic studies. It is important, in taking a history, to understand the presenting characteristic of pain. The five most important characteristics are:

1. Temporal qualities, including acute, recurrent or chronic; daily variation; onset and duration.
2. Intensity, including average pain; pain at its worst; pain at its least; pain at the time of history taking.
3. Topography, including localized versus regional pain; superficial versus deep pain; focal versus radiating pain.
4. Quality, including descriptors such as burning, aching, freezing, stabbing, electric shock–like, tooth achy, cramping, or knifelike.
5. Palliative and precipitating factors, including physical activities, emotional stressors, nutritional triggers, and circadian rhythms.

It is beneficial for patients to use a rapid rating scale such as the Brief Pain Inventory or the Visual Analog Scale [48]. Patients rate temporal aspects of pain from zero (no pain) to 10 (the worst imaginable pain). Such rating scales are helpful in following patients and aid in understanding the relationship between the patient and pain. Some patients rate their pain as a constant "10" but seem to be in no acute distress, suggesting a disassociation between their perception of pain and their physical manifestations.

Clinicians should spend considerable time trying to understand the inciting event of pain, which may provide insight into a disease state or injury that has been undiagnosed. In addition, it is critical to understand the patient's perception of the inciting event, which takes into account life experiences. Daily activities need to be considered, including physical limitations caused by pain and the amount of daily exercise. Some patients are so debilitated by pain that they are essentially homebound, performing little in the way of even sedentary activities. The support system must be explored, including the immediate family and the patient's work environment, if appropriate. Often, patients suffering with neuropathic pain feel alone and abandoned and essentially become imprisoned by pain. Many patients have discontinued all sexual activity as a manifestation of depression, rejection, or fear that such activity will further exacerbate pain.

In addition to a general past medical history, careful attention must be paid to any prior psychiatric conditions or prior episodes of prolonged pain-related conditions. This investigation may provide important insight into the patient's adaptive responses over time. Childhood trauma must be considered, although probing into childhood trauma must be done in a delicate and noninvasive manner. Even though there is a high incidence of childhood trauma and abuse in chronic pain patients, one cannot suggest or assume that a patient with chronic pain has experienced such trauma. Alcohol and drug histories are critical, because one facet of chronic neuropathic pain treatment may be the use of narcotic analgesics.

A careful search for comorbid medical conditions is important. The three most common comorbid conditions are depression, anxiety, and sleep deprivation. If these conditions are not managed properly, successful pain management is unlikely. Simple questions may suffice. For example, asking if the patient has felt depressed or hopeless or has lost pleasure may uncover an otherwise undiagnosed depression. Pain centers often use more formal depression scales as part of an initial assessment. Family history may provide a clue to possible genetic predispositions to psychiatric disease, pain syndromes, or both.

The patient's expectations of treatment must be assessed [23]. It is unrealistic to expect that a simple procedure or medication will completely alleviate pain. Realistic goals must be set. Too often, patients arrive with an expectation of obtaining a simple anatomic explanation and subsequent treatment of pain. Once the clinician begins to discuss neuropathic pain, patients may fail to understand that their pain is a result of a somewhat ill-defined dysfunction of the nervous system. Patients can feel a lack of validation, which can undermine future treatments. It is frequently helpful to end a discussion by asking the patient something such as the following: "Just so that I can be certain I have explained myself well, please summarize for me your understanding of your condition." Such a statement does not assume that the patient is not intelligent or was not paying attention but places the burden on the clinician for having satisfactorily explained the condition.

Once the patient understands that the pain is a chronic condition, the foundation for multidisciplinary, long-term treatment begins. Patients need to understand that the ultimate goal of treatment is to reduce pain, increase function, and improve quality of life. The focus on complete cessation of pain alone will lead to treatment failure. Patients should feel that they are an integral component of the treatment by actively participating in their pain management.

*Physical examination*

A careful physical examination should include vital signs, a focused musculoskeletal and extremity examination, and a neurologic examination. Patients with chronic pain generally do not present in acute distress, and vital signs should be stable. The musculoskeletal examination is important in many ways. First, some patients will demonstrate evidence of chronic maladaptation because of prolonged muscle spasm and avoidance-type behavior. Second, the musculoskeletal examination may reveal evidence of active mechanical signs of an entrapped nerve or of an irritated spinal segment. Third, the musculoskeletal examination may reveal evidence of psychologic maladaptation, in which patients claim pain when they are confronted directly with a musculoskeletal maneuver, but careful observation reveals that the patient is capable of such maneuvers when they are performing other tasks.

The extremity examination may demonstrate altered autonomic activity, for example a change in hair growth or nail bed pattern, a change in extremity color or temperature, or extremity swelling out of proportion to injury. Such changes are the hallmark of complex regional pain syndrome. Diabetic patients may present with diminution in peripheral blood flow, which can aggravate peripheral neuropathic pain. The findings in the neurologic examination may be normal in patients who have neuropathic pain but often point to dermatomal, regional, spinal, or brain dysfunction that correlates with the pain syndrome.

The sensory aspect of a neurologic examination is exceedingly important. In addition to testing for the presence or absence of primary sensory modality perception (vibration, proprioception, light touch, and pinprick), the examiner should test for alterations in sensory experience that are consistent with neuropathic pain. Allodynia is pain in response to a normally non-noxious mild stimulus. Hyperalgesia indicates an increased sensation of pain in response to a normally painful stimulus such as a pinprick. Hyperpathia is a prolonged painful experience following pinprick assessment.

Other findings of the neurologic examination may be abnormal, resulting either from a documented lesion or from a functional aberration caused by central nervous system dysfunction. For example, dystonia has been well described in complex regional pain syndrome or in patients who have a basal ganglia lesion [49]. Tremor may develop with peripheral neuropathy or may manifest as a physiologic aberration in patients who have chronic pain.

*Ancillary studies*

Ancillary studies should be used to exclude medical conditions that can either mimic or exacerbate the patient's clinical condition and to confirm or to aid in understanding the origin of pain. For example, deep venous thrombosis presents as extremity swelling with abnormal temperature sensation and can either mimic complex regional pain syndrome or coexist with this condition. Chronic low back and lumbar radicular pain, rarely, can be caused by a cauda equina tumor. Chronic extremity pain can coexist with active denervation in a nerve dermatome. Ultimately, all diagnostic tests are taken in conjunction with the history and examination to secure a diagnosis that then becomes the springboard for effective management.

## Management

As discussed previously, treatment for neuropathic pain should be multidisciplinary. Although many pain centers focus on anesthesiology-based procedures, such procedures are but one aspect of an important component of successful pain management. The following section presents a general discussion of the principles of multidisciplinary treatment. Such principles can be applied to any neuropathic pain state. Treatment must be individualized for the physical manifestation of pain and also for the patient's psychosocial adaptation.

### Psychotherapies

Because of the high prevalence of depression and anxiety with chronic neuropathic pain, psychotherapy is an important component of successful management. Even in patients who are not depressed, learning effective coping strategies for chronic pain is helpful. Although patients may be resistant to psychotherapy, sensing that the clinician views their pain as "psychosomatic," clinicians must stress the importance of psychologic intervention, because this intervention will help manage depression and coping skills and may uncover a previously undiagnosed, repressed trauma or other significant life event.

Cognitive behavioral therapy helps patients understand the interplay of pain perception, affect, and daily thought patterns. The focus is on developing positive expectations in patients [1]. Patients who have chronic pain are often resistant to insight-oriented therapy. It is the author's experience that many patients who have chronic pain are sufficiently disassociated from their emotions that such therapy is not possible. Insight-oriented therapy should be recommended only when there is a trusting bond between the patient and clinician and the patient expresses a desire to explore a possible relationship between previously unrecognized emotions and chronic pain. Group therapy is extremely beneficial, especially for patients who feel they are uniquely alone in their experience of chronic pain. Family therapy becomes important in helping other family members understand that chronic neuropathic pain is a real medical condition. Patients need to be validated within the family, and they also need to understand that at times they isolate themselves from the family because of pain.

In some cases, acute psychiatric intervention becomes necessary for chronic pain management. Long-term treatment is sometimes associated with a sudden insight or flashback into previously unrecognized trauma, severe depression, or poorly managed anxiety, and a skilled psychiatrist is required to help manage such conditions.

## Pharmacologic therapy

There are several pharmacologic strategies for treating chronic pain. No single drug effectively treats neuropathic pain. The following is a general discussion of various classes of drugs frequently used in chronic pain management. The best-studied conditions for using pharmacologic management are diabetic neuropathic pain and postherpetic neuralgia. The efficacy of pharmacologic therapy is less studied in other chronic neuropathic pain syndromes. Nonetheless, several generalizable treatment strategies exist.

## Anticonvulsants

Anticonvulsants have become first-line treatment for neuropathic pain syndromes [50–52]. Carbamazepine, phenytoin, valproate, and clonazepam were the first anticonvulsants to be well studied in treating patients who have neuropathic pain, especially with such conditions as trigeminal neuralgia and diabetic peripheral neuropathy [51]. Many well-controlled studies have shown that gabapentin is effective in treating postherpetic neuralgia and other neuropathic pain conditions [51–53]. The list has extended to newer anticonvulsants including topiramate, oxcarbazepine, lamotrigine, zonisamide, and levetiracetam [54–58]. The mechanism by which such drugs work is not completely clear and generally has to do with reduction in a hyper-excitability state, either peripherally or centrally. Interaction with GABA and other neurotransmitters may also be important.

The initial choice of drugs should be based on clinician comfort and relative indications. Only gabapentin is approved by the Food and Drug Administration for treating neuropathic pain, and this approval is limited to treatment of postherpetic neuralgia. Thus, the majority of anticonvulsant usage in treating neuropathic pain is off-label, a common practice in good clinical medicine. One can take advantage of the side-effect profile of some medications, for example topiramate for weight loss and zonisamide for sedative side effects. Anticonvulsants are administered using the dosing schedules commonly employed for treating epilepsy. Generally, only one anticonvulsant should be prescribed at a time, and upward titration should be based on efficacy and tolerability. Anticonvulsants may be used in conjunction with other medications described below.

## Antidepressants

Tricyclic antidepressants are much better studied in treating neuropathic pain than are the newer, more selective antidepressants [59–61]. Low-dose amitriptyline, in particular, has been shown in many well-controlled studies to be efficacious in treating various neuropathic pain conditions, independent of depression. The sedative side effects of amitriptyline often provide a useful adjunct in treating patients who have comorbid sleep deprivation. Tricyclic antidepressant dosage should begin at 10 mg/night, with an upward weekly titration in 10-mg increments as tolerated and needed.

Serotonin selective reuptake inhibitors, combined serotonin and norepinephrine reuptake inhibitors, and dopaminergic-mediated antidepressants are less well studied as medication adjuncts in treating neuropathic pain, but several studies demonstrate efficacy [62–66]. These agents become particularly useful when patients manifest with comorbid depression, anxiety, or both. Antidepressants may be beneficial because of their influence on descending serotonergic, adrenergic, and other pain inhibitory pathways and because of interaction with common pathways in depression and pain [67–69].

*Narcotic analgesics*

Narcotic analgesics (opioids) are the most potent prescription analgesics. Although there is wide acceptance for prescribing narcotic analgesics in patients who have cancer, acceptance is not so universal in treating patients with pain from other causes. Problems arise because of a lack of acceptance in using such medication long-term in these patients, combined with a fear of causing drug addiction. Narcotic analgesics take advantage of the innate opioid receptor system in the central nervous system. These medications mimic the action of endogenous opioids, providing a powerful pain signal transmission [70].

It is common practice in pain medicine clinics for patients to sign a narcotic agreement if they are to begin chronic narcotic analgesic treatment. Such agreements help provide clarity with regard to intent of narcotic usage and the manner in which medications will be used. The agreement usually stipulates that patients may obtain narcotics from only one physician, may use only one pharmacy, and may take medication only in the manner prescribed. Patients must return for monthly visits and are subject to random drug screening. Although a contract may seem harsh, the medical literature supports the use of such contracts, which help to minimize narcotic abuse by drug-seeking patients [1].

Initially, short-acting narcotics should be prescribed. When a patient's daily narcotic need is discerned, clinicians should switch to a long-acting medication that allows the patient to obtain sustained pain relief and to eliminate the sometimes intrusive behavioral pattern of taking a pain medication every 3 to 4 hours. Once a long-acting medication has been prescribed, short-acting medications can be used for breakthrough pain.

Tramadol hydrochloride is a unique narcotic-like medication. Tramadol does have weak mu opioid receptor agonism and enhances the inhibitory effect of descending serotonergic and adrenergic systems. Tramadol is efficacious in a variety of neuropathic pain conditions and can be used as a first-line medication before a more traditional narcotic analgesic is prescribed [1].

*Topical analgesics*

The best-studied topical analgesic is a 5% lidocaine patch [70]. This device may be especially useful in well-localized pain syndromes such as postherpetic neuralgia. Capsaicin may also be effective in relatively localized neuropathic pain conditions. Capsaicin leads to a depletion of substance P, a pain-generating neuropeptide in sensory afferent neurons. Capsaicin itself, however, may lead to a disquieting, burning pain, thus limiting its efficacy [71].

*Other adjunctive medications*

Tizanidine is a centrally acting alpha-2 adrenergic agonist with prominent antispasticity effects. This medication may be an important adjunct in patients who present with chronic muscle spasm or tension-type headache. Baclofen, a GABA agonist, may benefit patients who have chronic muscle spasm or paroxysmal pain. Mexiletine is an antiarrhythmic drug with demonstrable efficacy in treating some neuropathic pain conditions. Clonidine, another central alpha-2 adrenergic agonist, may be helpful in treating complex regional pain syndrome and related conditions when taken orally or transdermally [70].

Pulse therapy with corticosteroids or nonsteroidal anti-inflammatory drugs should be considered when patients develop acute musculoskeletal pain superimposed on chronic neuropathic pain. For example, some patients who have chronic back pain develop acute radicular pain with active, mechanical stretch signs on examination. In such patients, a 1- to 2-week course of nonsteroidal anti-inflammatory drugs or oral corticosteroids can help break the cycle of acute on chronic pain. Long-term corticosteroid and nonsteroidal anti-inflammatory drugs have little role in the treatment of chronic, neuropathic pain [70]. Neuroleptics and benzodiazepines are sometimes useful in and of themselves or in treating comorbid conditions [70,72].

There is some evidence that NMDA receptor antagonists ameliorate chronic neuropathic pain. Ketamine infusions have been studied, but the high rate of toxicity (causing hallucinations and anorexia) limits this medication's usefulness. Smaller doses of ketamine may be useful in select circumstances [73,74]. Oral NMDA receptor antagonist drugs have demonstrated little efficacy in treating chronic, neuropathic pain.

*Interventional strategies*

Several anesthesiology-based interventions are appropriate as one aspect of multidisciplinary pain management. It is a mistaken notion in some pain practices that management should be primarily intervention based. Indeed, in some practices, the failure of one intervention leads to an escalation in intervention strategies, often to the detriment of the patient [20].

Nerve blocks may be helpful for diagnostic purposes and sometimes may provide an important break in the chronic cycle of pain [75]. Once a successful nerve block is obtained, physical therapy and other strategies should be used immediately to help the patient overcome maladaptive postures. Sympathetic blockade, which by definition does not include primary sensory or somatic block, has been used both diagnostically and therapeutically in complex regional pain syndrome and related conditions [76]. (The lack of benefit from sympathetic blockade does not preclude the diagnosis of complex regional pain syndrome, however.) As with other nerve blocks, a successful sympathetic blockade should be followed immediately by progressive physical therapy.

Epidural and transforaminal corticosteroid injections may benefit patients who suffer with back conditions that have a demonstrable mechanical component, such as lumbar disc herniation and lumbar stenosis. Similarly, facet blocks may be exceedingly useful in breaking the cycle of chronic facet locking or in providing transient relief in patients who have segmental lumbar instability. Such relief allows the patient to begin more progressive physical therapy strategies.

Spinal cord stimulation relies on the principle that a stimulator, placed in the dorsal spinal cord, blocks central pain processing from a peripheral pain generator. Spinal cord stimulators should be considered only in patients who have relatively well localized extremity pain and who have exhausted all other treatment strategies [77]. Too often, spinal cord stimulators are placed as part of a rapid escalation in interventional techniques, when other multidisciplinary strategies have been neglected.

Intrathecal administration of narcotic analgesics takes advantage of a very-low-dose narcotic coupled with strong binding to spinal cord receptors, with minimal systemic side effects. Such strategies are particularly useful in patients who have demonstrated a positive effect to narcotic analgesics but who cannot tolerate systemic side effects [70,77]. These medications may be combined with intrathecal clonidine, which also has independent pain-alleviating effects, and baclofen, which may be useful in alleviating spasticity.

Other surgical interventions, including spinal surgery, must be approached with caution. Other than for trigeminal neuralgia, placing a lesion in the nervous system or performing decompressive surgery in an attempt to alleviate chronic, neuropathic pain has yielded equivocal results [20].

*Physical therapy*

Most patients who have neuropathic pain—especially patients who have chronic low back pain but also patients who have severe extremity neuropathic pain—have developed several maladaptive physical manifestations. Physical therapy should be an important consideration in treating chronic neuropathic pain [78].

Some physical therapy, such as craniosacral technique and myofascial release, is more intuitive and may help patients understand the link between physiology and the perception of physical pain. In these therapies, patients lie on a table, are extremely quiet, and the therapy is quite subtle. More conventional physical therapy includes the use of a transcutaneous electrical nerve stimulation unit, which may alleviate localized pain, as well as the employment of other modalities. In addition, range-of-motion, strengthening, and spine stabilization exercises help overcome chronic maladaptations.

*Complementary strategies*

Acupuncture is recognized by the World Health Organization as an effective treatment for pain. Several evidenced-based studies have demonstrated the efficacy of acupuncture in treating pain, although the difficulty of employing sham acupuncture leads to methodological flaws [79]. Acupuncture is not a stand-alone treatment but should be considered as part of a multidisciplinary approach, especially in patients who wish to explore nonpharmacologic strategies.

Nutritional counseling should be considered in patients who suffer with chronic neuropathic pain. Many such patients have poor eating habits, often because of chronic nausea or depression. In addition, many patients have a diet that is shifted toward high-carbohydrate and high-fat or junk foods. Such foods have an immediate gratifying effect, and poor eating habits often become part of a cycle of self-treatment underlying anxiety and depression [80].

Massage therapy can be used to desensitize areas of hyperalgesia and to help alleviate muscular and emotional stress. In some cases, massage therapy becomes a transition into developing greater insight into the interplay between physiology and physical pain perception [81].

**Summary**

Neuropathic pain is a neuropsychiatric condition in which pain is initiated or caused by a primary lesion or dysfunction in the nervous system. Understanding the complexity of neuropathic pain becomes the cornerstone for appropriate diagnosis and management. Diagnosis must take into account comorbid conditions. Successful management depends on realistic patient and physician expectations and an individualized, multidisciplinary approach.

**References**

[1] Staats PS, Argoff CE, Brewer R, et al. Neuropathic pain: incorporating new consensus guidelines into the reality of clinical practice. Adv Stud Med 2004;4(7B):S550–66.

[2] Merskey H, Bogduk N. Classification of chronic pain: descriptions of chronic pain syndromes and definitions of pain terms. 2nd edition. Seattle (WA): International Association for the Study of Pain; 1994.

[3] Melzack R, Casey KL. Sensory, motivational, and central control determinants of pain: a new conceptual model. In: Kenshalo D, editor. The skin senses: Proceedings of the First International Symposium on the Skin Senses. Springfield (IL): Charles C Thomas; 1968. p. 423–9.

[4] Treede RD, Kenshalo DR, Gracely RH, et al. The cortical representation of pain. Pain 1999; 79:105–11.

[5] Talbot JD, Marrett S, Evans AC, et al. Multiple representations of pain in human cerebral cortex. Science 2001;251:1355–8.

[6] Basbaum AI, Fields HL. Endogenous pain control systems: brainstem spinal pathways and endorphin circuitry. Annu Rev Neurosci 1984;7:309–38.

[7] Woolf CJ, Fitzgerald M. The properties of neurons recorded in the superficial dorsal horn of the rat spinal cord. J Comp Neurol 1983;221:313–28.

[8] Basbaum AI, Jessell TM. The perception of pain. In: Kandel ER, Schwartz JH, Jessell TM, editors. Principles of neural science. New York: McGraw Hill; 2000. p. 472–91.

[9] Duggan AW, Weihe E. Central transmission of impulses in nociceptors: events in the superficial dorsal horn. In: Basbaum AI, Besson JM, editors. Toward a new pharmaco-therapy of pain. Chichester (UK): John Wiley and Sons; 1991. p. 35–67.

[10] Hokfelt T, Johansson O, Ljungdahl A. Peptidergic neurons. Nature 1980;284:515–21.

[11] Meng ID, Manning BH. An analgesia circuit activated by cannabinoids. Nature 1998;394: 381–3.

[12] Peyron R, Schneider F, Faillenot MS, et al. An fMRI study of cortical representation of mechanical allodynia in patients with neuropathic pain. Neurology 2004;63:1838–46.

[13] Witting N, Kupers RC, Svensson P, et al. Experimental brush-evoked allodynia activates posterior parietal cortex. Neurology 2001;57:1817–24.

[14] Shih JJ, Cohen LG. Cortical reorganization in the human. Neurology 2004;63:1772–3.

[15] Mogil JS, Sternberg WF, Marek P, et al. The genetics of pain and pain inhibition. Proc Natl Acad Sci U S A 1996;93:3048–55.

[16] Katan W, Egan K, Miller D. Chronic pain: lifetime psychiatric diagnoses and family history. Am J Psychiatry 1984;142:1156–60.

[17] Dickinson LM, de Gruy FV, Dickinson WP, et al. Health-related quality of life and symptom profiles of female survivors of sexual abuse. Arch Fam Med 1999;8:35–43.

[18] Fillingim RB, Wilkinson CS, Powell T. Self-reported abuse history and pain complaints among young adults. Clin J Pain 1999;15:85–91.

[19] Goldberg RT, Goldstein R. A comparison of chronic pain patients and controls on traumatic events in childhood. Disabil Rehabil 2000;22:756–63.

[20] Scadding JW. Treatment of neuropathic pain: historical aspects. Pain Med 2004;5:S3–8.

[21] Dworkin RH, Backonja M, Rowbotham MC, et al. Advances in neuropathic pain; diagnosis, mechanisms, and treatment recommendations. Arch Neurol 2003;60:1524–34.

[22] Staats PS. Expanding the current management of neuropathic pain. Adv Stud Med 2004; 4(7B):S548–9.

[23] Nicholson B, Verma S. Comorbidities in chronic neuropathic pain. Pain Med 2004;5:S9–27.

[24] Romano JM, Turner JA. Chronic pain and depression: does the evidence support a relationship? Psychol Bull 1985;97:18–34.

[25] Keefe FJ, Wilkins RH, Cook WA, et al. Depression, pain, and pain behavior. J Consult Clin Psychol 1986;54:665–9.

[26] Krause SJ, Wiener RL, Tait RC. Depression and pain behavior in patients with chronic pain. Clin J Pain 1994;10:122–7.

[27] Grande LA, Loeser JD, Ashleigh OJ, et al. Complex regional pain syndrome as a stress response. Pain 2004;110:495–8.

[28] Frayne SM, Seaver MR, Loveland S, et al. Burden of medical illness in women with depression and posttraumatic stress disorder. Arch Intern Med 2004;164:1306–12.

[29] Asmundson GJ, Wright KD, Stein MB. Pain and PTSD symptoms in female veterans. Eur J Pain 2004;8:345–50.

[30] Otis JD, Keane TM, Kerns RD. An examination of the relationship between chronic pain and posttraumatic stress disorder. J Rehabil Res Dev 2003;40:397–405.

[31] Feldman JB. The neurobiology of pain, affect and hypnosis. Am J Clin Hypn 2004;46: 187–200.

[32] Liberizon I, Phan KL. Brain-imaging studies in posttraumatic stress disorder. CNS Spectr 2003;8:641–50.

[33] Saberski LR. When is it time for pain management? Pain Clin 2004;6:3–5.

[34] Sarno JE. Healing back pain: the mind-body connection. New York: Warner Books; 1991.

[35] Backonja M-M, Serra J. Pharmacologic management part 1: better-studied neuropathic pain diseases. Pain Med 2004;5:S28–47.

[36] Ochoa JL, Verdugo RJ. Reflex sympathetic dystrophy: a common clinical avenue for somatoform expression. Neurol Clin 1995;13:351–63.

[37] Hainline B. Reflex sympathetic dystrophy. In: Spivak JM, DiCesare PE, Feldman DS, et al, editors. Orthopaedics: a comprehensive study guide. New York: McGraw-Hill; 1999. p. 943–5.

[38] Stanton-Hicks M, Janig W, Hassenbusch S, et al. Reflex sympathetic dystrophy: changing concepts and taxonomy. Pain 1995;63:127–33.

[39] Max MB, Gilron I. Sympathetically maintained pain: has the emperor no clothes? Neurology 1999;52:905–7.

[40] Schwartzman RJ, Grothusen J, Kiefer TR, et al. Neuropathic central pain: epidemiology, etiology, and treatment options. Arch Neurol 2001;58:1547–50.

[41] Verdugo RJ, Ochoa JL. Sympathetically maintained pain I. Phentolamine block questions the concept. Neurology 1994;44:1003–10.

[42] Verdugo RJ, Campero M, Ochoa JL. Phentolamine sympathetic block in painful polyneuropathies. II. Further questioning of the concept of sympathetically maintained pain. Neurology 1994;44:1010–4.

[43] Deejeerine J, Roussy G. Le syndrome thalamique. Rev Neurol 1906;12:521–32.

[44] Boivie J, Leijon G, Johansson I. Central post-stroke pain: study of the mechanisms through analyses of the sensory abnormalities. Pain 1989;37:173–85.

[45] Leijon G, Boivie J, Johansson I. Central post-stroke pain: neurological symptoms and pain characteristics. Pain 1989;36:13–25.

[46] Woolsey RM. Chronic pain following spinal cord injury. J Am Paraplegia Soc 1986;9:39–41.

[47] Moulin DE, Foley KM, Ebers GC. Pain syndromes in multiple sclerosis. Neurology 1988;38: 1830–4.

[48] Cleeland CS. The Brief Pain Inventory, a measure of cancer pain and its impact. Quality of Life News Letter 2003.

[49] Schwartzman RJ, Popescu A. Reflex sympathetic dystrophy. Curr Rheumatol Rep 2002;4: 165–9.

[50] Namaka M, Gramlich CR, Ruhlen D, et al. A treatment algorithm for neuropathic pain. Clin Ther 2004;26:951–79.

[51] Wiffen P, Collins S, McQuay H, et al. Anticonvulsant drugs for acute and chronic pain. Cochrane Database Syst Rev 2000;3:CD001133.

[52] Tremont-Lukats IW, Megeff C, Backonja MM. Anticonvulsants for neuropathic pain syndromes: mechanisms of action and place in therapy. Drugs 2000;60:1029–52.

[53] Backonja M, Glanzman RL. Gabapentin dosing for neuropathic pain: evidence from randomized, placebo-controlled clinical trials. Clin Ther 2003;25:81–104.

[54] Chandramouli J. Newer anticonvulsant drugs in neuropathic pain and bipolar disorder. J Pain Palliat Care Pharmacother 2002;16:19–37.

[55] Vu TN. Current pharmacologic approaches to treating neuropathic pain. Curr Pain Headache Rep 2004;8:15–8.

[56] Guay DR. Oxcarbazepine, topiramate, zonisamide, and levetiracetam: potential use in neuropathic pain. Am J Geriatr Pharmacother 2003;1:18–37.

[57] Pappagallo M. Newer antiepileptic drugs: possible uses in the treatment of neuropathic pain and migraine. Clin Ther 2003;25:2506–38.

[58] LaRoche SM, Helmers SL. The new antiepileptic drugs: scientific review. JAMA 2004;291: 605–14.

[59] Max MB, Lynch SA, Muir J, et al. Effects of desipramine, amitriptyline and fluoxetine on pain in diabetic neuropathy. N Engl J Med 1992;326:1250–6.

[60] Kvinesdal B, Molin J, Froland A, et al. Imipramine treatment of painful diabetic neuropathy. JAMA 1984;251:1727–30.

[61] Max MB, Culnane M, Schafer SC, et al. Amitriptyline relieves diabetic neuropathy pain in patients with normal or depressed mood. Neurology 1987;37:589–96.

[62] Ansari A. The efficacy of newer antidepressants in the treatment of chronic pain: a review of current literature. Harv Rev Psychiatry 2000;7:257–77.

[63] Semenchuk MR, Sherman S, Davis B. Double-blind, randomized trial of bupropion SR for the treatment of neuropathic pain. Neurology 2001;13:1583–8.

[64] Mattia C, Paoletti F, Coluzzi F, et al. New antidepressants in the treatment of neuropathic pain. A review. Minerva Anestesiol 2002;68:105–14.

[65] Goldstein D, Iyengar S, Mallinckrodt C, et al. Duloxetine: a potential new treatment for depressed patients with comorbid pain. Pain Med 2002;3:177–81.

[66] Mattia C, Coluzzi F. Antidepressants in chronic neuropathic pain. Mini Rev Med Chem 2003;3:773–84.

[67] Mochizucki D. Serotonin and noradrenaline reuptake inhibitors in animal models of pain. Hum Psychopharmacol 2004;19:S15–9.

[68] Schreiber S, Rigai T, Katz Y, et al. The antinociceptive effect of mirtazapine in mice is mediated through serotonergic, noradrenergic and opioid mechanisms. Brain Res Bull 2002; 58:601–5.

[69] Delgado PL. Common pathways of depression and pain. J Clin Psychiatry 2004;65(Suppl 12):16–9.

[70] Caraceni A, Portenoy AC. Pain. In: Griggs RC, Joynt RJ, editors. Clinical neurology, 2004 edition [CD-ROM]. New York: Lippincott Williams & Wilkins; 2004.

[71] Hautkappe M. Roizen. Review of the effectiveness of capsaicin for painful cutaneous disorders and neural dysfunction. Clin J Pain 1998;14:97–106.

[72] Fishbain DA, Cutler RB, Lewis J, et al. Do the second-generation "atypical neuroleptics" have analgesic properties? A structured evidence-based review. Pain Med 2004;5:359–65.

[73] Schwartzman RJ, Goldberg ME, Dotson J, et al. Multi-day low dose ketamine infusion for the treatment of complex regional pain syndrome. Neurology 2004;Suppl5:A515.

[74] Correll GE, Maleki J, Gracely EJ, et al. Subanesthetic ketamine infusion therapy: a retrospective analysis of a novel therapeutic approach to complex regional pain syndrome. Pain Med 2004;5:263–75.

[75] Abram SE. Neural blockade for neuropathic pain. Clin J Pain 2000;16:S56–60.

[76] Boas RA. Sympathetic nerve blocks: in search of a role. Reg Anesth Pain Med 1998;23: 292–306.

[77] Hassenbusch SJ, Stanton-Hicks M, Covington EC. Spinal cord stimulation versus spinal infusion for low back and leg pain. Acta Neurochir Suppl 1995;64:109–15.

[78] Singh G, Willen SN, Boswell MV, et al. The value of interdisciplinary pain management in complex regional pain syndrome type I: a prospective outcome study. Pain Physician 2004;7: 203–9.

[79] Rosman SM, Hainline B. Complementary and alternative medicine. In: Hainline B, Devinsky O, editors. Neurological complications of pregnancy. 2nd edition. Philadelphia: Lippincott Williams & Wilkins; 2002. p. 307–16.

[80] Dallman MF, Pecoraro N. Chronic stress and obesity: a new view of "comfort food". Proc Natl Acad Sci U S A 2003;100:11696–701.

[81] Hasson D, Arnetz B. A randomized clinical trial of the treatment effects of massage compared to relaxation tape recordings on diffuse long-term pain. Psychother Psychosom 2004;73:17–24.

PSYCHIATRIC
CLINICS
OF NORTH AMERICA

ELSEVIER
SAUNDERS

Psychiatr Clin N Am 28 (2005) 737–751

# Neurobiologic Basis of Nicotine Addiction and Psychostimulant Abuse: a Role for Neurotensin?

Paul Fredrickson, MD[a],*, Mona Boules, PhD[b],
Siong-Chi Lin, MD[a], Elliott Richelson, MD[b]

[a]Department of Psychiatry and Psychology, Mayo Clinic College of Medicine,
4500 San Pablo Road, Jacksonville, FL 32224, USA
[b]Neuropsychopharmacology Laboratory, Mayo Clinic College of Medicine,
4500 San Pablo Road, Jacksonville, FL 32224, USA

Addiction is perhaps most succinctly defined as compulsive, out-of-control drug use despite serious negative consequences [1]. Many social, interpersonal, psychologic, and other variables contribute to this self-defeating set of behaviors, but the essence of addiction is that changes take place in the brain because of repetitive exposure to a drug [2]. Although considerable progress has occurred in devising effective interventions for various addictions, a lifelong susceptibility to relapse makes it clear that it is not known how to restore the brain to its former state, and that work toward understanding addiction is far from done [3]. This article focuses on what has been characterized as the keystone of the world of addiction, nicotine [4], and the psychostimulant drugs amphetamine and cocaine.

The scope of this article reflects the authors' clinical interests in treating nicotine dependence and amphetamine and cocaine abuse and the neurobiologic links with schizophrenia they have studied in their preclinical work. They briefly review animal models of addictive behaviors, discuss the neuroanatomic and neurochemical substrates of nicotine and psychostimulant addiction, and conclude with a brief summary of their work with an analogue of neurotensin as a putative therapeutic agent. This article is not a comprehensive review of a complex subject but rather gives the reader a sense of a possible role for neurotensin analogues as antipsychotic drugs and as treatments for addiction. Neurotensin is a neuropeptide that

---

* Corresponding author.
*E-mail address:* Fredrickson.Paul@mayo.edu (P. Fredrickson).

colocalizes with dopamine systems [5,6], behaves in certain paradigms like an atypical neuroleptic drug [7], and has been implicated in the psychomotor stimulant and reinforcing effects of drugs of abuse [8].

### Nicotine dependence and psychiatry

As public health efforts during the past few decades have succeeded in lowering the rate of smoking in the general population from 42% of adults in 1965 to a plateau of around 22% [9], a change in composition of the population of smokers has taken place. Psychiatric problems are more prevalent among smokers now than a generation ago. This prevalence has important implications for psychiatry's role in preventing the major morbidities and mortality associated with smoking. For example, as the rate of smoking has fallen in the general population, a strong positive association with depression has emerged [10]. Based on exposure to tobacco, patients with schizophrenia are most vulnerable to adverse health consequences.

Surprisingly, despite the high exposure to tobacco smoke, a number of reports suggest a lower rate of lung cancer and other malignancies in schizophrenic patients than in the population at large [11–15]. On the other hand, a recent study by Lichtermann [16] based on Finland's National Hospital Discharge and Disability Pension registers linked to the Finnish Cancer Registry, showed a higher rate of cancer (particularly of the lung) among schizophrenic individuals than in the population at large. The Finnish study also examined rates of illness among first-degree relatives of schizophrenic patients and found a lower-than-expected risk of cancer. Therefore, it is possible that a protective factor associated with schizophrenia does exist, as suggested by prior studies. In this well-designed study, the increased cancer risk for the patient cohort was consistent with increased smoking rates. Lichtermann hypothesizes that access to cigarettes (eg, smoking policies on psychiatric units), rates of institutionalization, access to medication, and population genetic variations may all contribute to differences with other published studies. Apart from cancer risk, individuals with schizophrenia suffer higher death rates from cardiovascular and respiratory disease [17–19]. Therefore, the weight of evidence points toward increased health risks from smoking as a result of increased smoking rates in schizophrenia.

Individuals with psychiatric illness are more likely to be smokers and to have a poorer prognosis for cessation [20]. Schizophrenic patients smoke at a prevalence rate two to three times higher than the general population [21]. These associations are of clinical relevance to the psychiatrist and raise the question whether patients with schizophrenia and other psychiatric illness use tobacco to self-medicate. For example, nicotine seems to ameliorate the attentional deficits and negative symptoms of schizophrenia [22–24].

Schizophrenic subjects demonstrate impaired sensory gating [25], a deficit improved by smoking [22]. These patients frequently display hypofrontality, or decreased activity in the prefrontal cortex, which correlates with negative signs and symptoms such as lack of goal-directed behavior, flattened affect, and diminished responsiveness to normally rewarding stimuli. Decreased activity in prefrontal cortex in the rat results in decreased burst firing in ventral tegmental dopaminergic neurons, an effect countered by nicotine [26,27]. In rats, nicotine enhances prepulse inhibition, a model of sensory gating [28]. Altered expression and function of the alpha 7 nicotinic receptor has been linked to the sensory gating deficit of schizophrenia [29]. More than 75% of schizophrenic subjects exhibit a sensory gating deficit, and evidence suggests decreased alpha 7 expression may affect gating in humans and in mice [30]. These studies support the hypothesis that psychotic patients smoke, in part, to alleviate the attentional deficits and negative symptoms of schizophrenia.

Several studies have demonstrated an increase in smoking after administration of haloperidol. This increase is thought to be a compensatory mechanism resulting from a partial blockade of nicotine's rewarding effects mediated by dopamine [31–34]. In one study [35], smoking decreased after haloperidol administration, although an initial reduction in the intercigarette interval suggested transient compensatory smoking behaviors. Although the conclusion thus far is tentative, classic antipsychotic drugs may have adverse effects on smoking behaviors by blunting reward pathways. Therefore, monitoring of smoking behaviors is warranted with changes in antipsychotic drug regimens.

Atypical antipsychotic drugs seem to have advantages over typical neuroleptics for smoking cessation. In a study by George and colleagues [23], 18 schizophrenic patients receiving atypical drugs were compared with 27 patients receiving typical antipsychotic medication. All subjects were prescribed nicotine transdermal therapy for 10 weeks along with random assignment to generic smoking cessation counseling or to a program tailored for schizophrenia. Although the tailored group therapy did not improve smoking cessation rates beyond standard counseling, there was a significant difference in smoking cessation at end of treatment for subjects in the atypical versus typical drug group (56% versus 22% abstinence). Smoking cessation rates at 6 months were much lower but remained higher in the atypical group (17% versus 7%). George and colleagues [36] reported similar results with respect to atypical and typical neuroleptics in a trial of bupropion for smoking cessation in schizophrenia.

Several investigators have reported a reduction in smoking in patients treated with clozapine compared with other neuroleptics [37–40]. Although smoking cessation rates are lower in schizophrenic subjects than in the general population when given standard smoking cessation treatment, patients receiving atypical antipsychotic drugs are at a relative advantage and are less refractory to smoking cessation efforts. Taken together, the available research indicates that successful management of addiction requires an awareness and understanding of special patient populations.

In summary, psychiatric syndromes are associated with a poorer prognosis for smoking cessation, particularly in patients who have schizophrenia. Existing smoking cessation strategies (nicotine replacement, bupropion, counseling) are more likely to be effective in conjunction with atypical rather than conventional antipsychotic drugs. Although cessation rates remain lower than for the general population, a significant proportion of schizophrenic patients do respond favorably. Given the changing trends of smoking and psychiatric illness, a greater role for the psychiatrist in achieving further reductions in the public health risk of smoking seems inevitable.

### Amphetamine and cocaine addiction—a need for new therapies

According to a United Nations report published in 2000 [41], more than 35 million people worldwide abuse amphetamines. The most recent surge of abuse involves methamphetamine. Its use reached epidemic proportions in parts of the United States during the last decade [42]. Cocaine abuse is estimated to involve at least 15 million persons worldwide. Cocaine played a prominent medicinal role in the late 1800s, but in the past century escalating abuse and addiction have dwarfed its therapeutic applications. Amphetamines and cocaine alter mental status by increasing excitatory neurotransmitters in the brain, resulting in short-term euphoria and addiction after repeated use.

Amphetamines and related psychostimulants are widely prescribed in the United States for attention deficit disorder, narcolepsy, and other forms of hypersomnia. Most patients tolerate therapeutic use of these drugs well and do not develop addiction. Psychiatric disorders frequently coexist with psychostimulant abuse, however, and can be aggravated by the drug abuse [43]. Pharmacotherapy trials using a wide variety of medications including antidepressants, carbamazepine, and dopamine agonists and antagonists have largely failed to show clear benefit or have suffered from high dropout rates [44].

Cocaine abuse has followed a cyclical pattern in the United States and in recent decades has reached high levels. Many pharmacotherapies have shown promise, but results of most randomized, controlled studies have failed to show efficacy for antidepressants, dopamine agonists, carbamazepine, or other agents [45]. Modafinil, a novel stimulant developed initially for treatment of narcolepsy, has shown early promise as a potential therapeutic agent and seems to blunt cocaine-induced euphoria [46], but confirmation of its role is needed. Additional pharmacotherapeutic options clearly are needed for management of cocaine and amphetamine addiction.

Cocaine and amphetamine increase extracellular levels of dopamine, serotonin, and norepinephrine. An increase in presynaptic release and inhibition of reuptake of these neurotransmitters, particularly dopamine, underlies their effects on reward pathways [47,48]. Intensity of stimulant-induced euphoria correlates with degree of dopamine release and dopamine receptor occupancy [49]. Psychostimulant activation of reward circuitry in humans has been observed with functional MRI in drug-naive subjects, demonstrating a direct drug activation of these pathways independent of craving or cued recall [50].

## Animal models of addiction

Attempts to model addiction in animals have yielded a wealth of data on brain mechanisms, but correlates to human behavior are not always obvious. Widely used models involve drug self-administration. Pleasurable experience is a typical initial response to a psychostimulant drug. That experience, however, does not lead invariably to addiction. Similarly, under certain conditions, animals self-administer a stable dose of drug but do not show escalation of dose or other features of addiction [51]. Thus, there is a difference between "liking" and "wanting" [52]. Avoidance of aversive experience (eg, drug withdrawal) can be modeled in animals and clearly affects human behavior. Negative reinforcement does not explain rapid reinstatement of drug use after long abstinence. In human smokers and psychostimulant addicts, cues to drug use develop and elicit powerful cravings, even in the absence of drug. Cue-controlled drug seeking can be modeled in laboratory animals [53]. The effect of drugs on the reward threshold also can be measured by intracranial self-stimulation, a technique that allows the animal to control electrical stimulation to brain reward pathways [54,55].

Repeated exposure to nicotine and other psychostimulants results in an interesting phenomenon called locomotor or behavioral sensitization [56–58]. Rats receiving daily or weekly injections show increasing activity over time in response to a fixed dose of drug. This response is unlike tolerance, in which an increased dose is required over time to achieve a given effect. Behavioral sensitization has been proposed as a model for the increasing incentive or motivational aspects of drug addiction [53,59]. Behavioral sensitization represents an enduring neural adaptation that may predispose to relapse long after the last drug exposure [60].

Knockout animals have been modified to delete a certain gene of interest (for example, a nicotinic acetylcholine receptor subunit) to allow assessment of the role a particular gene plays in various behaviors. One drawback is that these animals lack the gene from birth, and adaptive developmental processes may therefore affect neural systems [61]. A recent model of the alpha 4 nicotinic receptor results from a point mutation that produces animals displaying addictive behaviors to extremely low doses of nicotine [62]. These animals, termed knockin mice, have alpha 4 receptors that are hypersensitive to nicotine. In general, genetically modified animals may offer insights that cannot be obtained readily by traditional pharmacologic techniques. For example, mice lacking the gene for a phosphoprotein called DARPP-32 [63] allow study of the role this molecule plays in dopamine-mediated intracellular signaling, because suitable agonist and antagonist compounds do not exist for this pathway.

What conclusions can be drawn from animal models of addiction? They provide a means for screening potential therapeutic compounds and offer insights into mechanisms of addiction, but caution is warranted. A single model does not capture the complexity of human addiction, and a putative therapeutic drug that blocks self-administration in animals may prove ineffective in humans if it does not alleviate craving or cue-induced responses.

## Neuroanatomic and neurotransmitter correlates of addiction

Dopaminergic neurons in the ventral tegmental area of the mesencephalon projecting to the nucleus accumbens, medial prefrontal cortex, and amygdala form the mesocorticolimbic dopamine system. Functional changes in this system seem to underlie the actions of all drugs of abuse [64]. Dopaminergic neurons synapse on pyramidal excitatory amino acid (glutamatergic) neurons and nonpyramidal γ-aminobutyric acid (GABA) interneurons, with dopamine acting as a modulator of these circuits [65]. This reward circuitry undergoes profound changes with repeated psychostimulant exposure, resulting in a gain in the function of this neural circuit, thereby increasing behavioral responsiveness to subsequent drug exposure and drug cues [57].

Neuronal nicotinic acetylcholine receptors (nAChRs) are ligand-gated ion channels that stimulate release of dopamine, norepinephrine, GABA, glutamate, acetylcholine, and neuropeptides [66]. These channels are composed of five subunits forming an axis of symmetry around a membrane channel that provides a rapid cellular response when stimulated. Twelve subunit types have been identified [62], and their functional roles are being explored using genetic models (knockout and knockin mice). Nicotine strongly stimulates dopaminergic neurons in the ventral tegmental area and increases dopamine release in the nucleus accumbens. Release in the nucleus accumbens shell is greatest in nicotine-naive rats, whereas repeated exposure results in greater dopamine release in the nucleus accumbens core and reduction in the shell [67]. Thus, by acting on nAChRs, nicotine exerts powerful influences on brain reward circuits. Activation of nAChRs may also be crucial for development of addiction to amphetamine and cocaine [68].

One of the key mechanisms regulating levels of extracellular dopamine is the dopamine transporter (DAT). DAT is regulated actively in response to various stimuli, including the presence of DAT-blocking drugs [69]. Amphetamine interacts with DAT by competing for reuptake and by causing dopamine efflux (by reverse transport) and reduces cell surface expression of DAT [70]. In contrast, cocaine acts by preventing reuptake of released dopamine and increases surface expression of DAT. Thus, when cocaine is withdrawn, elevated DAT activity may cause extracellular dopamine to fall to lower-than-baseline levels, possibly a basis for the "crash" that occurs following cocaine highs [70]. Neurotensin mRNA expression in the brain is elevated in mice lacking the dopamine transporter. This increased expression may be a compensatory mechanism to counteract a hyperdopaminergic state [71].

In recent years, considerable progress has been made toward understanding the complex intracellular signaling processes that occur in response to receptor activation. Many receptors in the brain (eg, nAChRs) form a fast-response system, others (eg, dopamine receptors) mediate a slow synaptic response. Many psychotomimetic agents, including certain drugs of abuse, act through a final common intracellular pathway involving a molecule called adenosine 3′,5′-monophosphate-regulated phosphoprotein of 32 kilodaltons, or DARPP-32. DARPP-32, depending on its phosphorylation state, controls the activity of a variety of neuronal targets including ion pumps, receptors, and transcription factors [63]. DARPP-32 is necessary to mediate the action of dopamine. In animals with a genetic deletion of DARPP-32, behavioral effects of D-amphetamine are strongly attenuated [72]. Cocaine place preference in mutant animals is reduced but can be overcome by higher doses, suggesting that reward pathways are less sensitive but not blocked by deletion of DARPP-32 [73]. Nicotine's effect on motor activity does not involve the DARPP-32 pathway, but some transcription factors induced by nicotine do seem to depend on this pathway (Boules, unpublished data). Further studies using animal models of addiction should help clarify the role this important pathway plays in various aspects of addiction and recovery.

### A role for neurotensin?

Neurotensin is an endogenous peptide of 13 amino acids discovered more than 3 decades ago [74]. The amino acid sequence is pyroGlu-Leu-Tyr-Glu-Asn-Lys-Pro-Arg-Arg-Pro-Tyr-Ile-Leu-OH. Most, if not all, of the activity mediated by neurotensin is seen with the fragment NT-(8-13). The accumulated evidence has shown that neurotensin behaves as a neurotransmitter or neuromodulator in the central nervous system, and there are striking interactions between neurotensin, through its receptors, and central dopaminergic systems [5,75]. Neurotensin cell bodies are found in the ventral tegmental area, and most these neurons also contain tyrosine hydroxylase, the enzyme that is the rate-limiting step for dopamine synthesis. These dopamine/neurotensin neurons project to the nucleus accumbens, prefrontal cortex, and amygdala [76,77]. Neurotensin antagonizes dopamine and stimulant-induced transmission in mesolimbic pathways [78,79], although its effect may depend on the activation state of the dopaminergic system [80]. Thus, neurotensin participates in regulation of dopaminergic pathways implicated in addiction to nicotine, amphetamine, and cocaine.

A role for neurotensin in neuropsychiatric disease has been hypothesized for more than 2 decades [81]. Wolf and colleagues [82], in an autoradiographic study, found a 40% reduction in neurotensin receptors in entorhinal cortex of schizophrenic subjects compared with controls. In a large group of drug-free schizophrenic patients, those with lowest neurotensin concentrations in the cerebrospinal fluid had significantly higher levels of pretreatment psychopathology [83], particularly negative symptoms. Additionally, most antipsychotic drugs increase neurotensin transmission in the nucleus accumbens [84], thus lending support to the hypothesis that neurotensin may be a mediator of antipsychotic drug effects. Therefore, development of neurotensin analogues holds promise for the treatment of schizophrenia.

Neurotensin mediates its effects through receptors [85,86] that first were identified by radioligand-binding techniques [87,88]. There are two molecularly cloned receptors, one of high affinity (NTS1), and the other of lower affinity (NTS2). NTS1 and NTS2 are members of the superfamily of 7-transmembrane-spanning, G-protein–coupled receptors. NTS1, the most studied of the neurotensin receptors, activates intracellular $Ca^{2+}$ influx and regulates cyclic AMP, cyclic GMP, phosphatidyl inositol turnover, phospholipase C, protein kinase C, and $Na^+K^+$-ATP activity [89–92]. Additionally, NTS1 modulates dopamine receptors [93–95]. A third neurotensin-binding site, called NTS3, spans the membrane only once, and its functional response is unknown. This site shares 100% homology with the previously cloned human gp95/sortilin [96]. NTS3 may play a role in intracellular transport [97] and in apoptosis [98].

An advance in the study of neurotensin and its receptors came with the synthesis of the novel nonpeptide neurotensin receptor antagonists SR48692 [99] and SR142948A [100]. SR48692 has been shown to delay the development of behavioral sensitization to cocaine [101] and to block the development of sensitization to D-amphetamine [102]. These studies, however, required a high dose of antagonist and pre-exposure to the antagonist. Treatment had little effect once sensitization had developed. Because it can be assumed that abusers of psychostimulants are probably already in a sensitized state, use of neurotensin receptor antagonists for human psychostimulant addiction may be impractical.

Over many years, the authors' group has conducted extensive structure–activity studies of peptide and nonpeptide compounds that interact with neurotensin receptors. To affect the central nervous system, neurotensin must be injected into brain, because it is readily degraded by peptidases in the periphery. The authors have developed several brain-penetrating analogues that can be injected peripherally and cause neurochemical and behavioral changes similar to those caused by native neurotensin directly injected into brain. In addition, these analogues have high affinity for human neurotensin receptors. One of these analogues, called NT69L, is more potent and longer acting than any of the other analogues [103]. This analogue of neurotensin [8–13] incorporates a regioisomer of L-tryptophan [104].

Many of the authors' animal studies have focused on NT69L. This compound is presently in preclinical toxicology studies so that it can be tested in humans. After intraperitoneal injection in laboratory animals (rats and mice), this peptide causes profound hypothermia; antinociception; blockade of catalepsy caused by haloperidol; blockade of the climbing behavior caused by high-dose apomorphine; blockade of hyperactivity caused by cocaine, D-amphetamine, and nicotine; and blockade of initiation and expression of sensitization to nicotine [105–109]. In an animal model of Parkinson's disease, rats are lesioned unilaterally in the nigrostriatal pathway by the neurotoxin 6-hydroxydopamine. NT69L blocks the rotation caused by D-amphetamine and apomorphine in these animals. Therefore, this analogue of neurotensin shows efficacy in an animal model of Parkinson's disease and behaves as an atypical antipsychotic in other animal models [77,103]. NT69L effectively blocks the initiation and expression of nicotine-induced sensitization [108,109], a mechanism that is thought to underlie craving and risk for relapse to smoking. The authors expect the compound to have similar properties against amphetamine and cocaine [110]. NT69L itself is not self-administered by rhesus monkeys [111].

One of the confusing aspects of the neurotensin literature, as it relates to addiction, is that both antagonists and agonists are effective in animal models. Of the two nonpeptide neurotensin antagonists, SR48692 has higher affinity for NTS1 than for NTS2 [112] and very low affinity for NTS3. In vivo, SR48692 does not block all effects of neurotensin. The second neurotensin antagonist, SR142948A, has high affinity for both NTS1 and NTS2; its affinity for NTS3 is unknown. SR142948A has an inverted dose–response curve when blocking some effects of neurotensin. At low doses, some of the effects of neurotensin are blocked, whereas at higher doses of the compound the blocking effects are reversed [100]. Importantly, in vitro, at the molecularly cloned receptors, these antagonists activate NTS2 [113]. A unifying hypothesis emerging from the authors' laboratory is that activation of NTS1 blocks expression of sensitization (and the acute effects of psychostimulants), whereas activation of NTS2 blocks initiation of sensitization (E. Richelson, unpublished data). If these finding are confirmed, behavioral sensitization, an animal model for drug craving and risk for relapse, is caused by decreased transmission through neurotensin receptors. In turn, one would predict that neurotensin agonists hold promise for treating nicotine and other psychostimulant addiction.

## Summary

Addiction to psychostimulant drugs such as nicotine, amphetamine, and cocaine is a serious public health problem for which there is a paucity of accepted forms of pharmacotherapy. Nicotine dependence has become more frequently associated with psychiatric illness in recent decades, and patients who have schizophrenia are at highest risk and have the poorest prognosis for stopping their addiction. Possible mechanisms for this association include self-medication, with nicotine attenuating attentional deficits and negative symptoms. Neurotensin has been postulated to be an endogenous neuroleptic, and the performance of neurotensin analogues in animal models of addiction makes such compounds intriguing candidates for treatment of addiction in high-risk psychiatric populations.

## References

[1] Hyman SE, Malenka RC. Addiction and the brain: the neurobiology of compulsion and its persistence. Nat Rev Neurosci 2001;2:695–703.

[2] Nestler EJ, Aghajanian GK. Molecular and cellular basis of addiction. Science 1997;278: 58–63.

[3] Goldman D, Barr CS. Restoring the addicted brain. N Engl J Med 2002;347:843–5.

[4] Koop CE. Tobacco addiction: accomplishments and challenges in science, health, and policy. Nicotine & Tobacco Research 2003;5:613–9.

[5] Tyler-McMahon BM, Boules M, Richelson E. Neurotensin: peptide for the next millennium. Regul Pept 2000;93:125–36.

[6] Lambert PD, Gross R, Nemeroff CB, et al. Anatomy and mechanisms of neurotensin-dopamine interactions in the central nervous system. Ann N Y Acad Sci 1995;757:377–89.

[7] Jolicoeur FB, Gagne MA, Rivest R, et al. Atypical neuroleptic-like behavioral effects of neurotensin. Brain Res Bull 1993;32:487–91.

[8] Glimcher PW, Margolin DH, Giovino AA, et al. Neurotensin: a new reward peptide. Brain Res 1984;291:119–24.

[9] No authors listed. Cigarette smoking among adults. MMWR Morb Mortal Wkly Rep 2003;54:509–13.

[10] Murphy JM, Horton NJ, Monson RR, et al. Cigarette smoking in relation to depression: historical trends from the Stirling County study. Am J Psychiatry 2003;160:1663–9.

[11] Gulbinat W, Dupont A, Jablensky A, et al. Cancer incidence of schizophrenic patients. Br J Psychiatry 1992;161(Suppl):75–83.

[12] Mortensen PB. The occurrence of cancer in first admitted schizophrenic patients. Schizophr Res 1994;12:185–94.

[13] Baldwin JA. Schizophrenia and physical disease. Psychol Med 1979;9:611–8.

[14] Tsuang MT, Perkins K, Simpson JC. Physical diseases in schizophrenia and affective disorder. J Clin Psychiatry 1983;44:42–6.

[15] Harris AE. Physical disease and schizophrenia. Schizophr Bull 1988;14:85–96.

[16] Lichtermann D, Ekelund J, Pukkala E, et al. Incidence of cancer among persons with schizophrenia and their relatives. Arch Gen Psychiatry 2001;58:573–8.

[17] Tsuang MT, Woolson RF, Fleming JA. Premature deaths in schizophrenia and affective disorders. Arch Gen Psychiatry 1980;37:979–83.

[18] Allebeck P, Wistedt B. Mortality in schizophrenia. A ten-year follow-up based on the Stockholm County inpatient register. Arch Gen Psychiatry 1986;43:650–3.

[19] Buda M, Tsuang MT, Fleming JA. Causes of death in DSM-III schizophrenics and other psychotics. Arch Gen Psychiatry 1988;45:283–5.

[20] Lasser K, Boyd JW, Woolhandler S, et al. Smoking and mental illness. A population-based prevalence study. JAMA 2000;284:2606–10.

[21] Dalack GW, Healy DJ, Meador-Woodruff JH. Nicotine dependence in schizophrenia: clinical phenomena and laboratory findings. Am J Psychiatry 1998;155:1490–501.

[22] Adler LE, Hoffer LD, Wiser A, et al. Normalization of auditory physiology by cigarette smoking in schizophrenic patients. Am J Psychiatry 1993;150:1856–61.

[23] George TP, Ziedonis DM, Feingold A, et al. Nicotine transdermal patch and atypical antipsychotic medications for smoking cessation in schizophrenia. Am J Psychiatry 2000; 157:1835–42.

[24] Smith RC, Singh A, Infante M, et al. Effects of cigarette smoking and nicotine nasal spray on psychiatric symptoms and cognition in schizophrenia. Neuropsychopharmacology 2002;27:479–97.

[25] Adler LE, Pachtman E, Franks RD, et al. Neurophysiological evidence for a defect in neuronal mechanisms involved in sensory gating in schizophrenia. Biol Psychiatry 1982;17: 639–54.

[26] Tung CS, Grenhoff J, Svensson TH. Nicotine counteracts midbrain dopamine cell dysfunction induced by prefrontal cortex inactivation. Acta Physiol Scand 1990;138: 427–8.

[27] Nomikos GG, Schilstrom B, Hildebrand BE, et al. Role of alpha 7 nicotinic receptors in nicotine dependence and implications for psychiatric illness. Behav Brain Res 2000;113: 97–103.

[28] Acri JB, Morse DE, Popke EJ, et al. Nicotine increases sensory gating measured as inhibition of the acoustic startle reflex in rats. Psychopharmacology (Berl) 1994;114: 369–74.

[29] Adler LE, Olincy A, Waldo M, et al. Schizophrenia, sensory gating, and nicotinic receptors. Schizophrenia Bull 1998;24:189–202.

[30] Leonard S, Breese C, Adams C, et al. Smoking and schizophrenia: abnormal nicotinic receptor expression. Eur J Pharmacol 2000;393:237–42.

[31] McEvoy JP, Freudenreich O, Levin ED, et al. Haloperidol increases smoking in patients with schizophrenia. Psychopharmacology 1995;119:124–6.

[32] Caskey NH, Jarvik ME, Wirshing WC. The effects of dopaminergic $D_2$ stimulation and blockade on smoking behavior. Exp Clin Psychopharmacol 1999;7:72–8.

[33] Caskey NH, Jarvik ME, Wirshing WC, et al. Modulating tobacco smoking rates by dopaminergic stimulation and blockade. Nicotine Tob Res 2002;4:259–66.

[34] Dawe S, Gerada C, Russell MA, et al. Nicotine intake in smokers increases after a single dose of haloperidol. Psychopharmacology 1995;117:110–5.

[35] Brauer LH, Cramblett MJ, Paxton DA, et al. Haloperidol reduces smoking of both nicotine-containing and denicotinized cigarettes. Psychopharmacology 2001;159:31–7.

[36] George TP, Vessicchio JC, Termine A, et al. A placebo controlled trial of bupropion for smoking cessation in schizophrenia. Biol Psychiatry 2002;52:53–61.

[37] Procyshyn RM, Ihsan N, Thompson D. A comparison of smoking behaviours between patients treated with Clozapine and depot neuroleptics. Int Clin Psychopharmacol 2001;16: 291–4.

[38] George TP, Sernyak MJ, Ziedonis DM, et al. Effects of clozapine on smoking in chronic schizophrenic outpatients. J Clin Psychiatry 1995;56:344–6.

[39] Combs DR, Advokat C. Antipsychotic medication and smoking prevalence in acutely hospitalized patients with chronic schizophrenia. Schizophr Res 2000;46:129–37.

[40] McEvoy JP, Freudenreich O, Wilson WH. Smoking and therapeutic response to clozapine in patients with schizophrenia. Biol Psychiatry 1999;46:125–9.

[41] United Nations Office of Drug Control and Crime Prevention. World drug report 2000. Oxford (UK): Oxford University Press; 2000.

[42] Office of National Drug Control Policy. Methamphetamine: facts and figures. Washington (DC): Office of National Drug Control Policy; 1998.

[43] Narrow WE, Rae DS, Robins LN, et al. Revised prevalence estimates of mental disorders in the United States. Arch Gen Psychiatry 2002;59:115–23.

[44] Grabowski J, Shearer J, Merrill J, et al. Agonist-like, replacement pharmacotherapy for stimulant abuse and dependence. Addict Behav 2004;29:1439–64.

[45] Silva de Lima M, Garcia de Oliveira Soares B, Alves Pereira Reisser A, et al. Pharmacological treatment of cocaine dependence: a systematic review. Addiction 2002; 97:931–49.

[46] Dackis CA, Lynch KG, Yu E, et al. Modafinil and cocaine: a double-blind, placebo-controlled drug interaction study. Drug Alcohol Depend 2003;70:29–37.

[47] Seiden LS, Sabol KE, Ricaurte GA. Amphetamine: effects on catecholamine systems and behavior. Annu Rev Pharmacol Toxicol 1993;33:639–77.

[48] Fleckenstein AE, Gibb JW, Hanson GR. Differential effects of stimulants on mono-aminergic transporters. Eur J Pharmacol 2000;406:1–13.

[49] Volkow ND, Wang G-J, Fowler JS, et al. Reinforcing effects of psychostimulants in humans are associated with increases in brain dopamine and occupancy of $D_2$ receptors. J Pharmacol Exp Ther 1999;291:409–15.

[50] Vollm BA, de Araujo IE, Cowen PJ, et al. Methamphetamine activates reward circuitry in drug naive human subjects. Neuropsychopharmacology 2004;29:1715–22.

[51] Ahmed SH, Koob GF. Transition from moderate to excessive drug intake: change in hedonic set point. Science 1998;282:298–300.

[52] Robinson TE, Berridge KC. The neural basis of drug craving: an incentive-sensitization theory of addiction. Brain Res Brain Res Rev 1993;18:247–91.

[53] Everitt BJ, Dickinson A, Robbins TW. The neuropsychological basis of addictive behaviour. Brain Res Brain Res Rev 2001;36:129–38.

[54] Schulteis G, Markou A, Cole M, et al. Decreased brain reward produced by ethanol withdrawal. Proc Natl Acad Sci U S A 1995;92:5880–4.

[55] McBride WJ, Murphy JM, Ikemoto S. Localization of brain reinforcement mechanisms: intracranial self-administration and intracranial place-conditioning studies. Behav Brain Res 1999;101:129–52.

[56] Domino EF. Nicotine induced behavioral locomotor sensitization. Prog Neuro-Psycho-pharm Biol Psychiatry 2001;25:59–71.

[57] Pierce RC, Kalivas PW. A circuitry model of the expression of behavioral sensitization to amphetamine-like psychostimulants. Brain Res Brain Res Rev 1997;25:192–216.

[58] Kalivas PW. Interactions between dopamine and excitatory amino acids in behavioral sensitization to psychostimulants. Drug Alcohol Depend 1995;37:95–100.

[59] Deroche V, Le Moal M, Piazza PV. Cocaine self-administration increases the incentive motivational properties of the drug in rats. Eur J Neurosci 1999;11:2731–6.

[60] Miller DK, Wilkins LH, Bardo MT, et al. Once weekly administration of nicotine produces long-lasting locomotor sensitization in rats via a nicotinic receptor-mediated mechanism. Psychopharmacology (Berl) 2001;156:469–76.

[61] Picciotto MR, Caldarone BJ, King SL, et al. Nicotinic receptors in the brain: links between molecular biology and behavior. Neuropsychopharmacology 2000;22:451–65.

[62] Tapper AR, McKinney SL, Nashmi R, et al. Nicotine activation of alpha 4 receptors: sufficient for reward, tolerance, and sensitization. Science 2004;306:1029–32.

[63] Greengard P. The neurobiology of slow synaptic transmission. Science 2001;294:1024–30.

[64] Koob GF, Sanna PP, Bloom FE. Neuroscience of addiction. Neuron 1998;21:467–76.

[65] Steketee JD. Neurotransmitter systems of the medial prefrontal cortex: potential role in sensitization to psychostimulants. Brain Res Brain Res Rev 2003;41:203–28.

[66] Leonard S, Bertrand D. Neuronal nicotinic receptors: from structure to function. Nicotine Tob Res 2001;3:203–23.

[67] Di Chiara G. Role of dopamine in the behavioural actions of nicotine related to addiction. Eur J Pharmacol 2000;393:295–314.

[68] Schoffelmeer A, De Vries TJ, Wardeh G, et al. Psychostimulant-induced behavioral sensitization depends on nicotinic receptor activation. J Neurosci 2002;22:3269–76.

[69] Kimmel HL, Carroll I, Kuhar MJ. Withdrawal from repeated cocaine alters dopamine transporter protein turnover in the rat striatum. J Pharmacol Exp Ther 2003;304: 15–21.

[70] Kahlig KM, Galli A. Regulation of dopamine transporter function and plasma membrane expression by dopamine, amphetamine, and cocaine. Eur J Pharmacol 2003;479:153–8.

[71] Roubert C, Spielewoy C, Soubrie P, et al. Altered neurotensin mRNA expression in mice lacking the dopamine transporter. Neuroscience 2004;123:537–46.

[72] Fienberg AA, Hiroi N, Mermelstein PG, et al. DARPP-32: regulator of the efficacy of dopaminergic neurotransmission. Science 1998;281:838–42.

[73] Zachariou V, Benoit-Marand M, Allen PB, et al. Reduction of cocaine place preference in mice lacking the protein phosphatase 1 inhibitors DARPP-32 or inhibitor 1. Biol Psychiatry 2002;1:612–20.

[74] Carraway R, Leeman SE. The isolation of a new hypotensive peptide, neurotensin, from bovine hypothalami. J Biol Chem 1973;248:6854–61.

[75] Binder EB, Kinkead B, Owens MJ, et al. The role of neurotensin in the pathophysiology of schizophrenia and the mechanism of action of antipsychotic drugs. Biol Psychiatry 2001;50: 856–72.

[76] Kinkead B, Binder EB, Nemeroff CB. Does neurotensin mediate the effects of antipsychotic drugs? Biol Psychiatry 1999;46:340–51.

[77] McMahon BM, Boules M, Warrington L, et al. Neurotensin analogs. indications for use as potential antipsychotic compounds. Life Sci 2002;70:1101–19.

[78] Kalivas PW, Nemeroff CB, Prange AJ. Neurotensin microinjection into the nucleus accumbens antagonizes dopamine-induced increase in locomotion and rearing. Neuroscience 1984;11:919–30.

[79] Ervin GN, Birkemo LS, Nemeroff CB, et al. Neurotensin blocks certain amphetamine-induced behaviours. Nature 1981;29:73–6.

[80] Brun P, Leonetti M, Sotty F, et al. Endogenous neurotensin down-regulates dopamine efflux in the nucleus accumbens as revealed by SR-142948A, a selective neurotensin receptor antagonist. J Neurochem 2001;77:1542–52.

[81] Nemeroff CB. Neurotensin: perchance an endogenous neuroleptic? Biol Psychiatry 1980; 15:283–302.

[82] Wolf SS, Hyde TM, Saunders RC, et al. Autoradiographic characterization of neurotensin receptors in the entorhinal cortex of schizophrenic patients and control subjects. J Neural Transm 1995;102:55–65.

[83] Sharma RP, Janicak PG, Bissette G, et al. CSF neurotensin concentrations and antipsychotic treatment in schizophrenia and schizoaffective disorder. Am J Psychiatry 1997;154:1019–21.

[84] Kinkead B, Shahid S, Owens MJ, et al. Effects of acute and subchronic administration of typical and atypical antipsychotic drugs on the neurotensin system of the rat brain. J Pharmacol Exp Ther 2000;295:67–73.

[85] Le F, Cusack B, Richelson E. The neurotensin receptor: is there more than one subtype? Trends Pharmacol Sci 1996;17:1–3.

[86] Vincent JP, Mazella J, Kitabgi P. Neurotensin and neurotensin receptors. Trends Pharmacol Sci 1999;20:302–9.

[87] Uhl GR, Snyder SH. Neurotensin receptor binding, regional and subcellular distributions favor transmitter role. Eur J Pharmacol 1977;41:89–91.

[88] Kitabgi P, Carraway R, Van Rietschoten J, et al. Neurotensin: specific binding to synaptic membranes from rat brain. Proc Natl Acad Sci U S A 1977;74:1846–50.

[89] Slusher BS, Zacco AE, Maslanski JA, et al. The cloned neurotensin receptor mediates cyclic GMP formation when coexpressed with nitric oxide synthase cDNA. Mol Pharmacol 1994;46:115–21.

[90] Yamada M, Yamada M, Watson MA, et al. Neurotensin stimulates cyclic AMP formation in CHO-rNTR-10 cells expressing the cloned rat neurotensin receptor. Eur J Pharmacol 1993;244:99–101.

[91] Watson MA, Yamada M, Yamada M, et al. The rat neurotensin receptor expressed in Chinese hamster ovary cells mediates the release of inositol phosphates. J Neurochem 1992; 59:1967–70.

[92] Poinot-Chazel C, Portier M, Bouaboula M, et al. Activation of mitogen-activated protein kinase couples neurotensin receptor stimulation to induction of the primary response gene Krox-24. Biochem J 1996;320:145–51.

[93] Fuxe K, O'Connor WT, Antonelli T, et al. Evidence for a substrate of neuronal plasticity based on pre- and postsynaptic neurotensin-dopamine receptor interactions in the neostriatum. Proc Natl Acad Sci U S A 1992;89:5591–5.

[94] Li XM, Ferraro L, Tanganelli S, et al. Neurotensin peptides antagonistically regulate postsynaptic dopamine $D_2$ receptors in rat nucleus accumbens: a receptor binding and microdialysis study. J Neural Transm Gen Sect 1995;102:125–37.

[95] Von Euler G, Fuxe K. Neurotensin reduces the affinity of $D_2$ dopamine receptors in rat striatal membranes. Acta Physiol Scand 1987;131:625–6.

[96] Mazella J, Zsurger N, Navarro V, et al. The 100-kDa neurotensin receptor is gp95/sortilin, a non-G-protein-coupled receptor. J Biol Chem 1998;273:26273–6.

[97] Sarret P, Krzywkowski P, Segal L, et al. Distribution of NTS3 receptor/sortilin mRNA and protein in the rat central nervous system. J Comp Neurol 2003;461:483–505.

[98] Nykjaer A, Lee R, Teng KK, et al. Sortilin is essential for proNGF-induced neuronal cell death. Nature 2004;427:843–8.

[99] Gully D, Canton M, Boigegrain R, et al. Biochemical and pharmacological profile of a potent and selective nonpeptide antagonist of the neurotensin receptor. Proc Natl Acad Sci U S A 1993;90:65–9.

[100] Gully D, Labeeuw B, Boigegrain R, et al. Biochemical and pharmacological activities of SR 142948A, a new potent neurotensin receptor antagonist. J Pharmacol Exp Ther 1997;280: 802–12.

[101] Horger BA, Taylor JR, Elsworth JD, et al. Preexposure to, but not cotreatment with, the neurotensin antagonist SR 48692 delays the development of cocaine sensitization. Neuropsychopharmacology 1994;11:215–22.

[102] Rompre PP, Perron S. Evidence for a role of endogenous neurotensin in the initiation of amphetamine sensitization. Neuropharmacology 2000;39:1880–92.

[103] Boules M, Fredrickson P, Richelson E. Current topics: brain penetrating neurotensin analog. Life Sci 2003;73:2785–92.

[104] Fauq AH, Hong F, Cusack B, et al. Synthesis of (2S)-2-amino-3-(1H-4-indolyl)-propanoic acid, a novel tryptophan analog for structural modification of bioactive peptides. Tetrahedron Asymmetry 1998;9:4127–34.

[105] Tyler-McMahon BM, Stewart JA, et al. Highly potent neurotensin analog that causes hypothermia and antinociception. Eur J Pharmacol 2000;390:107–11.

[106] Cusack B, Boules M, Tyler BM, et al. Effects of a novel neurotensin peptide analog given extracranially on CNS behaviors mediated by apomorphine and haloperidol. Brain Res 2000;856:48–54.

[107] Boules M, Warrington L, Fauq A, et al. A novel neurotensin analog blocks cocaine- and D-amphetamine-induced hyperactivity. Eur J Pharmacol 2001;426:73–6.

[108] Fredrickson P, Boules M, Yerbury S, et al. Blockade of nicotine-induced locomotor sensitization by a novel neurotensin analog in rats. Eur J Pharmacol 2003;458:111–8.

[109] Fredrickson P, Boules M, Yerbury S, et al. Novel neurotensin analog blocks the initiation and expression of nicotine-induced locomotor sensitization. Brain Res 2003; 979:245–8.

[110] Richelson E, Boules M, Fredrickson P. Neurotensin agonists: possible drugs for treatment of psychostimulant abuse. Life Sci 2003;73:679–90.

[111] Fantegrossi WE, Ko MCH, Woods JH, et al. Antinociceptive, hypothermic, hypotensive, and reinforcing effects of a novel neurotensin receptor agonist, NT69L, in rhesus monkeys. Pharmacol Biochem Behav 2005;80:341–9.

[112] Betancur C, Canton M, Burgos A, et al. Characterization of binding sites of a new neurotensin receptor antagonist, [$^3$H]SR 142948A, in the rat brain. Eur J Pharmacol 1998; 343:67–77.

[113] Vita N, Oury-Donat F, Chalon P, et al. Neurotensin is an antagonist of the human neurotensin NT$_2$ receptor expressed in Chinese hamster ovary cells. Eur J Pharmacol 1998; 360:265–72.

ELSEVIER
SAUNDERS

PSYCHIATRIC
CLINICS
OF NORTH AMERICA

Psychiatr Clin N Am 28 (2005) 753–761

# Index

*Note:* Page numbers of article titles are in **boldface** type.

# Changing Your Address?

Make sure your subscription changes too! When you notify us of your new address, you can help make our job easier by including an exact copy of your Clinics label number with your old address (see illustration below.) This number identifies you to our computer system and will speed the processing of your address change. Please be sure this label number accompanies your old address and your corrected address—you can send an old Clinics label with your number on it or just copy it exactly and send it to the address listed below.

We appreciate your help in our attempt to give you continuous coverage. Thank you.

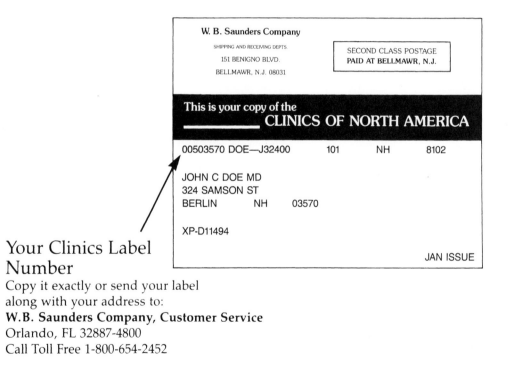

**Your Clinics Label Number**
Copy it exactly or send your label along with your address to:
**W.B. Saunders Company, Customer Service**
Orlando, FL 32887-4800
Call Toll Free 1-800-654-2452

Please allow four to six weeks for delivery of new subscriptions and for processing address changes.